THE TOTAL SERVICE MEDICAL PRACTICE

17 Steps to Satisfying Your Internal and External Customers

Vicky Bradford, Ph.D.

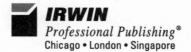
IRWIN
Professional Publishing®
Chicago • London • Singapore

Dr. Vicky Bradford can be reached at:
The Bradford Company
1177 Race Street, Suite 202
Denver, CO 80206
Phone: 303-832-5776
Fax: 303-832-5767

This publication is designed to provide accurate and
authoritative information in regard to the subject matter
covered. It is sold with the understanding that neither the
author nor the publisher is engaged in rendering legal, accounting,
or other professional service. If legal advice or other expert
assistance is required, the services of a competent professional
person should be sought.

From a Declaration of Principles jointly adopted by a Committee
of the American Bar Association and a Committee of Publishers.

Library of Congress Cataloging-in-Publication Data

Bradford, Vicky.
    The total service medical practice : 17 steps to satisfying your
internal and external customers / Vicky Bradford.
       p.   cm.
    ISBN 1-55738-645-5
    1. Medicine—Practice   I. Title.
R728.B69 1997
610′ .68—dc20   96–41980

Printed in the United States of America
1 2 3 4 5 6 7 8 9 0 DOC 3 2 1 0 9 8 7 6

This book is dedicated to the healthcare providers in my life who have dedicated their lives to helping others:
Lori Sexton Markham, RN, BSN, CCN
David Markham, RN, BSN, CCN
Jill Tompson Sexton, RN, CNN
Gregory Chess, CCJS, CACII

It is also dedicated to all of the physicians, practice administrators, and clinical and nonclinical staff members in medical practices around the country, who each day extend their knowledge and their hearts to serve.

CONTENTS

PREFACE

"Amy, This Book's For You"

She wasn't an especially memorable woman . . . at first glance anyway. Sitting in the middle of the fourth row in one of my seminars for physicians, office managers, and staff, she seemed like a rather typical participant in these workshops which I'd been conducting for the past several years. During my presentation, she appeared to listen carefully enough, and she even took a few notes as I talked. She was smiling at my funny stories and participating willingly during the exercises. At the break, I noticed her approaching me, and, as she neared, I saw that the smile had vanished from her lips and her eyes had filled with tears. I waited to see what nerve I had touched; what long ago pain I had inadvertently brought to the surface.

"Dr. Bradford," she began.

"Yes, Amy," I replied and waited.

"I . . . I want to thank you."

"For what?" I queried, uncertain as to the specific cause of her appreciation.

"For understanding. For knowing how badly we need to hear these things."

I remained silent, believing that perhaps she was giving me more credit than I deserved. My participant continued. "It's tough out there. We try hard, and we are so overwhelmed. So much is changing."

"It must be difficult," I murmured.

"Difficult! Some days it feels downright impossible. And that is why we need to hear what you are saying. You have helped me put things in perspective. You have started me thinking about the way we do things in my office, on my job. I only hope that you can do the same for others."

The tears were not mentioned by either of us. While I never knew exactly what had caused them, they and her words stayed with me. I contemplated her comments and I hypothesized about her tears. Then, in a sudden burst of decision, I realized that I wanted to write this book, to commit to paper the things I had shared with Amy and her colleagues. Although I knew that not all, nor even most, medical-practice personnel had reached Amy's obvious level of frustration, I felt she had been right about the need for these concepts to be presented in a tangible form. So you see, it was not by any great design, nor to fulfill any grand plan, that I set on this project. I merely hoped to convey to a broader audience what Amy's words and even her tears had told me needed to be conveyed. And so, "Amy, this book's for you."

It is also for you, my reader. *You* are a physician, an office manager, or a staff member. You are from a small specialty-practice in a big city, a bustling family-practice in a farming community, or a large multispecialty-practice in a medium-sized town. You have completed medical school or nurse's training, a graduate program in medical management or a course of study in a technical skill, or you've been busy learning and gaining experience on the job. You are either frustrated with the changing healthcare scene, or you have accepted and perhaps embraced it—or you are stuck somewhere in between. You are a male or a female representing a single ethnic background or an interesting mixture. You are different from many of my other readers, and yet, so like them in one very important way: You share with them a dedication to helping others.

Now I'd like to help *you* understand a few unique features about this book. First, it is not just a philosophical discussion about service. Rather, it offers a specific 17-step process for creating a Total Service Medical Practice. By incorporating some techniques you may already know with others that I'm certain will be new to you, I have attempted to organize a breadth of disparate information into a coherent whole. By relying on original focus-group and depth-interview research, an extensive review of the literature, as well as comments and observations made by my workshop participants, I have attempted to bring your daily life into this discussion. In each chapter, I cover the specific topic at hand, and, where appropriate, I make suggestions for how to use the information. In the Appendix, you will find several forms that pertain to specific content items. As you can see, I want to offer you a hands-on approach presented in a book that you will pick up again and again as you complete the process toward Total Service. (A separate workbook containing worksheets that will help you implement the 17 steps is also available).

You also will notice that some chapters address specific segments of practice personnel—physicians, managers/administrators, staff. I hope that you will read them all! For this 17-step process to work, each person in the practice must be aware of what everyone else is doing, and why. Also, reading those chapters that are not targeted specifically for you may help you gain greater empathy and appreciation for your colleagues and for what they experience in the performance of their roles in your medical practice.

Another unusual feature of this book is that the chapters vary considerably in length. There is a simple reason for this. Because each chapter represents a different step in the process, I was not guided by page or word count. Rather, I focused on the step under discussion and what I felt needed to be said about it. Sometimes that took only 10 pages, and, as in the case of Chapter 14, *Handle the Difficult Moments of Truth,* it required almost five times as many. I was asked by my editor how I arrived at 17 steps and, thus, 17 chapters, and my answer was similar to the above: Because that's how long it takes. The content of this book, then, is driven not by some artificial standard but by the ideas themselves.

Since I wanted you to feel involved as much as possible, I made an important stylistic decision. I chose to write in the first person speaking to the second person: In other words, from *I*, the author, to *You*, the reader. By so doing, I hope to make this a personal conversation between the two of us. I want you to feel as though we have just seated ourselves in the conference room at your office or on your living-room couch at home. My goal is to be your coach, albeit from a distance, for bringing these concepts to your practice. I want us to go together on this journey toward creating a Total Service Medical Practice. It's a trip well worth taking.

"Ya Can't Get No Where on a Ten-Dollar Horse"

By what means do we transport ourselves into the world of the Total Service Medical Practice? I discovered my answer to that question in a most unexpected place. Late one evening during the early phases of writing this book, I found myself wakeful. I had spent the day organizing ideas and correlating concepts, seeing in my mind's eye the content take shape. Not all of the sharp edges of my ideas were smoothed out yet, and something seemed to be missing. I decided I needed time away from *it* for a while. A chronic night person, I prepared a cup of herbal tea, leaned back in my recliner, and opened my newly acquired copy of *How to Argue and Win Every Time* by famed trial attorney Gerry Spence.[1] And there, as fate or the writing gods would have it, in the middle of Mr. Spence's eloquent prose was the missing piece from my own.

When describing Part I of his book on argument, Mr. Spence relied on one of his well-known stories. He told of a cowboy from somewhere out West, Wyoming no doubt, who stood one day watching a dude ride awkwardly into town. The dude was dressed in typical fine duds, and he sat astride a spectacular black leather saddle, with shiny silver trim. But the horse he rode was an unremarkable nag, swayed in the back and splayed of hoof. The cowboy said to the dude with amused disgust, "Look at ya. Ya got a thousand-dollar saddle on a ten-dollar horse. Ya can't get no where on a ten-dollar horse, no matter how fancy a saddle ya put on 'im!" Tying this tale to his point, Mr. Spence concluded, no matter how clever the orator, no matter how many slick tricks of argument he or she has mastered, technique in the end is nothing more than the thousand-dollar saddle. "To win, " he wrote, "we need a saddle all right, but we need to mount it on a powerful horse." The steed to which Mr. Spence referred was a reader freed from the traditionally negative teachings about argument, and a reader open in mind as well as spirit to the positive possibilities of arguing well.

As I read the preface to Mr. Spence's book, I realized that his point was remarkably pertinent to my own, and it provided the missing link I had been looking for. Just as his book needed a reader who was deeply committed to viewing argument in a positive light, I too needed such a dedicated recipient for my ideas. I realized the limitations of what *I* had to offer, and I gained clarity on what *you* must bring to the reading of this book. The truth is that I can provide all of the models and strategies and methods— the *techniques* of service—and you can even put them into practice. However, if you do so without the belief in the value of and the *rightness* of service in the healthcare environment, most especially in the medical practice, you will be just like the dude on the ten-dollar nag. The kind of steed I need for the ideas in this book is represented by the physicians, the office managers, and staff members who truly embrace the concepts of service.

The fact that you have picked up this volume and have read this far is a very positive indication of your interest in this topic. Before you continue any farther, however, I ask you to pause a moment and consider four pertinent questions, questions that will help you ascertain the extent of your commitment to creating and maintaining a Total Service Medical Practice. The answers will help you come to know the kind of horse that will carry your Total Service saddle to the finish line.

Question 1: Do I really believe that service has a place in healthcare?

If you answered *Yes*: Move on to Question 2.

If you answered *No*: At least read Chapter 2 before rejecting the idea completely.

Question 2: Do I really want to serve?

If you answered *Yes*: Advance to Question 3.

If you answered *No*: Please return this book to the bookstore and get your money back! But before you do that, ask yourself the next question.

Question 3: Am I free of any personal barriers to serving others?

If you answered *Yes*: You are ready and willing to embrace the concepts offered in this book! Skip the next question.

If you answered *No*: Since you are probably experiencing some of Amy's frustrations, I urge you to acknowledge that these feelings have begun to block your desire to serve, and then go on to Question 4.

Question 4: What do I need to do to remove the barrier(s) so that I can open up my desire to serve?

Whatever needs to be done, I urge you to do it. Sometimes it means confronting your reluctance to accept the new paradigms that are foreign to the image you had of the practice of medicine when you were in medical school or in nurse's training. Sometimes it means recognizing that you have allowed the stress of the job to detach you from the very people you are trying to help. Sometimes it is simply accepting the old adage, "The only thing that is constant is change itself." Ultimately, removing the barriers means just deciding to do it—deciding to stop being blocked and to risk being opened.

A Total Service Medical Practice is characterized by people who truly want to serve. This commitment must be felt at a deep and personal level. When that happens, then the thousand-dollar saddle can be placed on the back of a very powerful horse. Just think of the possibilities when your medical practice is composed of a team of these wonderful creatures! There is no load you can't pull, no race you can't win, no hill you can't climb!

So, as we say out here in the West, "Giddyup! Let's go!" Oh, and with your permission, I'd like to bring Amy along for the ride!

END NOTE

1. Gerry Spence, *How to Argue and Win Every Time* (New York: St. Martin Press, 1995), pp. 5–7.

ACKNOWLEDGMENTS

Even though writing is a solitary activity, it is very much a team effort, and my team is composed of winners!

Professionally, I have been supported by three outstanding editors at Irwin Professional Publishing, Jeffrey Krames who saw the value of this project at its inception; Kristine Rynne who knew exactly when to extend her generous patience and when to pull in the reins; and Pat Muller who was my expert guide through the often confusing maze of publishing. Also, my thanks to Carrie Sestak, who brought this project through to completion.

I have received invaluable assistance from the fine folks at the Medical Group Management Association (MGMA): Fred Graham, executive vice president, who envisioned the win-win idea of co-publishing; ACMPE director Andrea Rossiter, who has championed me and my ideas throughout MGMA; former head librarian Barb Hamilton; and the MGMA's superior staff of knowledgeable librarians (especially Cynthia, Mary, Donna, and Jeff), who put *service excellence* into practice each and every day.

I have had other professional champions, too: Kim Gawart of Hoechst Marion Roussel Pharmaceuticals (HMR), my most special friend and client; and several of her colleagues at HMR, especially Pattie Aspenleiter, Jeff Ball, Joe Canny, Jim DiPaolo, Mark Fluitt, Buzz Harrell, Pamela Hawtalker, Cindy Heidt, Mikel Hill, Michael Hunt, Jim Johnson, Kathleen McHugh, Dave Melanaphy, Matt Mincweksi, Mara Phillips, Tom Rice, Kirk Schamp, Scott Sutter, Tony Severoni, Darrell Simms, Cortney Spezia, Carol Wells, Ken Wentzel, and Gary White. Other professional colleagues have encouraged and assisted me, including Les Powell of Boehringer Manheim Pharmaceuticals; Karen Linden, vice president of Columbine Medical Group, Denver, Colorado; Sue Phillips, director of provider relations for Capital Community Health Plan, Washington, D.C.; and William Ries, president of Lake Forest Hospital, Chicago, Illinois.

I am indebted to all those who gave of their time and knowledge for this book, especially office managers Mary Frances

Bills, Deborah Goodyear, Marilyn Haley, and Arlene Stolte; and my personal physicians Neil Sullivan, M.D., Debra Gussman, M.D., and Nurses Jill Tompson Sexton, Lori Sexton Markham, and David Markham; case manager Gregory Chess; and attorney Frank Plaut. I also wish to acknowledge June Griener for her wise counsel during the early days of the project, and Julie Clayton for her able assistance in the final preparation of the manuscript.

On a personal level, I have so many to thank that I cannot begin to name them all. However, a few deserve special recognition: Greg, whose presence in my life is my foundation; Joanne and Roni, who supported me, celebrated with me, and even fed me when I had no time to cook! Mike and Dave, who cheered me on when I was stuck, and whose opinions I always trusted; Marnie, who helped me ask the right questions and discover my own answers; Helen, who provided not only her belief in me but also a quiet haven in which I could make one last big push to completion; Ellen, who helped nurse me back to health after my injury; Brooke, who gave me back the use of my arm; and my friend Mary, as well as the Genva Group, who were always there in spirit.

I also want to thank my family: Betsy Sexton and Janice and Lewis Bossing, whose belief in me has never wavered; my parents LaVerne and Pete Hesser, who instilled in me the value of serving others; my aunt Nora Bartine, who taught me how to live; and my grandmother Cora Geeslin, who taught me how to tell a story. I also want to thank my nephew Brian Sexton, who long ago made me believe that I could do anything; my nephews Lewis and Bill Bossing, who have shown me through their own lives the value of listening to your heart. And, of course, I want to thank the nurses in my family, most especially Lori, who has always seemed more like a little sister than a niece. Their dedication and commitment has served as an inspiration when I needed it. Last, I have to thank Sojie who went through the tough times of my life by my side, and Elizabeth and Nicki whose collective devotion has provided irreplaceable support even during those lonely hours between 1:00 and 4:00 A.M.

Yea team! And thank you!

ONE

PREPARING FOR THE JOURNEY

Before you can actually start the journey to a Total Service Medical Practice, you need to spend a little time planning the trip. The Preface and chapters in Part I are designed to help you do just that.

Perhaps you are like many readers of any book, and you have skipped over the Preface. If that's the case, I urge you to go back and read it now; the perspective that you will need for implementing the 17 steps is contained within those pages. When you finish the Preface, return to this page and start your preparation for the journey to Total Service.

Now that you've gained an understanding of why this book was written and what you need to bring to the reading of it, you are ready to move on to the chapters in Part I.

Chapter 1 defines key concepts that will help you understand where you are going. Chapter 2 provides the rationale you should consider before embarking on this trip. Chapter 3 explains the lessons about service learned by those who have traveled this route before you. Reading these chapters carefully and formally discussing the ideas therein will provide the background and the insights that you and your colleagues will need in order to cast off and to stay on course.

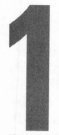

CHAPTER

Step One—Understand the Key Concepts

One of my favorite photographs from my own personal travels depicts me standing below a road sign in New Zealand. Shoulders shrugged, I am looking helplessly at the camera as I reflect my confusion over which way to go next. Above my head towers the road sign—a tall wooden pole with no less than 20 little plaques, each bearing the whimsical Maori name of a New Zealand town and each pointing in a slightly different direction. Expecting more of a British flavor to the language and not the heavy influence of the native inhabitants, my confusion was understandable; everything about the New Zealand road sign was strange to me. It is no wonder I could not interpret its meaning.

There are some communication situations, however, where breakdowns occur for no apparent reason. The language, the topic, even the surroundings are familiar. Why, then, does the message from one person to another become garbled and unclear? Actually, it is rather simple to explain.

There is an old adage in communication theory that goes like this: "Meaning is not in words; it is in people." So, if my meaning differs from your meaning, and it very often can, we will frequently arrive at vastly different interpretations of any given message. Because of this phenomenon, it is helpful to begin any discussion with a definition of key terms. By so doing, the chances of a mutually understood message can be increased. While this entire book operationally defines the phrase *The Total Service Medical Practice*, a few key terms require a more targeted approach. Even though the words themselves may not be new to you, the specific meaning I have for them is important to your understanding of the concepts in this book. By defining them for you now, I hope to avoid confusion for you later. I want your journey to a Total Service Medical Practice to be a smooth one.

MEDICAL PRACTICE

In the good old days, when a patient talked of "going to the doctor," a certain, rather specific image came to mind. The small one-man shop was the rule and the term *medical practice*, if used at all, referred to actual treatment and diagnosis. Then, gradually the one-physician office expanded to include two or three or more, and group practices were born. Also, as medical knowledge increased so did specialization, and today the AMA recognizes 25 specialities and numerous subspecialties.[1] Regardless of the size or type of the practice, however, the model and concepts presented in this book apply to them all. The common denominator is simple: Where human beings are involved in providing healthcare for other human beings, this approach will work for you.

As I have watched the organizational structures of medical practices change over the last several years, I have begun to realize that this book and its focus on service are not only well-timed, but perhaps are needed more than ever. As practices join together in one of many structural manifestations, the accompanying stresses and strains from diminishing autonomy, as well as the increasing focus on cost containment, can push the concept of service to the background. In times such as these the *conscious* focus on service, *people helping people*, is key to the continued providing of quality care. By tracing the history of these structural changes for you now, I also want to illuminate the potentially negative effects they can have on service, effects which can be minimized if recognized and responded to appropriately.

One big motivator for the merging of small practices into larger ones has been the need for physicians to gain strength through unity. This need to influence decisions more effectively regarding the direction of healthcare delivery resulted in a wide range of different organizational structures. Beginning with the traditional group practice (with its geographical centralization and the integration of management and financial operations), some unique structures have emerged that cover the gamut of possibilities.

Perhaps the first alternative to the traditional group practice was the Independent Practice Association (IPA). Arising out of the need for a larger power base, but also a desire to retain autonomy, the IPAs provided legal negotiating ability that physicians felt they needed. The impact has been mostly positive, although the potential for a negative effect exists. When medical practices are placed in a somewhat adversarial position with one of their important secondary customer populations (HMOs, PHOs, etc.), the service relationships between the two entities can be forgotten. Avoiding this problem requires vigilance and conscious effort.

IPAs paved the way for another manifestation of joining: the Clinic Without Walls (CWW). A blend of the traditional group practice and an independent practice association, CWWs offer the following essential features: multispecialty representatives on the panel, multiple locations, centralized 800 phone number for easy access, centralized billing and collection and authorization, peer consultation, quality assurance programs, computerized information systems, and marketing/practice development capabilities. The attraction of the CWWs can be summed up this way: "CWWs allow members independence while providing a needed marketing advantage . . . Since physicians do not have to share office space with others, they feel they maintain more autonomy than in a traditional group practice or clinic setting. At the same time the CWWs are able to actively market the skills of the group and members."[2]

More recently, the emergence of the Management Service Organization (MSO) has provided yet another way for physicians to gain strength through affiliation. In an MSO, physicians join together administratively. Either the physicians create this entity themselves, or they are approached by an independent management company designed to provide these services to medical practices. The services offered by an MSO include all administrative functions—billing, group purchasing, contracting, and staffing. The Medical Group Management Association conducted an information exchange, asking its subscribers to respond to the following question: "Does your group contract for services with an MSO?" Eighty-one groups responded "Yes;" 781 said "No ." When asked how effectively the MSO was working, almost all responded "Too early to tell."[3] Obviously, the MSO is a current attempt to provide autonomy and yet also offer the advantage of group affiliation.

The major impact of the CWWs and MSOs on service revolves around the diminished direct control over certain key nonclinical service areas of the practice. When billing and claims and even scheduling are handled offsite, it becomes more difficult to control these functions, to be certain that they are reflecting the practice's commitment to service. Thus, when selecting a CWW or MSO with which to affiliate, questions regarding service issues should be asked and satisfactorily answered. Also, delineated processes for correcting service errors should be clarified. In short, even though the administrative duties may be handled offsite, the customer will hold the physician's practice accountable for them. Problems with those functions can impact the customer's perceptions of the service delivered by that practice. Careful up-front scrutiny and planning can counter the potential negative impact on service.

Changes have not stopped with the CWWs and MSOs, however. When the Clinton commission on Health Care Reform entered the picture, suddenly the entire healthcare field found itself under fire. One recommendation that emerged from that body was the creation of Integrated Delivery Systems (IDS), sometimes also known as Community Care Networks (CCN). Combining medical groups, physicians, hospitals, and health plans, these entities offer a coordinated continuum of health services for a defined population. When the furor over the commission and all of its recommendations quieted down, the healthcare field realized that this was merely a lull in the storm. The realization, for some the fear, was that if they did not make some changes voluntarily, the government would do it for them. The IDS appeared to be an idea with merit, and its increasing viability was documented in the *MGM Journal*, the official publication of the Medical Group Management Association.

According to the opinions of 580 healthcare industry experts representing virtually all healthcare organizational forms, the IDS is the wave of the future. The panel predicts that the free-standing medical practice may well become a thing of the past as early as 1999.[4]

How far from the traditional practice will the IDS model wander? The jury is still out on that question. Some believe that the IDSs will closely resemble the staff-model HMO, with all healthcare needs being housed under one or at the most two roofs. Others say the changes will result in the disappearance of the small two- and three-physician practices and the increased emergence of larger multispecialty clinics. Still others think such joint efforts will be on paper only, as has occurred in the IPAs and to a lesser extent the CWWs and MSOs.

Regardless of these and future organizational manifestations, however, one fact is clear: the image of the medical practice has become increasingly fuzzy and the challenges for service only heightened. These alternate structural forms can bring with them a loss of identity and a blurring of purpose. To avoid these reactions, medical practices need to reach out and embrace the concepts of service. This focus will remind them of their reason for existing at a time when it might be easy to forget.

Regardless of the form that your practice takes, the purpose of medical care has not and will not ever change. Medical care can be defined as the providing for the physical and mental well-being of one human being by another. It doesn't matter if your practice is a free-standing solo entity, a part of an established legal group, a member of an IPA, a PHO, a CWW, an MSO, an IDS, or a CCN. People will still be coming through your doors to receive treatment for their illnesses, solace for their pain, encouragement in making healthy life choices. Their need for you will be as real as it has always been, maybe even more, as the healthcare field rockets out of their control. How your medical practice responds to the pressures of your ever-changing environment and how effectively you deal with the major customer populations you serve will directly impact the physical and mental well-being of all concerned.

For the purposes of this book, then, I will be defining *medical practice* as follows: The setting in which one or more physicians provide healthcare to patients in an office environment, including any off-site nonclinical (and occasionally clinical) functions associated with that care. Today, perhaps more importantly than ever before, the practice in which that care occurs must be a combination of top-notch technical expertise and quality nonclinical service.

SERVICE

Several years ago, when the concept of *service* in healthcare was first discussed, many healthcare workers were unsure how it could apply. The differences between medical care and car sales seemed very real. The doctors as well as their staffs questioned the validity of applying these concepts, which worked well in retail sales, to their profession. Also, they were unsure how to give the customers (usually defined as patients) what they wanted and thought they needed, while still practicing solid medicine. As patients became more and more informed about the new medical technologies, they also became more and more demanding. Yet, not all of these technologies are appropriate to each patient. Physicians and their staffs found themselves in the awkward position of having to say no, while at the same time they were hearing from many sources that they had to give the patients what they wanted and thought they needed. Another change that has impacted the provision of service in the medical practice has to do with managed care and the realization that many aspects of the practice are now being influenced more strongly than ever by outside entities. The introduction of IDSs creates a renewed risk of the loss of autonomy.

All of this creates an atmosphere in which medical practice personnel of all types begin to question many things, among them, "In this environment how can I provide quality service? Does it even matter?" To the second question I cry a resounding "Yes!" To answer the first, let's begin with an understanding of what is meant by the word *service* in the context of the medical practice.

As it pertains to the process described in this book, *service* refers to the nontechnical aspects of healthcare, sometimes called the *psychosocial* or *nonclinical aspects of care*, the *practice development issues*, or, almost poetically, the *art of caring*. Whatever they are labeled, service issues are not *directly* involved in the technical diagnosis or treatment of illness, nor in the specification of preventive measures prescribed for maintaining good health. They are, however, aspects of the customers' experience in the medical practice that can and do impact the success of any treatment or health maintenance regimen.

Service aspects of healthcare cover three basic areas: the interpersonal interactions between practice personnel and the customers, the systems (including policies, procedures, and processes) in which all must function, and the customers' impressions based on nonrelational interactions with the practice (parking, appearance of the office, etc.). These aspects can and do impact the practice in many ways, and will be discussed in much greater detail throughout this book. However, at this point in time, it is important to note that when I speak of *service* in the medical practice, I mean all of the above and will refer to them as the *nonclinical* aspects of care.

I begin this next discussion with some fear of being misunderstood, so allow me to precede it with a qualifier: The goal of any Total Service Medical Practice should be to give the customers what they want and even more. Having said that, however, I realize that in reality this is not always possible or even advisable. Customers don't always make reasonable requests; sometimes the very thing they want can even harm them. So, there are instances, especially in healthcare today, when customers must be told "No." It is how they are given that message that makes the difference between a Total Service situation and one that is not. In Chapter 14, I describe a specific process for delivering that message while remaining consistent with the service goals and philosophy of a Total Service Medical Practice.

An important and relatively recent distinction needs to be made when talking about service, and that is the difference between customer satisfaction and service quality. The early research on customer service focused its attention of the notion of meeting customer expectations and thus creating satisfaction. In the mid-1980s Parasuramn, Zeithaml, and Berry developed a scale known as SERVQUAL, said to measure the perceived quality of consumer services.[5] This scale has been applied to healthcare in the form of patient satisfaction surveys which measure the following determinants: reliability, responsiveness, competence, availability, courtesy, communicativeness, credibility, security, understanding (empathy), and physical environment.[6]

In the early 1990s, however, Taylor and Cronin made an important observation. They wrote of a distinction between customer satisfaction and attitudes about service quality: "The distinction appears to revolve around the arguments that (1) service quality is a form of attitude representing a long-run overall evaluation, whereas (2) satisfaction represents a more short-term, transaction-specific measure."[7] Thus, according to this distinction, *customer satisfaction* refers to a response to a specific experience. *Service quality*, on the other hand, refers to a customer's long-term favorable or unfavorable attitudes regarding the nonclinical aspects of his or her *repeated* experiences with the practice.

To obtain the complete picture of the customer's perceptions of service, a practice needs to maintain a balanced approach. Reliance on short-term reactions alone is not enough. A patient, for example, may give negative feedback about a given service-episode but may still hold a positive attitude about the overall service provided by the practice. While the problematic situation encountered by the patient needs to be resolved for that individual and compared against feedback from other patients to determine generalizability, it is helpful to know long-term attitudes about service in the practice as well. Such comparisons can also place a given incident and/or customer in perspective. A medical practice should measure both perceptions of customer satisfaction and attitudes about service quality. In Chapter 6, I discuss how this can be done, and sample questionnaires for each are provided in the Appendix.

In this book, then, when referring to *service*, I will be speaking of the nonclinical aspects of care that lead to a high level of customer satisfaction (reactions to specific episodes of service) and positive customer attitudes of service quality (long-term attitudes about the nature of service provided by the practice). When I use the phrase *quality service*, I am referring to both.

CUSTOMERS

The introduction of the notion of *customers* into healthcare has not been immediately embraced by all concerned. Some fear that the use of that term will violate the very nature of the doctor/patient relationship. Still others who have accepted the idea of the patients as customers have stopped with that acceptance. In fact, the literature concerning issues in healthcare is replete with references to *patients* in the customer role, but very little has been written from a broader point of view.

To those holding the first concern, let me reassure you. The principles covered in this book in no way are designed to denigrate nor deny the special nature of the doctor/patient relationship. In fact, any physician who applies the concepts in this book will find that this unique relationship is only enhanced. If patients are being treated as valued customers, then they are being given the physician's undivided attention, are being listened to effectively, and are made to feel cared about as individuals—all attributes to be found in the best doctor/patient relationship.

Regarding those who already have included patients in their definition of *customers*, I ask you to stretch yourselves even further. The term *customers* will be used quite widely in this approach to Total Service. First, the distinction between internal and external customers is key to the successful implementation of the concepts in this book. The internal customers are all of those who actually work in the medical practice, from the physician to the receptionist to the billing clerk and more. These people are involved daily in bringing quality service to external customers. However, if they do not feel respected, understood, and valued by those with or for whom they work, then it becomes extremely difficult for them to provide quality service to those outside the practice.

Traditionally, the definition of the term *customers* has been focused externally, specifically on the users of a product or on the recipients of a service. In the Total Service Medical Practice, the definition of *external customers* breaks with tradition. Of course, the primary customers are the patients, and a great deal of the discussion in this book will focus on that population. However, other secondary customers are key to the success of the medical practice and to the successful treatment of that primary customer group. Jean Trygstad, the referral services director of Park Nicollet Medical Center in Minneapolis, said that focusing on patients as your only customers "is like training on an indoor track when the race is to be held on a hilly terrain in July; you may finish the race but you won't win. Other customers must be considered."[8]

During my workshops for medical practice personnel, the participants complete an exercise in which they list their external customers. Based on those responses as well as on a thorough review of the literature, I have identified at least four additional, secondary customer populations: family members of patients, other physicians, insurance carriers, and hospitals. (An inter-dependence exists between your practice and these groups—you need each other in order to provide quality care to the patients). When I speak of *customers* in this book, often I will be talking of the *patients*. However, I will frequently make correlations to members of these additional populations as well. Also, much of what I say regarding service to one population is pertinent to providing service to another. Just remember, to become a Total Service Medical Practice, the word *customers* takes on new and different meanings.

During the interviews that I conducted with office managers in preparation for writing this book, I asked the following question: "Do you believe that service is important to the medical practice today?" Given the history of healthcare's reluctant acceptance of this concept, I was pleased to hear their responses. "Medicine is service driven." "Medical care is, first and foremost, a service business." "If we want to stay in business we have to deliver in the nonclinical as well as the clinical." Perhaps a sixteen-year veteran of medical practice office management summed it up best. When describing her view of service to the patients as customers, she explained, "In the first place, maybe 30 percent of the people who come to see you are well and come in for a well exam. The others are already sick. They don't know what they have, they don't know what you are going to tell them while they are there, and they are already worried. You better have someone at the front desk who is responsive to these patients, someone in the back office who can take care of them, a doctor who is willing to listen to them, and someone in the billing department who can bill them correctly. I think it has to go all the way through the process. I believe that customer service is one of the most important aspects of a medical practice. Our patients deserve no less." I would only add, the same is true for all the customers you serve!

For our purposes, then, *customers* of a medical practice will be defined as all individuals or groups, either inside or outside the practice, with whom that practice has an interdependent relationship.

TOTAL

This word implies that I am discussing something more than smile-training and slogans . . . and I am. I am talking about a deep commitment to a way of life, not just a quick fix to problems. *Total*, in the context of this book, refers to proactive steps, not defensive reactions. The Total Service Medical Practice will not merely react to problems after they have occurred. Rather, through a specifically outlined process, it will take the lead in preventing difficulties before they exist and will have developed a carefully structured process of service recovery for any problems that may occur. The Total Service Medical Practice will neither engage in isolated efforts of acknowledging the importance of service nor will it be only vaguely aware of the importance of the nonclinical aspects of care. Rather, it will embrace a complete and comprehensive process of inquiry, analysis, and action, leading to the creation and maintenance of the Total Service perspective. So, although the word *total* is short, containing but five simple letters, it represents a great deal: the proactive, complete, conscious process of delivering quality service to all internal and external customers. That is what the Total Service Medical Practice truly means, and that is what will be covered in this book.

END NOTES

1. *The Official ABMS Directory of Board Certified Medical Specialists*, 27th ed. (New Providence, New Jersey: Marquis Who's Who, A Reed Reference Publishing Co., 1995, pp. xxxvii–xlvii.

2. Fred McCall-Perez, "Emerging Practice Patterns: Clinics without Walls," *Journal of Medical Practice Management* 9, no. 4 (March/April 1994), p. 222.

3. "MSOs-Management Firms," MGMA Information Exchange #4749, March 1995.

4. Timothy M. Rotarius et al., "Integrated Delivery Systems/Networks in the Uncertain Future," *MGM Journal* 42, no. 4 (July/August 1995), p. 22.

5. Joby John, "Improving Quality through Patient-Provider Communication," *Journal of Health Care Marketing* 11, no. 4 (December 1991), p. 53.

6. Ibid.

7. Steven A. Taylor and J. Joseph Cronin, Jr., "Modeling Patient Satisfaction and Service Quality," *Journal of Health Care Marketing* 14, no. 1 (Spring 1994), pp. 34–44.

8. Jean Trygstad, "Winning the Referral Marathon," *Group Practice Journal* 39, no. 6 (November/December 1990), p. 48.

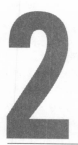

CHAPTER

Step Two—Understand the Whys of Service

WHY A SPECIFIC, STRUCTURED APPROACH TO SERVICE?

Most people who have chosen careers in healthcare realize that they are in a helping profession. As such, they are aware, at some level, of the service orientation that must accompany that choice. However, the application of specific service principles to this field, particularly to medical practices, has not been universal. I have found that this is not usually due to a lack of caring personnel, but rather it is attributable to a lack of specific focus.

When a practice does not have a conscious service commitment and has not implemented a structured service approach, it will not only miss opportunities to serve its customers well but may also even create negative experiences. Daniel Gottovi, M.D., a pulmonologist in Wilmington, North Carolina, explained what happened in his practice. In the latter part of 1989, the 27-doctor clinic with which he is affiliated decided to assess a charge for clinical phone calls, without any advance consideration of the impact of this decision on the customers. The new policy was communicated through an insert in January billings. Soon after the mailing had been distributed, the office switchboard was swamped with angry callers, and even a radio talk show blasted the practice. The newspaper ran an article ending with this comment from a former patient: "How would you like to call your doctor, ask for a new prescription, and get charged $3.50 for it? There are many ways of making money. Making one [phone] call . . . is not a good one." Dr. Gottovi explained: "We goofed! It was an honest mistake, but one that was costly in lost patient revenue and even community goodwill."[1] This clinic's well-meaning but unconscious actions emphasize the importance of formalizing your practice's commitment to service. Quality service does not just happen. It requires a managed process with well-defined steps and outcomes.

WHY DOES SERVICE MATTER?

Of course, there are humanistic responses with which to answer this question. In my workshops for medical practice personnel, participants often say, "It's just the right thing to do!" and I agree with that completely. It takes that kind of belief and attitude to provide the powerful horse I referred to in the Preface. Without that commitment to helping and serving people, no plan, model, or method will provide the kind of service your customers want and expect.

However, there are other reasons for consciously creating a Total Service practice. They make sense from both the business perspective as well as, perhaps surprisingly, from the clinical. Divided into practice development rationale and clinical rationale, these reasons are worth consideration as you embark on your journey toward a Total Service Medical Practice.

Practice Development Rationale

Practice Development Reason #1: Quality service
increases the attraction of new patients.
How does your practice attract new patients? If medical practices were like most businesses, the answer would include advertising. It is not uncommon to see a movie theater or a clothing store engage in a campaign that announces or emphasizes its commitment to service. In my part of the country, the Men's Wearhouse television commercials say very little about the quality of the clothing product. Rather the emphasis is on George Zimmer, the company president, and his personal service guarantee.

However, such a campaign for a doctor's office is difficult to justify. The secret of effective advertising is repetition, and the staying power of a single ad, in any kind of medium, is minimal. Thus, potential customers must be exposed to the message over and over so that it stays in their minds. George Zimmer is on one Denver television channel no fewer than 10 times a day, and that kind of exposure costs money. Big money. It is not the most cost-effective way for a medical practice to get its message across. Carol Mullinax, as director of the communications department for the Ohio State Medical Association, is responsible for that association's media relations, and she has reached the following conclusion: "An effective, well-thought-out campaign may create a warm fuzzy feeling toward physicians—temporarily. But when someone goes to the doctor and feels that he or she has been treated insensitively, kept waiting, or subjected to any of the host of other things people complain [about], any benefit from the paid message would be cancelled out. In short, money can't buy you love! Personal experience counts the most."[2]

There is an old rule of public relations: The best promotion comes through word of mouth. For medical practices, that is very much the case. The attraction of new patients comes from people talking to people, and the two primary sources for this spreading of the word are current patients and referring physicians. Even within the confines of a managed care network, word-of-mouth recommendations are still heavily relied on.

People will talk, and when patients talk to each other they don't usually discuss the doctor's technical expertise. Sometimes they might include the physician's diagnostic or surgical skills, but most often when asked by a friend or family member to make a recommendation, patients usually discuss the nonclinical aspects of their experiences with a given practice, including the courtesy of the receptionists and ancillary staff; waiting time, especially for physicians; and telephone etiquette. One physician, Richard Abrams, M.D., an internist in Denver, is a firm believer that his efforts to provide exceptional service have been rewarded with word-of-mouth referrals. Dr. Abrams makes it a practice to make unsolicited, follow-up phone calls to patients to ask how they are feeling after surgery or after beginning a new treatment or prescription. He reports, "I [make the calls] first thing in the morning. It takes less than 60 seconds per call. I can't begin to tell you how many patients I've gotten referred to me as a result of these phone calls."[3] One woman who has been a practice manager for fifteen years responded to my question, "What is the nicest compliment that you've ever heard about your practice?" by saying, "When somebody said 'so and so recommended you.' It felt good to know that our patients are happy enough with our practice to recommend us to someone else. And it's just good business."

The other major source of new patients is other doctors. Probably the most common referral process occurs between primary care physicians, to use the parlance of managed care, and specialists. Again, even within the constraints of a participating physicians' network, PCPs usually have a choice of doctors to whom they can and do refer their patients. Marilyn Haley, the office manager of a busy multisited asthma practice, understands this fact: "Certainly it is different in today's healthcare environment. A specialty practice like ours is a referral practice. So it's just as important for us to keep the referring doctor happy as it is to keep the referred patient."

Why does one doctor refer a patient to another doctor? Of course, technical expertise and previous experience are key criteria. But referrals are also based on service issues: How does that practice interact with his or her practice? How accessible is the doctor for consultation? How quickly can the referred patient be seen? Referring doctors also consider patients' reports about a particular office. Office manager Arlene Stolte explained it this way: "A positive experience in a physician's office is the best way to ensure future referrals."

It is clear, then, that one important consideration in the choice of your practice by either patients or other physicians is the quality of the service you offer. To gain new patients, your practice must be consciously on top of its service game.

Practice Development Reason #2: Quality service increases the retention of existing patients.

"It's not what it used to be," stated David Chube, M.D., of Gary, Indiana. Dr. Chube was describing the difference in patient loyalty from the days before he joined his father's family practice. He explained, "If patients are not satisfied with the service they're getting, not only from the physician but from the staff, they'll walk. They go find somebody else."[4] Years ago, it wasn't that way; patients stayed with one doctor, often for a lifetime. Now, due in some degree to the enforced changes resulting from shifts in employers' benefits packages and to the emphasis on specialization in the medical profession during the last few decades, patients are quite likely to experience several different medical practices during their life spans. The old feelings of commitment and personal affiliation are harder to establish and maintain. The truth is that patients are becoming more independent; some doctors call them *fickle*. They have become more consumer-oriented than ever before. The old mystique of the godlike nature of their physician and the old Marcus Welby image of the kindly, house-calling, neighborhood doc has been replaced in their minds. Instead they often refer to physicians as their partners in healthcare, and they seek a more active role in their treatment regimen. While this change is not inherently bad, and can result in increased patient responsibility, it also can lead to a more tenuous doctor/patient relationship.

Patients will leave a practice for service reasons. The Technical Assistance Research Project (TARP), the widely respected consumer research project conducted for the U.S. Office of Consumer Affairs, examined customer complaint behavior. An examination of the study's results reveals that regardless of the type of business involved, the primary reason people stopped using a particular company was because they had encountered a problem or unpleasant surprise in a transaction with that company.[5] The same is true of patients in a medical practice.

Specifically, patients report difficulties with their doctors as one of the major reasons for taking their business elsewhere. While interviewing patients during the research phase of writing this book, I was told quite directly, "Doctors aren't gods. They are human beings like the rest of us. I expect to be treated with respect and caring or I will take my business elsewhere." Ken Terry, senior editor for *Medical Economics*, referred to this problem as well when he cited the following results of a telephone survey conducted by the Miles Institute of Health Care Communication: "a fourth of the one thousand respondents said that they have left the care of a doctor because of communication problems."[6] In the good old days, that issue might never have even been raised, and, if it had been, the number of errant patients would have been much, much smaller.

Difficulties with staff members are also cited by some patients as reasons for changing practices. A patient I interviewed explained the impact of the staff in her orthopedic surgeon's office on her choice to see another doctor. "The attitude of the staff was so bad. They were negative, uncaring, and mean. That's no way to treat a patient!" Other patients reported the following staff-related factors as significant to their decisions to leave specific practices: lack of staff professionalism, petty staff bickering, lack of attentiveness, too much social conversation among staff members, and lack of confidentiality.

Given the increasingly independent nature of patients and the increasingly transitory nature of healthcare itself, the old feelings of commitment and personal affiliation with one physician and his or her practice are harder to establish and maintain. It can be done, however, and the purpose of this book is to give you one specific process for facilitating that affiliation. Even specialists' practices, who will always have a more transitory relationship with their patients, are not relieved from the responsibility of creating a service focus. As has been discussed, their repeat business comes from the referring doctors who do listen as patients describe their experiences with a specialist's office. For primary care doctors, the retention of their patient load is vital to their business success, and patients *doctor shop* much more than they used to. Robert Taylor, M.D., explained, "A colleague in a long-established primary care practice reports: 'Over the past few years I've learned that patient loyalty can be fragile and that as physicians we've got to extend ourselves farther than ever before to meet patients' needs.' "[7] This extending also includes the patient's relationships with the practice staff as well as with the systems in which medical care is delivered.

Practice Development Reason #3: Quality service increases attraction and retention of service-oriented personnel.

"It takes a special kind of person to work in a medical practice. That person needs to care about people and to love the medical environment. Finance can't be the paramount consideration, because nobody gets rich working here. Our staff have to really want to help people; they have to really want to serve." With these words, an office manager in a workshop described the kind of employee any medical practice would be pleased to have.

I confess to being surprised when I learned that not all people understood the importance of service. In fact, some actually saw it as pandering to the customer's whims, or so I was told. In preparation for one of my workshops, I was asked by the coordinator to be sure to cover the reasons a medical practice would want to focus on service. She confided that she had heard some of the office personnel discussing this very issue, and they concluded that the customers were making unreasonable demands and that to cave into them would be a loss of their own dignity. I, of course, honored her request and thus the preliminary draft of this chapter was created. My consciousness was also raised regarding the importance of finding and keeping staff who are committed to service and understand its value; it's not as easy to replace them as it might appear.

Losing practice personnel is also expensive. Office manager Deborah Goodyear explained, "The whole philosophy around practice personnel has changed. It used to be that you just replaced the person. That just isn't true any more. You hire well to begin with and train them and mold them and work with them, but don't get rid of them. It's way too costly, on many levels, to throw them away!" Ms. Goodyear related another economic reason for staff retention: "When an office is in transition all the time, when you go through a lot of practice personnel and the patients have been here longer than the staff, things seem to be in upheaval. Patients like to know who they are talking to, what their nurse's name is, and if the nurse remembers who they are. If patients constantly see new faces every time they walk into the office, this could eat away at their trust and comfort level and that could result in high patient turnover." So pragmatically it is wise to hire good people, and in a medical practice those people have to care, and be aware of the importance of service.

In addition, the practice personnel who are committed to providing quality service don't just *want* but *need* to work in an environment where that is not only rewarded but valued. They cannot be happy nor thrive in a situation where the concepts of service are not consciously stated, internalized, and operationalized. One staff member told me: "I love it here! We do everything we can to put our customers first." Then she paused a moment and continued reflectively, "I have to have this." The medical practice that provides the space and place for its staff to find fulfillment is the one that will retain these employees. It is also the one that will consistently provide the kind of experiences that will keep the customers satisfied and happy.

Practice Development Reason #4: Quality service decreases the likelihood of malpractice suits.

Perhaps the very mention of the word *malpractice* makes the hair on the back of your neck stand up, or it might bring a sick and sinking feeling to the pit of your stomach. Perhaps you feel like Billy J. Davis, M.D., a general practitioner from Harwell, Georgia, when he said, "We've been drilled, admonished, warned, and advised [about malpractice] so many times!"[8] I'm certain that is true. In today's litigious society, medical malpractice suits account for a great deal of court time and a huge chunk of attorneys' fees. Although a large percentage of the suits are hospital-related, a significant proportion are based on perceived or real problems in the medical practice. In fact, The Physicians Insurers Association of America reported that 26 percent of 90,000 malpractice claims started with incidents that took place in the physician's office.[9]

Thus, I sympathize with what you must be experiencing; I can only imagine how it must feel to be constantly looking over your shoulder to see who is preparing to file suit, to say nothing about the huge insurance premiums that must be paid in order to protect a physician from that dreaded possibility. And yes, in spite of all of that, I am going to talk about malpractice anyway. However, I hope to be able to bring you some good news rather than bad. The truth is this: a medical practice that provides quality service has a smaller likelihood of being sued than a practice that does not!

An interesting phenomenon exists in the decision-making process regarding the filing of a malpractice suit. James Orlikoff, former director of the American Hospital Association's Institute on Quality of Care and Patterns of Practice, explained, "Many sue who have no reason to do so, legally. Many have legal reasons to sue but choose not to . . . What motivates a patient to become a plaintiff? All you're left with [if you rule out medical negligence] is patient interaction, how the patient feels about the provider . . ."[10] Charles Wold, the past president of the Society of Medical-Dental Management Consultants observed, "For every successful malpractice claim there are probably hundreds more that never arose. What's the difference? In most cases, the patient was too well disposed toward the physician and the practice to seriously consider suing."[11] Barbara Brown, Ph.D., R.N., head of the risk management division of Virginia Professional Underwriters, Inc., also has observed this phenomenon. She wrote, "Patients will accept error but they will not accept the feeling that they have not been seen, haven't been heard, and haven't been accepted. We've had cases where patients seemed to have sued primarily because of a feeling that no one cared about them."[12]

It really doesn't take much to avert a suit with many patients. Sometimes all it requires is listening and honoring a simple request. For example, there was the case of the man who required leg surgery and asked his physician to complete a form for his employer explaining that he couldn't work. The form had to be signed within 15 days, the patient explained, or else he could be fired from his job. The physician accepted the form for his secretary to complete. The patient made repeated calls to the physician and the secretary during the following week to learn if the form had been mailed. Despite promises that it would be mailed, it wasn't until after the deadline. The patient was fired. He then sued the physician. Closer attention to detail and really listening to the patient's request could have averted this entire situation, which incidentally involved no complaints about the medical care the patient received.[13]

Frank Plaut, the former president of the Colorado Bar Association, told this story of a client who went into the hospital for back surgery. After she seemed to be very slow to recover, a second surgery was performed and an 11-inch sponge left from the first operation was found in the wound. Mr. Plaut explained: "If ever there was a legitimate case for malpractice, this was it." During the time in which they discussed her case, Mr. Plaut advised his client to name everyone who might have been remotely involved in providing substandard care in the suit. In spite of his advice, she steadfastly refused to include one of the physicians. When pushed to reveal her reason for not wanting to name this doctor in her suit, she explained, "He was the only person who came by to see me. He was the only one who tried to find out what was wrong with me. He was the only one who cared. If I have to include him, then I won't sue anyone."

Malpractice is primarily a problem in human relations. The first key relationship where such difficulties can be found is that between the doctor and the patient. John-Henry Pfifferling, Director of the Center for Professional Well-Being, in Durham, North Carolina, stressed, "The source of malpractice claims, contrary to widely held views, is not simply improper or inadequate medical care . . . High on the list of nonclinical causes are faults in the physician/patient relationship. Patients who are unhappy with the manner in which they have been treated by physicians are much more likely to sue when the outcome is even moderately untoward." He continued by advising, "Key to reducing the incidence of malpractice suits is helping physicians understand that attention has to be paid to their behavior."[14] In his article on how to reduce malpractice risks, Inge K. Winer, Director of Quality Assurance for the University of Chicago Hospitals and Clinics, cited a survey of malpractice defense attorneys that found that 70 percent of suits were attributed to failures in doctor/patient relationships.[15] In Chapter 13, specific suggestions for establishing and maintaining positive patient/physician relationships are discussed. By being open to exploring these suggestions, physicians will not only assure that they are demonstrating effective customer-service behaviors, but will also reduce their likelihood of being sued.

Physicians are not the only individuals in a medical practice who can and do impact a patient's decision to file suit. Andrew M. Scherffius, who practices law in Atlanta and represents the plaintiffs in malpractice suits, made the connection directly to the staff in the practice as well. "I've been involved in many cases in which an attentive office staff helped keep a suit from proceeding." He also has seen cases where office staff have seriously hurt a doctor's position.[16] In Chapter 9, I cover some specific guidelines for hiring and retaining an effective, customer-focused staff. In Chapter 12 and Chapter 13, I explain specific skills for establishing and maintaining effective customer interactions (Moments of Truth). Also, in Chapter 10, I offer advice to staff members on the importance of their role in the office in creating satisfying and positive patient relationships. As with the suggestions to the physicians, if medical practice personnel implement these ideas, the possibilities of litigation can be significantly reduced.

What about those situations in which the patient perseveres and the case goes to court? Again, the physician from a Total Service Medical Practice will be in much better shape to sway the jury than one who is not. Charlotte Miller, director of practice assessment and quality improvement for the American Medical Association in Chicago, said, "Juries feel that physicians are more responsible than their patients. What's more, juries aren't prone to be sympathetic toward a doctor unless they can see solid proof that both the doctor and staff made 'reasonable attempts' to ensure good patient care."[17] Included in that *good patient care* is a substantial dose of effective service behaviors.

Practice Development Reason #5: Quality service increases a practice's attractiveness for group or network affiliation.

As I mentioned in Chapter 1, physicians are increasingly aware of the advantages of voluntarily coming together in one of a wide variety of group structures. As the pressures to join increase, the competition for membership does too, thus making acceptance into a group more and more selective. A number of factors are considered when applications for affiliation are evaluated, and high among them are the service aspects of practices seeking to join.

In the last few years, all types of managed care organizations have also increased their scrutiny of physicians' practices in their networks. An area of particular interest to these companies is member-patient satisfaction with the providers and their staff. Solicited through surveys that are more completely discussed in Chapter 6, these member-patient reactions focus on the nonclinical aspects of the visit to the doctor's office. Probably because it is assumed that most lay people do not have enough expertise to evaluate the technical aspects of their medical experiences, the surveys concentrate on such issues as waiting time, personal concern shown by the doctor, and attitudes of the receptionist and other practice personnel.

This increasing health plan interest in member-patient perceptions has occurred for two reasons. The first has to do with the retention of members. Although employees are usually limited in the choice they themselves have about which plans are included in their employers' benefits packages, they can and do influence their employers' decisions. Although benefits managers consider cost and coverage, they also listen to what their employees say about the plan. When interviewing benefits managers for a research project I was conducting a few years ago, one of them provided this succinct summary: "When our members are unhappy with a plan, we look for another one."

There is a direct link between the members' satisfaction with a health plan and what happens to them in their doctors' offices. While conducting some member focus groups for an IPA client, I made the following query: "What is important to you about the service you receive from a health plan?" Their responses focused on the attitude of the staff in their doctors' offices. I asked again, thinking that perhaps they hadn't understood my question, and again they talked about the physicians' practices. Then, I realized that, to these members, the doctor's office *is* the health plan. This realization has since been reinforced by participants in my workshops for medical practice personnel. They have a very keen sense of the connection in their patients' minds between the doctors' offices and their patients' insurance carriers. This realization is also not lost on the managed care companies themselves. If the plan's members are happy with the visits to the practices in their network or the doctors on their staffs, then the employer is much more likely to stay with that carrier. If not, then the plan may well lose business (and so would any practice or physician dropped from the plan due to such patient dissatisfaction).

The health plans' own certification processes provide the second reason for this focus on service issues in the medical practice. To be competitive in their industry, managed care companies need to be certified by the National Commission on Quality Assurance (NCQA). Two significant standards in that accreditation process are patient satisfaction and quality improvement. Low ratings can directly impact the plan's ultimate certification. Thus, member-patient satisfaction surveys are used by the health plan to flag practices or physicians or their staff that may be having difficulties and to provide them with feedback on how to improve. In addition, positive responses are used during the NCQA certification process to demonstrate and document the company's emphasis on quality.

The same member-patient satisfaction data are used by the health plans during the recredentialing process when network physician's are up for review; patients who are consistently dissatisfied—whether with doctors or with their staff—can result in a physician's dismissal from the panel. Staff-model HMOs consider patient satisfaction during the times of performance appraisals, and the results can literally affect retention decisions. The director of provider-relations for a major managed care company confirmed, "Of course, if problems are discovered we will work with the doctors and their practices to correct the difficulties. But if things don't improve, we will consider this the next time they come up for review."

So, whether doctors are seeking inclusion or retention in a physician-formed group, in a managed care network, or on an HMO staff, patients' evaluations of the service aspects of their care have become increasingly important.

Practice Development Reason #6: Quality service reduces stress for everyone!

What causes stress in the medical practice? Ask a different person and you'll get a different answer. Office managers and staff report the following: "Differing policies among insurance carriers." "The paperwork!" "The telephone!" Doctors report: "The schedule!" "The loss of autonomy." "The pressure of diagnosis and treatment." Add to these the stress brought on by negative service interactions and you've got an environment that pushes the stress meter off the scale.

Patients report a wide variety of reasons for their stress in a doctor's office: "Waiting!" "Uncaring attitude of staff." "Doctors who don't listen." Even "Outdated magazines!" These may all be contributors to the patients' stress levels, and on occasion may indeed be the initial causes. However, in the healthcare field, your primary customers are often dealing with another inherent stressor, simply expressed by one focus group member: "I'm afraid of what's wrong with me." Another described the same reaction as he explained more fully, "When I go to a doctor's office, I'm usually sick or have been injured. I don't feel good and sometimes I'm afraid. Then almost anything that happens is going to upset me and make me mad." Even patients who come in for a wellness visit relate experiencing a certain level of anxiety. The kind of fear and at times what appears to be inexplicable anger resulting from varying levels of patient anxiety only add to the already taxing elements of daily life in the physician's practice.

None of these stressors for either practice personnel or their customers can be completely eliminated. The telephone will keep ringing, doctors' schedules will continue to be full, and patients will always experience medical problems that concern them. So, in Chapter 14, I discuss some specific suggestions for dealing with stress on both a short-term and long-term basis. For now, the point that needs to be made is this: Positive service situations are less stressful than negative ones. By providing positive service experiences for your customers in a medical practice, you can and will reduce the stress for all parties, and this is a goal worth striving for.

Clinical Rationale

At first, some people have been surprised to find this next section included in my discussion of rationale for service. They have previously considered why service makes good sense from a business standpoint, but they haven't really pondered the connections between service issues and diagnosis, treatment, and healing. Let's explore these now.

Clinical Reason #1: Quality service leads to improved diagnoses.

At first glance, service and diagnosis may seem unrelated. However, it requires only a moment's pause to recognize their connection. First, even the biological data needed for accurate diagnosis can be affected by the patient's service experiences. One focus group participant explained what happens to him when he is not recognized by the receptionist on arrival and must wait to be acknowledged: "Nothing makes me angrier than to walk up to a counter and have someone look at me and go back to doing something on the computer, like I'm not even there. That really burns me! Literally, my blood pressure goes up if I have someone who will just leave me hanging." Patients in this state do not provide useful diagnostic data because their bodies are producing unreliable physiological reactions.

In addition to the scientific tests and physical examinations, important diagnostic information is obtained through other means as well, most especially through effective patient interviews. When patients feel listened to and cared about, two of the service issues listed as important by most patients, they also feel relaxed. Then they are able to listen better and can understand questions asked by the physician or other providers. When they are feeling calm, patients can also think more clearly and can thus recall more and better information for consideration, information that can be used in making the most accurate and complete diagnoses. And what about that angry patient cited above? He expressed it best: " If I'm already mad at the world when the physician gets to me, I don't even hear what he asks me!" So, diagnosis can be assisted by having a calm, relaxed patient who has been treated well out front, was not kept waiting too long in the exam room, and is listened to and made to feel cared for by the physician. These are all service aspects of the patient's experience with the practice that can impact the quality of the diagnosis.

Clinical Reason #2: Quality service improves compliance with treatment.

A textbook used in a required course at the University of Colorado Medical School defines compliance as ". . . the degree to which a patient carries out the clinical recommendations of the treating physician. Examples include keeping appointments, entering into and completing a treatment program, taking medications correctly, and following recommended changes in behavior or diet."[18]

A rather puzzling phenomenon occurs regarding patients and their compliance with treatment: Many of them don't do it. In general, only one-third comply with treatment completely, while another one-third sometimes comply with only certain aspects of treatment, and still another one-third never comply at all.[19]

In an attempt to understand why such a high percentage of patients fail to comply regularly, a number of variables have been investigated. Although not the only factors, certainly two of the most important are the doctor/patient and the staff/patient relationships which are operationalized by how well parties communicate with each other. As the above-mentioned textbook put it: "Simply stated, when there are communication problems, compliance decreases."[20]

One reason patients do not comply with treatment, which can be directly traced to communication difficulties, is that they literally do not understand what has been prescribed. Often the lack of understanding is created by what's happening inside the patients themselves. In communication theory, emotional upsets such as anger or fear are called *noise*, and they can often block the sender's message from getting through to the receiver. So, when patients who are suffering from communication noise-blocks interact with their physicians, they cannot attend to the messages as they are being sent and thus literally do not comprehend all, if any, of what their physicians are saying. Many patients are angered by being ignored, or left to wander the halls in search of the exam room, or abandoned while attired in odd little gowns. As these angry patients wait in cold, sterile environments, they will be experiencing some internal noise. One patient explained, "If you get me cross-ways, [get me angry] then I'm going to be down your throat and I'm probably going to misinterpret what you tell me."

It also can be argued that a calm, caring approach by the physician, and also the staff, can reduce the patient's focus on another type of internal block, the physical noise. When patients do not feel well or are experiencing pain, they will find it more difficult to focus on what is being said. Although not 100 percent effective, the simple belief that someone is there to help facilitates their relaxation, which often lessens their pain, thus enabling them to focus more successfully on what is being said. One patient summarized it this way: "When I am hurting, I need reassurance. I literally feel better if I know someone cares." Positive service behaviors can and do create a communication environment in which patients experience much less internal emotional or physical noise and thus can better comprehend the treatment as explained, allowing them to process the information well enough to ask clarifying questions.

Of course, not all treatment-comprehension problems are caused by communication noise within the patients! Physicians and/or staff also can contribute to this problem by speaking too quickly, using technical terms without explanation, and not verifying the patient's understanding before terminating the conversation. One elderly patient told me, "My doctor went through it so fast and used such big words, I got lost! And I was afraid to ask him to repeat." Age of the patient is not the critical variable here! Based on what they report, most patients have experienced this phenomenon at one time or another.

An additional reason for noncompliance is the influence from outside sources, something the physician will not realize if he or she does not know about patients as people. As much as possible, the physician should encourage patients to open up about their lives in general. Sometimes patients are more comfortable sharing this kind of information with assistants or other staff. Robert Bright, M.D., of Bremerton, Washington, realizes this and encourages his staff members to gather pertinent information about what's going on in the patient's life in the course of conversation. For example, a staff member may learn that a patient who is not supposed to be exerting herself at home is not getting any help from her husband or family. Once the doctor is alerted, he or she can address the situation in a tactful discussion with the patient and her husband or family.[21] This kind of inquiry, regardless of who is conducting it, not only reveals important factors that impact the patient's compliance, but is perceived by the patient as "Here is someone who really cares." Caring is, after all, one of the criteria patients use to determine their satisfaction with the service they have received in a medical practice.

Continued compliance can be greatly increased by praise from the physician, a behavior that is indicative of a Total Service orientation. Alan Rockoff, M.D., a dermatologist, told of a young man who was being treated for cystic acne and had very high blood lipids. "I explained the importance of getting them down and how to do it, not only for his skin but for his general health and appearance. On the next blood workup, they'd dropped significantly. I praised him highly, asking how he'd managed [to follow instructions] when so many people can't. He was extremely proud of following my advice to avoid fast foods, most sweets, etc. . . . His skin is much better. I continue to praise him."[22] People respond well to positive reinforcements, and the praise of a physician means a great deal to most patients.

Not just the doctor's praise is important, however. Staff, both medical and nonmedical, also can have an impact. A patient who had endured a long and painful recovery process from an automobile accident described the way the enthusiastic support and praise of the orthopedics physician's assistant and receptionist helped her keep going in her difficult period of rehabilitation. "When I showed them how well I was walking, the PA said, 'Wow! You are doing so well!' The receptionist was equally supportive, praising me for my progress. When I left that office, I felt like I could do anything!" This patient in fact continued with her therapy, and in spite of the metal plate and six screws holding her injured hip in place, today walks without a limp. She credits the positive support provided by the entire staff with the successful outcome of her treatment and her willingness to stick with it even when it hurt.

Compliance with treatment is important to the clinical outcomes desired by the physician and the patient. The kinds of behaviors that will facilitate compliance are also the kinds of behaviors that will be interpreted as signs of quality service by the patients. Thus, the rationale for doing them meets important service and clinical goals. (Specific suggestions for increasing compliance are offered in Chapter 14. Several of the Twelve Steps To Effective Patient Interviews covered in Chapter 13 will also be helpful).

Clinical Reason #3: Quality service facilitates the clinical outcomes.

In addition to their impact on patients' compliance with treatment, the service behaviors of physicians and their staff affect clinical results as well. Although somewhat controversial, there is substantial evidence that feelings of positiveness and peace can and do facilitate the healing process. Your practice represents the one place where patients should be able to find peace of mind and even hope. Any tension or anxiety they might experience as a result of visiting your practice is felt even more intensely. The Texas Back Institute has carefully documented the connection between service and clinical outcomes. Each year for the past several years, a random sample of 500 to 800 patients have been interviewed by a marketing firm, providing results with a confidence level of 95 percent. Robert Reznik, vice president of the clinic, stated, "[Patient] satisfaction related to nontechnical psychosocial aspects of these service encounters can influence a patient's technical clinical outcome, especially if pain relief is a measure of clinical outcome for a clinic."[23] He also concluded that, "Clinical outcome may be adversely influenced when the customer is not satisfied on a psychosocial level with the service encounter."[24]

Clinical Reason #4: Quality service increases the opportunity for continuity of care.

I first heard the term *continuity of care* when my niece was in nurse's training, and since that time I have grown to understand its importance in the treatment of patients. This concept makes sense even to a layperson such as I. In most instances, the longer any given patient can be seen and cared for by the same healthcare provider, the more complete the knowledge of medical history, treatment regimen, medications, etc. One family physician explained, "When I have the patient over an extended period of time, I know firsthand what health problems she has experienced and what treatment plans I have used to address them. Although this information can be factually gained through patient interviews and the transfer of charts, I can't help but believe my own personal knowledge affords that patient better healthcare ."

So, clinically, a goal for many doctors is to retain the patient as long as possible. In a Total Service Medical Practice they will have a much better chance of doing so. In spite of the changing times, patient loyalty can still be developed, and service issues are the keys to creating that kind of relationship.

All of the above clinical reasons for providing quality service have been focused exclusively and appropriately on the primary customer. It should be remembered, however, that positive relationships between a medical practice and its secondary customers often can impact these clinical issues as well. Family members and other physicians, for example, are frequently needed to provide additional important diagnostic information about patients. If the relationships the practice has with these customers are not positive, and thus do not allow for open and honest communication, then the result can be inaccurate and erroneous information. Secondary customers are often also needed to administer, monitor, or encourage treatment plans, thus having a direct impact on the patient's compliance, yet the examples of ignored family members and uninformed hospital staff abound. We even know that family members often call the shots for patients when it comes to choosing and remaining with a physician. Hospitals, managed care companies, and other physicians can exert varying degrees of influence on this decision as well, meaning continuity of care for the patient can be interrupted by a source outside the doctor/patient or even staff/patient relationships. In order to provide the best kind of clinical care to the patients of your practice, the secondary customers must also be nurtured and valued.

The practice of medicine has long been known as the *art of healing* and many people refer to the service aspects of the medical experience as the *art of caring*. I would like to combine the two in such a way as to express the real meaning behind the rationale for quality service: The *healing art of caring*. *Healing* is the essential component of diagnosis, treatment, and healing of patients. *Caring* is shown in many ways, and the exploration of these ways will provide the content for the remainder of this book.

END NOTES

1. Daniel Gottovi, M.D., "The Best Experts of All Help Run Our Practice," *Medical Economics* 68, no.9 (May 6, 1991), pp. 56–57.

2. Carol Mullinax, "Can the Luster Be Restored?" *The Internist* 35, no. 1 (January 1994), p. 12.

3. Richard Abrams, M.D., quoted by Anne-Marie Nelson and Stephen W. Brown, "Do You Know What Your Patients Expect?" *Family Practice Management* 1, no. 5 (May 1994), pp. 52–53.

4. David Chube, M.D., quoted by Robert McCoppin, "Service Is the Key to Healthy Practice," *American Medical News* 35, no. 11 (March 18, 1994), p. 12.

5. John Goodman, of the Technical Assistance Research Programs Institute, "Consumer Compliant Handling: An Update Study for the U.S. Office of Consumer Affairs (Washington, D.C., 1986).

6. Ken Terry, "Telling Patients More Will Save Your Time," *Medical Economics* 71, no 14. (July 25, 1994), pp. 40, 43.

7. Robert Taylor, M.D., "What Do Patients Look for in Their Physicians?" *Physician's Management* 31, no. 10 (October 1991), p. 54.

8. Billy J. Davis, M.D., quoted by Stu Chapman, "Get with the Program: Malpractice Prevention 2000: Targeting Who's at Risk," *Physician's Management* 37, no. 7 (July 1994), p. 45.

9. "Don't Let Staff Push Patients into Malpractice Suits," *Medical Office Manager* 7, no. 1 (January 1993) p. 3.

10. James Orlikoff quoted by Flora Johnson Skelly, *American Medical News* 35, no. 25 (June 29, 1992), pp. 25–26.

11. Charles R. Wold, "The Art of Malpractice Risk Management," *Physician's Management* 33, no. 2 (February 1993) p. 57.

12. Barbara Brown quoted by Skelly, see note 10.

13. Paul Gerber and Marjolin Bijlefeld, "Ways Your Staff Can Lead You down the Malpractice Path," *Physician's Management* 33, no. 1 (January 1993), p. 94.

14. John-Henry Pfifferling, "Ounces of Malpractice Prevention," *Physician Executive* 20, no. 2 (February 1994), p. 36.

15. Inge K. Winer, "What Physicians Can Do to Reduce the Risks of Malpractice Litigation," *Journal of Medical Practice Management* 8, no. 3 (Winter 1993), p. 214.

16. Andrew M. Scherffius, quoted in "Don't Let Staff Push Patients into Malpractice Suits," see note 9.

17. Charlotte Miller quoted in "Don't Let Staff Push Patients into Malpractice Suits," see note 9.

18. Harold I. Kaplan and Benjamin J. Adock, *Synopsis of Psychiatry: Behavioral Sciences, Clinical Psychiatry*, 6th ed. (Baltimore: Williams and Wilins, 1991), p. 9.

19. Ibid.

20. Ibid.

21. Robert Bright, M.D., cited by Nelson and Brown, pp. 51–52, see note 3.

22. Alan Rockoff, M.D., "An Easy Way to Boost Patient Compliance," *Medical Economics* 71, no. 24 (December 26, 1994), pp. 54–56.

23. Bob Reznik, "How Customer's Satisfaction Can Influence Clinical Outcome in a Back Specialty Clinic," *MGM Journal* 41, no. 1 (January/February 1994), p. 78.

24. Ibid., 54.

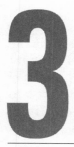

CHAPTER

Step Three—Learn the Lessons of Service

In the mid-1980s, Karl Albrecht's and Ron Zemke's book *Service America* placed major focus on a systematic process for making service the core philosophy of an organization.[1] Since that time, a wide variety of different industries, including healthcare, have embraced those concepts and implemented the accompanying methods. The road traveled by those organizations has revealed some important lessons from which we all can learn. In this chapter, I have incorporated those lessons, and others, into the process of creating a Total Service Medical Practice. The combined result is offered here as a way to help you start your journey on solid footing.

LESSON 1: CREATING A TOTAL SERVICE MEDICAL PRACTICE STARTS AT THE TOP.

No organization that has chosen to implement the Total Service philosophy can be successful in its efforts without the complete buy-in and commitment of those in leadership positions. In the medical practice this starts with the physicians. Howard Levine, M.D., a specialist in nose and sinus surgery at the Academy of

Medicine of Cleveland, explained, "It comes from the top. If the physician doesn't set the service standard as a role model, it won't be performed by the staff. People who work for a physician, I think, will take on the behavior of the physician."[2] Patients tend to believe this too; as one focus group participant expressed, "It all starts with the doctor. If he cares, the staff cares. It's just that simple."

Although physicians are really the key to how practice personnel respond to service issues, others are in positions of leadership that impact employees as well. Office managers or practice administrators provide the essential link between the doctors and the staff. In larger practices, supervisors have the responsibility of directing the work in specific areas, and they too are part of the leadership to whom employees look for examples of how to serve.

Before the other practice personnel are introduced to specific service concepts and methods, all of these leaders need to have a clear understanding of what it means to be a Total Service Medical Practice and of what their accompanying respective responsibilities are. Then, they will be in a position to be effective role models for their employees and to make the kinds of decisions that demonstrate their commitment. To create and maintain a Total Service Medical Practice, the physicians, practice managers, and supervisors must be willing not only to *talk the talk but walk the walk* of service. Specific suggestions to help physicians operationalize this popular saying are offered in Chapter 8. (These same suggestions can be modified for office managers and supervisors as well). For now, it is important for you to understand that it is only by witnessing this kind of behavior that the employees will realize that their leaders are serious about commitment to service.

LESSON 2: CREATING A TOTAL SERVICE MEDICAL PRACTICE MEANS PUTTING EMPLOYEES FIRST.

While browsing in my local book store one day, I encountered a small volume that leapt from the shelf into my awareness. Entitled *The Customer Comes Second*, it jolted me to pick it up. What did the author mean by this provocative title? On closer examination, my question was answered. Written by Hal Rosenbluth, the CEO of the global professional travel agency that bears his name, the thesis was quite simple: The key to effective external service starts within. Mr. Rosenbluth explained, "We put our people first . . . We hire nice people, encourage them to bind emotionally with the company, train them continuously, and equip them with the best technology. The customers and profits will follow." This philosophy worked well for Rosenbluth Travel as they experienced a phenomenal 7,500 percent growth increase in fifteen years and maintained a 96 percent client retention rate. Rosenbluth summed it up this way: "Everyone around us wanted to work in an environment like ours. Our people were happy, fulfilled, and excelling, and it showed. Clients enjoyed working with our people and they let us know it."[3]

The philosophy that worked for Rosenbluth Travel can and will work for you. In the medical practice grounded in internal service, employees feel respected, understood, and valued. They like to come to work every day, feel that they have significant contributions to make no matter what their jobs, and experience a high level of job satisfaction. When they are satisfied, then they will be able to satisfy customers. When they are not, the task is almost impossible.

No medical practice can provide quality service without the enthusiastic support of all clinical and nonclinical staff members. It is up to the leaders (physicians, managers, and supervisors) to provide the kind of environment in which their employees and service can thrive. (Part III of this book offers specifics of how this can be done.)

LESSON 3: CREATING A TOTAL SERVICE MEDICAL PRACTICE MEANS EMPOWERING ALL PRACTICE PERSONNEL.

Empowerment has become a key term in organizations of the 1990s. It represents more than a trendy concept, however, especially for medical practices. What does this term mean? Basically, it refers to a feeling of being valued, respected, trusted, and appreciated, as discussed in Lesson 2. It also means being accorded the appropriate power or authority to make decisions without fear of reversal.

When asked to explain this notion of empowerment, practice personnel have some very definite ideas. Staff members are perhaps the most vocal, describing *empowerment* as: the acknowledgment of contributions to the success of the practice, appreciation for work done, authority to make certain decisions within their knowledge and expertise, and the assurance that these decisions will not run the risk of frequent reversal.

Practice managers also have operationalized this concept. They too explain it as a need to be trusted to make appropriate nonclinical decisions. They seek a clearly defined area of supervision and management that will not be micromanaged by the physicians. Also, they indicate a desire for their expertise to be respected and valued.

Although less vocal about their desire for empowerment, or perhaps more accurately re-empowerment, physicians also have their own needs. They express a sense of loss of control and the need to somehow regain it. Just as any other practice employee, they want to feel valued, respected, and appreciated. Doctors also indicate a need to be involved in the process of change and not to be merely passive recipients of it.

A Total Service Medical Practice can and does bring practice personnel into their full potential. From the physicians to the managers to the staff—all will be accorded the respect, trust, appreciation, and value they deserve. They will also be given the authority to make clearly specified, appropriate decisions. Even if the policies of managed care seem to direct some decisions, many others, both clinical and nonclinical, are still within the purview of the practice, and these need to be clearly delineated and understood. The practice with empowered personnel is the practice that will not merely react to, but will *respond to* and even *anticipate*, the changes in its environment. In addition, empowered personnel will have the confidence, knowledge, and enthusiasm to provide not just good but exceptional service.

LESSON 4: CREATING A TOTAL SERVICE MEDICAL PRACTICE TAKES TIME.

"Are we there yet?" This is a question asked often by children in the backseat of a car as well as by employees and even leaders of an organization that has started down the road to Total Service. Eager to start reaping the benefits of the new approach to business, and sometimes just eager to be finished with the process itself, along about mile ten or week five they begin to wonder "Are we there yet?" You will probably find yourself doing the same. When and if it happens, please remember that change such as this takes time.

Time must be spent learning about the model of a Total Service Medical Practice, and time must be spent implementing the 17 steps. As you will see, many of these steps simply cannot be rushed. It takes time to talk to customers and determine their wants and needs, and to conduct surveys to measure how effectively your practice is meeting those desires. Time is also required to examine how you are functioning as a practice team and to learn ways to function more effectively. No system, cycle, or process has ever been examined both quickly and thoroughly. Time is required for just the *doing* of the implementation.

Time also is required to move all practice personnel through the change process. To begin with, everyone, including physicians, practice managers, and staff, will have to learn some new ways of doing things. Even if your practice is already providing good service to its customers, this systematic, organizationally based, philosophical approach is new, and it will require breaking some old habits. As Mark Twain once wrote, "Habit is habit, and not to be tossed out the window by any man; but coaxed down the stairs one step at a time." (In Chapter 9, I describe a specific process common to anyone who experiences change.)

So, don't get in a hurry. Take your time and take the time to make this process work for you. This lesson can save you frustration and confusion as you work your way toward Total Service.

LESSON 5: CREATING A TOTAL SERVICE MEDICAL PRACTICE MEANS STAYING CLOSE TO YOUR CUSTOMERS.

This lesson presents a special challenge to the medical practice of today. As previously discussed, the lifelong relationship between physician and patient is no longer the norm, and secondary customer populations are growing less and less familiar as well. Changes in medical practices themselves have also contributed to this feeling of increasing distance between practices and their customers.

We have already covered the changes in structural forms faced by medical practices today. As any practice loses some of its autonomy, it will also face nearly automatic feelings of distance from its customers, particularly from its patients. Increasing work loads also contribute to this push away. The self-imposed financial pressure to see more patients by practices experiencing capitation, and the organizational pressure placed on some staff-model physicians to do the same, have resulted in increasing patient loads. Physicians are probably the first to really feel the crunch, but the impact soon filters to all office personnel as well. As practice employees begin to experience the pressure that accompanies such growth, it becomes easier and easier to get farther and farther away from the customers.

Another reason why some practices have drifted from their customers is that they have become complacent. This can happen when you've been practicing medicine a long time or are finishing your 17th year of managing an office. It also happens as you draw the one thousandth vial of blood or file the one millionth insurance claim. You begin to think, "I've been in this so long and I know my customer so well that I don't need to ask." This attitude can lull you into a false sense of security that can cause you to miss some very important issues for today's customers of medical practices.

Some factors outside the control of the practice also contribute to the feeling of distancing. As employers change health plans and patients continue to doctor-shop, it becomes increasingly difficult to stay close to your customer. This transitory nature of healthcare that we have already explored carries with it the same distancing effect brought on by the actions of some practices themselves.

So, with all of these forces pushing medical practices away from their customers, it is not as easy to stay close to customers as it might first seem. To work against this almost automatic movement away requires conscious, systematic, and continuous efforts. It means using a well organized and structured process for talking with your customers and measuring their reactions to the service provided. Without this information, your practice will drift as time and increased work load push you away from the constantly changing attitudes and opinions of your customers. (Chapter 6 describes a range of methods for getting close to your customers and staying there.) It should also be noted that the hectic pace kept in most medical practices makes it increasingly difficult to stay close to the customers within, meaning that internal service can also suffer.

LESSON 6: CREATING A TOTAL SERVICE MEDICAL PRACTICE WILL IMPROVE YOUR BOTTOM LINE.

Customers behave in some odd ways at times. One of their oddest behaviors is their response to what they perceive as poor or unsatisfactory service. As many as 96 percent of unhappy customers don't complain; they just leave.[4] In healthcare today, the official leave-taking may not happen immediately, because the patients have to wait until the next benefits package is offered. However, they can leave in other ways. For example, some patients report that they avoid seeking medical care rather than go back to the practice that offended them. This not only has a negative impact on the practice's bottom line, but also a dangerous effect on the patients' health. Others withdraw emotionally, becoming passive recipients of treatment rather than active partners in their healthcare. This can lead to misdiagnosis, ineffective treatment, and lack of informed consent—all of which lead not only to poor healthcare but to potentially expensive malpractice suits. Still other patients seem to take leave of their senses by becoming chronically angry or even hostile. It's almost as if they have decided that, if they are forced to stay in this situation, then they will make things as difficult as possible. The impact of emotional upsets such as these on diagnosis, treatment, and healing processes has already been discussed in Chapter 2. The hidden, but real, costs due to staff stress, such as illness and absence, caused by trying to handle these difficult situations cannot be underestimated either.

Customers also engage in another odd behavior as a result of poor service. Research has found that although most dissatisfied customers will not tell anyone in the offending organization or business about their problem, they will tell eight to ten other people about that bad experience; 13 percent tell more than 20.[5] For medical practices, the receivers of these complaints are usually other current patients, potential new ones, referring physicians, and benefits managers. The above research covered consumer-oriented industries generally, but if we were just looking at healthcare, the figures would be even higher, for patients at least. When patients are dealing with their health, everything becomes magnified, heightening the intensity of their feelings when dissatisfied. Plus, people tend to talk about their healthcare experiences more often than about other events in their lives. Thus, they will be more likely to voluntarily initiate conversation about problems encountered in a medical practice than about problems in a retail store.

The Cleveland Clinic conducted a study to determine the costs of a dissatisfied patient. After factoring in the number of people one unhappy patient would tell (nine) and assuming that 25 percent of those people and that patient would choose to seek hospitalization elsewhere, the Clinic concluded that the potential lifetime revenue loss as a result of one dissatisfied patient was about $400,000.[6] Although it typically costs more for a patient to be hospitalized than to make an office call, the greater frequency of visits to a given practice over a lifetime tends to even things out, meaning that this figure may not be that far away from the cost of losing one of your patients through poor service.

Phillip Crosby, a well-known leader in the field of total quality management, reports that in service industries, 35 percent of the sales dollar is lost to poor service quality.[7] Thus, it makes sense that doing it right the first time will save cold hard cash for your medical practice.

LESSON 7: BECOMING A TOTAL SERVICE MEDICAL PRACTICE WILL DISTINGUISH YOUR PRACTICE IN THE MARKETPLACE.

Medical practices today find themselves facing increasing competition, many for the first time. As I mentioned in Chapter 2, selection for affiliation in groups and networks is causing comparisons that may not have been made even a few years ago, and membership in these entities is becoming essential to practice survival. Also, as mentioned earlier, patients are more consumer-oriented than ever before. The term *doctor shop*, which understandably sets most physicians' teeth on edge, aptly describes what often occurs.

So, how does a practice gain the edge in this new competitive environment? Thomas C. Royer, M.D., the chairman of the board of governors for Henry Ford Medical Group, provided the answer: "Today, service standards are the hallmark of marketing a group practice."[8] Specifically referring to competition for patients, he continued, "Previously patients 'became prisoners of our technological services.'"[9] For example, at Henry Ford in the 1970s, 60 percent of the technological services offered were considered unique in the market. In 1995, only 3 percent were. Dr. Royer urged all practices to set, define, and market service standards, saying that this would be one of the most important tasks a practice can undertake.[10]

LESSON 8: BECOMING A TOTAL SERVICE MEDICAL PRACTICE MEANS BEING WILLING TO CHANGE THE WAY YOU DO THINGS.

Karl Albrecht pointed out that systems are often the enemy of service.[11] When I mention this lesson in my workshop, heads nod vigorously all around the room. During consultations, I hear more frustration expressed by employees who want to provide quality service but must implement policies and procedures that make it almost impossible to do so. Customers in focus groups complain about the difficulties of "working with the practice." The Total Service Medical Practice must be willing to examine and change any system, policy, procedure, or process that prevents employees from providing quality service.

Why do I say *willing*? Because I have found that of all the old habits organizations are reluctant to change, these *ways of doing things* are the most difficult. For example, I've seen organizations cling to old policies for no better reason than, "We've always done it that way." Don't allow yourself to stop with that response. Instead, ask, "Why did we start doing things this way in the first place?" If you don't know, then it is time for reevaluation. If you can trace the origin, then ask if the conditions have changed since that time. If so, then you should consider making alterations to fit current conditions. The Total Service Medical Practice will never allow itself the easy answer of "We have always done it that way!"

LESSON 9: A TOTAL SERVICE MEDICAL PRACTICE IS PROACTIVE AND POSITIVE, NOT DEFENSIVE.

The term *defensive* is used in two related but different ways in this lesson. First, too often organizations wait until there is a service problem before they decide to act, and then they are in the defensive or reactive mode of attempting to put out fires. Don't wait until then. Even if your practice is already doing a good job in service, you can make the best better.

If your practice is already facing service problems, then be wary of experiencing the second type of defensiveness as well. Theoretically, *defensiveness* in this context is defined as the attempt to protect one's personhood from attack. When people in any organization discover that they have unsatisfied and thus unhappy customers, they often feel the desire to defend themselves. Without a conscious effort to behave otherwise, they are likely to respond to this news in one of the following ways:

Denial:	"I did not treat the customer that way!"
Excuses:	"Well, if the weather wasn't so bad, I'd be in a better mood."
Anger:	"That customer is the biggest jerk I've ever seen."
Apathy:	"So you're sick!"
Blaming:	"I don't know why the receptionist told you doctor could see you at 5:15. She's always making mistakes like that!"
Condescending:	"What's the matter, can't you read!"
Giving Up:	"I don't care what you do. It won't matter anyway."

Employees in a Total Service Medical Practice would not demonstrate any of these responses to the discovery of service problems. Rather, the personnel would all be actively involved in the process of inquiry and would understand that problems are not weaknesses, but are opportunities for improving service to their customers. Any organization that responds to criticism with "I'm so glad you told me about that. Now I have a chance to fix it" is on its way to being a service champion. Those who add, "And how can I make things right for you now?" are already there!

FIGURE 3–1

The Total Service Medical Practice

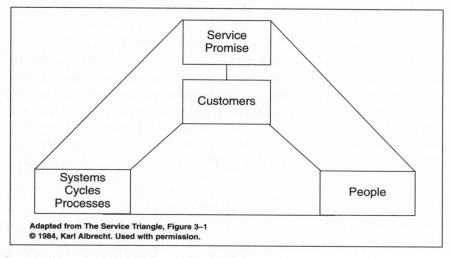

Adapted from The Service Triangle, Figure 3–1
© 1984, Karl Albrecht. Used with permission.

LESSON 10: CREATING A TOTAL SERVICE MEDICAL PRACTICE IS AN ON-GOING PROCESS.

The Total Service Medical Practice is not a figment of my imagination. The model in Figure 3–1, adapted from the well-known image of the Service Triangle first designed by Karl Albrecht, gives a glimpse of what such a practice looks like. To think that this model is your goal, however, would be incorrect. The creating and maintaining of service is not a thing; it is a process. What this model allows us to do is to pause a moment to study the parts, much as athletic coaches do by using a freeze-frame approach when studying a film of an athlete in action. Just as any shooter going up for a basket cannot pause to be studied, neither can a Total Service Medical Practice be halted in its continuous process of providing service. The only way either can be analyzed and thus understood is to artificially stop the action in mid-air, so to speak. That is what Figure 3–1 does. It provides a stationary image, albeit a temporary one, of what a Total Service Medical Practice looks like.

Becoming and remaining a Total Service Medical Practice, however, is a process that never ends. Once we cover the 17 steps, you will need to return to the beginning and start again. This time your journey will be smoother than the first and the process will go more quickly. In Chapter 17, I will also give you some additional suggestions for making this return trip an easier one. You will repeat these 17 steps (or slightly modified versions of them) over and over again, and as you do, they will become the natural way your practice does business. You and your colleagues will find yourselves going through them with all of the skill and grace of Michael Jordan as he floats skyward to make that winning basket. Then, you will find that the Total Service perspective has become not a series of separate steps, but a deeply ingrained way of life. When that occurs, you can truly say, "We are a Total Service Medical Practice!"

END NOTES

1. Karl Albrecht and Ron Zemke, *Service America* (Homewood, Illinois: Dow Jones–Irwin, 1985).
2. Howard Levine, M.D., quoted by Robert McCoppin, "Service Is Key to a Healthy Practice," *American Medical News* 34, no. 11 (March 18, 1991), p. 14.
3. Hal Rosenbluth, *The Customer Comes Second* (New York: William Morrow, 1992).
4. Randall Luecke, Virginia Rosselli, and Judy Moss, "The Economic Ramifications of 'Client Dissatisfaction,'" *Group Practice Journal* 40, no. 3 (May/June 1991), p. 10.
5. Ibid.
6. Randall Luecke, Virginia Rosselli, and Jody Moss cited by Steven Koger, "Service Management" *College Review* 10, no. 1 (Spring 1993), p. 6.
7. Phillip Crosby, *Quality Without Tears* (New York: McGraw-Hill, 1990).
8. Brenda Hull, "Service Standards Hallmark for Practice Marketing," *MGM Update* 34, no.11 (November 1995), p. 7.
9. Ibid.
10. Ibid.
11. Karl Albrecht, *At America's Service* (Homewood, Illinois: Dow Jones–Irwin, 1988), pp. 4–5.

TWO

FOCUS ON
THE CUSTOMER

You are now ready to turn your attention to the customers themselves, and the chapters in Part Two lead you through this process. Chapter 4 discusses the key customer populations that a medical practice serves and describes how yours can identify its own. Chapter 5 offers several factors that should be discussed prior to seeking customer feedback. Chapter 6 provides a range of specific methods that your practice can use for getting close to its customers and staying there.

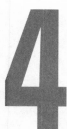

CHAPTER

Step Four—Identify Your Customers

As I mentioned in Chapter 1, not so long ago the idea of having *customers* seemed quite foreign to those in the healthcare field. It brought to mind only images of the person waiting on line at a gas station or browsing in a clothing store. The idea of healthcare actually being involved in *customer service*, as it is known in the business world, was difficult for some to accept. Today the situation is changing, however. Hospitals, insurance carriers, laboratories, and yes, medical practices all are beginning to realize that the healthcare picture is not like it used to be.

THE NEW TERMINOLOGY MAY NOT BE SO NEW AFTER ALL

While many concepts from the business world have been incorporated into the healthcare scene, none shine their light more brightly and with greater familiarity on the picture of healers and their patients than do the principles involved in Total Service. Why? Because the basic foundation of both healthcare and service is *people helping people*. Every concept, every idea, every method and technique that I have to offer in this book is tied to that basic principle. Total Service allows doctors and their office personnel to do what they have always wanted to do: put the patient first. Let's begin at the beginning—with the expanded definition of the term *customers*.

WHO ARE YOUR CUSTOMERS?

In Chapter 1, I described the break with tradition that a Total Service Medical Practice makes when it defines its *customers* as *all individuals* or *groups*, either inside or outside the practice, with whom that practice has an interdependent relationship. As is clear from this definition, the scope of the word is broadened significantly. The next step in becoming a Total Service Medical Practice, then, is to identify who your customers are, using this expanded definition.

Internal Customers

In order to provide quality service to the external customers, a Total Service Medical Practice must begin within; the practice in which the personnel do not treat each other as valued customers will not provide quality service to anyone else.

In my workshops, after defining *internal customers* as "all those who are employed by the practice," I ask the participants to name all individuals or groups they can think of who fit that definition. The lists vary, but those most often included are: receptionists, filing clerks, billing clerks, appointment clerks, nurses, nurse practitioners, physician's assistants, physicians, office managers, insurance coordinators, as well as janitorial and mail room personnel.

Why take the time to actually make this list? Wouldn't it just be easier to answer the question "Who are your internal customers?" with "Everybody who works here!" Yes, it would be easier and even faster, but there are two reasons for not settling for the simplest, quickest response. First, by taking the time to think of and actually write down those who fit the definition of *internal customer*, you underscore the importance of *all* practice personnel. Second, the listing process helps make sure that no one is forgotten. Frequently there are individuals who are very important to the practice but who actually work at a different location; sometimes just down the hall. In addition, practices with multiple sites must take care not to forget their colleagues across town. All of these individuals play key roles in the successful functions of the practice, and they should be included.

When a medical practice places emphasis on internal service, an interesting chain reaction is set in motion. In such a practice, coworkers treat each other as valued customers. This leads to happy employees who enjoy their jobs, which in turn creates an environment where everyone works together in a cooperative and efficient manner, providing quality service internally to each other. As this occurs, then the external service is also invariably of a high standard. External customers can tell you if your practice works well together or not, and they are almost always accurate. The importance of internal service cannot be underestimated.

A focus on internal service also helps any employees who have limited or no contact with external customers to understand their part in providing quality service. The traditional definition of *customer* seemed to limit service concerns to those personnel who were directly involved with providing a service or selling a product. The people behind the scenes could not see their connection to the service perspective. By broadening the definition to include *internal service*, these people can more readily see that what they do matters. Karl Albrecht and Ron Zemke coined an important saying about internal service: "If you're not serving the [external] customer, then you better be serving someone who is."[1]

External Customers

Now it is time to shift your focus outside the practice, to those external customers who are vital to your success. Defined as "individuals or groups not employed by the practice but with whom that practice has an interdependent relationship," this explanation also broadens the traditional meaning of *customer*. The same workshop exercise that asks for a list of internal customers also requests a similar list of external ones. Although these lists can become quite long and each practice should formulate its own, five external customer groups seem essential to the survival of any medical practice: patients, patients' families, other physicians, managed care companies, and hospitals. The medical practice that

possesses a customer orientation to each of these groups will be a
thriving one.

Primary Customers

Although all customer populations are important, not all are equal
in weight. There is one customer population without whom all
others and even the practice itself would have no reason to exist.
In any organization, the primary customers are those who fit the
old traditional definition: those who use the service or buy the
product. In the medical practice, the primary customers, then, are
the patients.

Within the broad category of *patients*, several specific
populations should be recognized. Age differences provide
important subgroupings to be considered: babies and children
have different healthcare and service needs than do people much
farther along in the aging process, especially those euphemis-
tically called *the seniors*, while the needs of teenagers and young
adults vary from each of the groups at either end of the aging
continuum. Men and women also present subgroupings with
unique healthcare needs that should be recognized and
addressed, but often are not. In addition, different ethnic groups
also can present special challenges, and the diversity in our
society is growing rapidly, placing an even greater importance on
understanding the unique characteristics of the patients in these
populations. A Total Service Medical Practice will have a keen
understanding of any and all of these or other patient subgroups
which it serves.

Secondary Customers

In addition to these primary customer populations, there are other
groups or entities with whom the practice has an interdependent
relationship and who also help the practice provide quality
healthcare to its patients. The first of these key secondary external
customer populations is closely related, both figuratively and
literally, to the primary customers. In fact, in pediatric, geriatric,
and high acuity cases, they often become surrogates, speaking for
and making healthcare decisions for actual patients. I'm referring
of course to the family members of your patients. Not necessarily
family members who are also patients of your practice, these folks

are caretakers or merely interested relatives who care about what is happening to their loved ones.

Beyond their surrogate patient role, the family members are important to a medical practice for some very specific reasons. In Chapter 2, I talked about their connection to the effective diagnosis and treatment of patients' illnesses and injuries through the information they provide to the physicians and the support they give to the patients. There are also some practice development reasons for serving this customer population well. Unhappy family members can and do generate as much negative word-of-mouth advertising as patients, maybe even more. Also, evidence supports the fact that many patients are pushed into malpractice claims by upset members of their families. By the same token, satisfied family members are often eager to spread the good news about the patient's positive healthcare experiences and also, where appropriate, often will become new patients of the practice themselves. The Total Service Medical Practice will recognize patients' families as members of a distinct customer population with their own unique wants and needs, and will establish positive relationships with them.

The next external customer population is composed of other physicians and their practice personnel. In healthcare today, this relationship has become more than just a collegial one. Given the medical management function of primary care physicians, specialists need these referring doctors in order to stay in business. By the same token, primary care physicians need specialists in order to provide specific medical care to their patients. Physicians of both types, as well as their office personnel, depend on cooperative, supportive relationships with their colleagues in other practices, and all need to have user-friendly systems in place for the literal and figurative moving of their mutual patient load. Even within the somewhat restrictive networks of managed care and the potentially more restrictive networks in the IDSs, there is and will continue to be the need for one physician to refer patients to another. By viewing each other as valued customers, these physicians and their practices will ensure that the relationships between them are positive and that the way things are done within each practice promotes quality service.

Managed care companies make up the next secondary external customer population. I am not unaware of the changes that managed care has brought to the healthcare field and the resulting tensions that can exist between medical practices and these organizations. Yet, in spite of all of that, I am going to make perhaps a startling claim: If you view these organizations and the people in them as *customers*, and treat them accordingly, your relationship with them will improve and your life will be easier. This does not mean that you will stop questioning decisions or policies that you think should be questioned, nor does it mean that you become the passive observer of the continuing changes that will occur. What it does mean is, just as with any customer population, you will take the time to discover what this customer wants and needs from you and will do all you can to meet those needs. The truth is that managed care is here to stay. So, the Total Service Medical Practice will accept this fact and will discover ways to work with these organizations successfully.

The fifth and final secondary external customers I will discuss in detail are the hospitals. Just as with insurance companies, the relationship between medical practices and this customer population has been in a constant process of change. In the book *Management of Hospitals*, this evolution is described in four stages: The Trustee Period (1900–1920s) was a time when most hospitals were established by philanthropists and religious orders, and doctors were independent practitioners receiving low pay, if any. The Physicians' Period: (1920–1960) was a time when the doctors and medical technology ruled and was characterized by rapid growth as well as development in medical technology and specialization. In the Administrative Period (1960–1980s) the hospital administration began to be more influential in the decision-making processes around the business aspects of healthcare, which were becoming more and more prominent. The fourth period stretches from the 1980s forward and is optimistically called the Team Period. It is described as the time when trustees, physicians, administrators, and nurses must pool their skills and work as a team in order to make the most effective use of available resources.[2]

Although many hospitals and physicians are reflecting the spirit of the Team Period in their collaborative and joint ventures together, this is not always the case. Even though physicians and hospitals have long been interdependent—one cannot exist without the other—these two groups are often at odds. There are many reasons for this conflict, but perhaps even ten years ago Frederick Wenzel, then Executive Director of the Marshfield Clinic in Marshfield, Wisconsin, grasped its basic nature: "The ultimate conflict results from the professionals' [physicians'] need for freedom and the organizations' [hospitals'] need for integration."[3]

In spite of this seemingly almost inherent conflict, however, both sides are calling for more than a truce. They are calling for a partnership. The *MGM Journal* published a two-person forum on this very issue. Speaking for the hospitals, Janet Reich, president of Marketing, Management, and Imaging, expressed her desire for a meeting of the minds: "What is key, and will be found in the most successful hospital-affiliated group practices, is a true partnership, where both parties' interests become the interests of the whole."[4] Sandra Reifsteck, associate administrator of the Carle Clinic Association, represented the medical practice's point of view and brought all of this back to service. "No longer can we abide by the 'us versus them' attitude. We must remember that we each are a customer of the other, and the patient is the customer of both."[5] The Total Service Medical Practice will recognize this need for collaboration and will move to make it happen.

An additional population that belongs in the Secondary Customer category is the *vendors*. Medical practices rely on this group of people to supply essential equipment, supplies, and services. The vendors, in turn, need the practices to buy what they are selling. Although I include no further discussion of vendors in this book, I urge you to keep this group in mind. In order to meet many of the wants and needs of your other customer populations, your practice relies on what the vendors have to offer. By establishing and maintaining positive relationships with this key group of secondary customers, your service capabilities will be enhanced.

Identifying the Customers of Your Practice

Now it is time to sit down as a practice, or as appropriate representatives thereof, and identify your customers. Begin by making a list of internal customers and then do the same for the external ones, including both primary and secondary customer groups. Once the lists have been created, examine them even more closely by asking appropriate questions, such as (1) What are the demographics of this group? (2) What are their unique healthcare needs? (3) What roles do members of this group play in the healthcare process? (4) What, if any, subgroups should be considered, and why? Your practice will no doubt want to create its own questions. Whatever it chooses to ask, however, the purpose should be kept in mind: To identify *who*, in the larger sense of that word, your internal and external customers really are. Then you will be ready to listen to what they have to say.

Also you need to spend some time reflecting on the interdependence that characterizes the nature of any customer relationship. Internally, you need each other to carry out tasks, complete processes, and, most important, to provide quality service to your customers. Externally, you need your primary customers—the patients—in order for your practice to exist, while the patients need your practice and its personnel to provide for their healthcare. The secondary external customer populations rely on you just as much as you rely on them. Family members need you to care for their loved ones, and you need their help in that process. Other physicians, managed care companies, and hospitals depend on medical practices like yours for clinical and clerical expertise, and you depend on them to assist you in providing quality, cost-effective care to your patients.

One final thought: Identifying your customers as groups does not mean that you do not need to know them as individuals. Nothing could be farther from the truth. *Each person* with whom you interact deserves your interest and understanding. Throughout this book you will find many references to ways in which you can convey both to each and every customer you serve.

END NOTES

1. Karl Albrecht and Ron Zemke, *Service America* (Homewood, Illinois: Dow Jones–Irwin, 1985), p. 96.

2. Rockwell Schulz and Alton C. Johnson, eds., *Management of Hospitals*, 2d ed. (New York: McGraw-Hill, Inc., 1983), pp. 3–12.

3. Frederick Wenzel, "Conflict: An Imperative for Success," *Journal of Medical Practice Management* 1, no. 4 (April 1986), p. 254.

4. Janet Reich, "Recognizing and Overcoming Barriers: Physician/
Hospital Relationship Building," *MGM Journal* 38, no. 4
(July/August 1991) pp. 60, 71.

5. Sandra W. Reifsteck, "Through the Eyes of a Group Practice
Administrator: Physician/Hospital Bonding," *MGM Journal* 38, no. 4
(July/August 1991) p. 76.

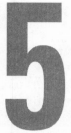

CHAPTER

Step Five—Prepare For Feedback

"I have my finger on the pulse of what my customers want and need," one workshop participant told me, "I don't need to *ask* them what they think!" While I enjoyed the unintentional pun and recognized that in some rare instances this statement might possibly be accurate, more often than not nothing could be farther from the truth. In fact, one of the biggest challenges faced by the medical practice of today is staying in touch with its customers.

In Chapter 3, I discussed the forces both inside and outside the practice that provide an almost automatic *push away from* rather than *pull toward* your various customer populations. Therefore, a well organized, planned, and carefully implemented process of soliciting feedback from your customers must be undertaken. The specifics of how to seek this input are covered in Chapter 6. However, before leaping immediately to the implementation of that step, the proper framework for feedback needs to be established. If it is not, feelings can be hurt, anger can be inflamed, and defensive behaviors will almost inevitably follow, resulting in the worsening of service rather than the improving of it.

Establishing the proper framework for receiving feedback from your customers is important. By taking the time to talk about what you are doing and why and how it fits into the big picture, everyone in the practice can approach the solicitation of feedback with a more positive attitude. A discussion of the seven factors covered in this chapter is a key part of becoming a Total Service Medical Practice; the first six deal with the "whys" of actively seeking customer feedback, and the last two cover how to enhance its positive reception. The goal in implementing this step is simple: to help all practice personnel prepare for receiving customer feedback in the most positive manner.

FACTOR 1: IN ORDER TO OBTAIN COMPLETE AND ACCURATE DATA, CUSTOMERS NEED TO BE *ASKED* FOR THEIR FEEDBACK.

Regardless of your role, the chances are quite good that you don't have a clear picture of the service perceptions of your practice's customers. If you have any information, it is very likely only a piece of the puzzle. Let's focus on your patients for a while. I am willing to bet that no one in your practice sees the complete picture regarding this group's service attitudes and perceptions.

Research shows, typically and rather ironically, that physicians are often the least informed of all. The most frequently quoted study on this issue was conducted in 1989 by Steve Brown and Teresa Swartz. Their empirical research found that the understanding that physicians had of patient expectations tended to be inaccurate.[1] O'Connor's study of a 500-employee multispecialty clinic agreed with these findings.[2]

Patients report several reasons for not talking with their doctors about service issues. A most common one is the differing status that some patients perceive between themselves and their doctors. Citing the vastly different income, education, and career choices that exist between their doctors and themselves, some patients explain their reluctance to discuss service issues with their physicians in this way: "I just can't relate to the doctor—I don't think he could understand what I am saying."

The high esteem some patients accord their physicians is another reason they are reluctant to speak to their doctors about service issues. "I don't want to bother him with these things," said one patient. "He has more important things to think about." Most often these patients do not mean to convey that service issues are unimportant to *them*; rather, they don't believe that physicians would find them so.

Frequently cited by patients and yet often surprising to physicians, fear is another reason for the patients' reluctance to talk to their doctors about service problems. Rightly or wrongly, some patients are afraid that telling a doctor about a service issue would adversely affect the quality of their technical care. Otherwise outspoken people have reported feeling so unexpectedly vulnerable during their times of illness or injury that they have been reluctant to bring service problems to the attention of their doctors. One patient put it this way: "I don't want him mad when he sticks that needle in me!" This fear issue is even described by some patients as their reason for filing malpractice suits; they fear facing the doctor so much that they prefer to let the court do the complaining for them.

Still another reason why patients do not discuss service issues with their doctors is that doctors often seem so rushed. While most physicians realize that their schedules are overflowing, they may not be totally aware of the impact this has on voluntary patient feedback. One woman reported, "I would like to talk to my doctor more, but he is so busy. I go in with my list of *medical* questions and feel lucky if we get to most of them. When do I have time to talk to him about service?" I admit that this was the reason I did not bring my own service concerns to the attention of a doctor who treated me once. As she dashed from examination room to examination room, this physician did not appear to have the time for conversation about anything other than the technical business at hand, and even that was rushed.

Some physicians erroneously believe that a doctor's technical expertise is all that matters and that is why patients don't bring up service issues. One surgeon stated, "My patients don't care about service! All they care about is how skilled I am when I make that incision." This perception, in many cases, is not totally correct. While technical expertise may be given a higher priority, patients still report that service issues do matter. After pondering this point a moment, one woman rather poignantly observed, "Maybe that's how poor service in the medical practice has been perpetuated. We put up with poor service because the technical expertise *is* so important. We allow them to treat us poorly as people, because they have the medical knowledge and expertise we need."

Some patients do talk to their physicians, and when they do, their feedback takes some interesting and often incomplete forms. Not wanting to step on any toes, sometimes they will only comment about the elements of the practice that are not person-related. They may express a desire for improvement in the physical environment of the practice, such as expanded parking facilities or more convenient office hours. However, research shows that these issues, although important to patients, do not head their lists. Thus, physicians who do hear from their patients often hear about issues that in many instances trouble the patients the least. Because of this, physicians may well have a skewed impression of what is important.

Patients are even more reluctant to talk to physicians about problems in the doctor/patient relationship. Whatever the rationale—be it status differences, elevation of status, fear, or some other reason—many patients report that it is almost impossible for them to discuss with their doctors their need for the physicians to spend more time with them, to listen more carefully to them, or to show them that they care.

When patients report problems with practice staff to their doctors, many physicians confess that they really don't want to know. While at some level they understand that, as the owners of the business they should know, in all honesty they would rather not be bothered. Doctors want to practice medicine! Hiring and firing and correcting staff behaviors are not why they went to medical school. So, these physicians usually end up turning over any such service complaints to someone else in the practice, most often the manager.

Whether receiving a handoff from a physician or a staff member, or responding to a patient's insistence on *going to the top*, office managers do handle most of the more severe service problems in a practice. While resolving many service complaints is the job of any effective office manager, this feedback should not be construed as the complete service picture, because it is not. A complaint, by its very nature, does not focus on the positive. Thus the office manager, after hearing a series of these comments, may think that service in the practice is worse than it is. Conversely, since most patients don't *voluntarily* voice their complaints, many service problems will not be heard at all.

Although usually dealing with complaints, office managers report that they also are aware of satisfied customers, but their awareness is usually based on an intuitive sense and the occasional, random patient comment. The verifiable and specific reasons for the patients' satisfaction often are not known. Thus, relying on the office manager's often oddly distorted image of service will not provide the complete picture needed to make service decisions in the practice.

Clinical and nonclinical staff also often have a partial image of service. Although they may hear grumblings about physicians or may bear the brunt of a patient's anger, these staff members are seldom able to gain a complete and accurate impression. Perceived as having no authority to change things, patients usually either ask to talk to someone else or they explode with no rational reason offered, often leaving staff unclear about the specifics.

Moreover, staff members do not have a clear image of how important they are to the patients' satisfaction with and attitudes about service in the practice. Staff members who are open and caring and service-oriented add significantly to the patients' experiences, yet they are not often told of their value directly by the patients. Compliments and even complaints about the staff are usually given to the practice manager or sometimes to the physicians.

Voluntary patient communication about the practice is not, then, a reliable source for data. In fact, physicians are often kept in the dark about how patients feel, office managers deal most often with those who are extremely upset, and the staff members tend to function in an information vacuum. Thus, your practice needs to seek other methods for discovering how your patients perceive the service aspects of their experiences.

Regarding the attitudes and perceptions of the secondary customer populations, medical practices again have little if any information. The main reason is that very few practices have actually asked these customers for their opinions. It is not because the practices do not care about input from these customers, but rather because until recent years they have not been included in the definition of that term. Also, although some specialists' practices have made attempts to ask the referring practices about service issues, others have not solicited feedback because of a concern that such inquiry would be considered a bother. Typically, the dialogue between practices and their secondary customers regarding service issues has not been actively sought. Thus, what is important to these key customer populations is usually not known and their perceptions or attitudes about service in a given practice have not usually been determined.

In preparation for the active solicitation of patient feedback about service, everyone in the practice needs to have the opportunity to reflect on this fact: You won't really know what the customers think unless you ask them.

FACTOR 2: WHEN ASKED WHAT IS IMPORTANT TO THEM ABOUT NONCLINICAL ASPECTS OF CARE, CUSTOMERS OFTEN COME UP WITH SOME SURPRISING ANSWERS.

Some practices have already begun the kind of solicited data collection that I will be discussing in the next chapter. The results of these studies have revealed, once again, the importance of talking with the customers in a structured way. Jane Anderson, a consultant for Vantage Institute and the administrator of Tempe Dental Group, described the kind of unexpected information that can be found when customers are officially queried. She reported, "If you [talked to] your patients you might be surprised to find that the number-one reason for [their] returning to [your] dental office is not the quality of dentistry, the cleanliness and warm colors of the reception room, the cost of treatment, or even your location. The top reason is the way they are treated by staff members."[3] One office manager I interviewed told of the unexpected reactions patients had to the major office renovations her practice had undertaken. Anticipating positive responses, she was surprised when patients said, "Gee, you know, I liked it better the way it was."

Pediatrics Management surveyed 636 readers of *Parents* magazine to determine the traits parents value most in their children's doctors and in those physicians' practices. While a pediatrician's clinical competence and willingness to take time with a patient counted for a lot, surprisingly, according to this study, much of what shaped the parents' perceptions of a practice was unrelated to the physician's demeanor or skill. Office staffers' friendliness and professionalism were considered extremely or very important by 84 percent of the parents surveyed, while two-thirds of the poll's participants gave the same importance to the staff's helpfulness with health records. Parents gave considerably less weight to office decor, as well as to the availability of books and toys in the pediatricians' waiting rooms.[4]

So, the bottom line here is: Ask! You might well learn something you don't know!

FACTOR 3: SERVICE CANNOT BE IMPROVED WITHOUT CUSTOMER FEEDBACK.

The feedback you receive from customers should not be allowed merely to fall on deaf ears. The next step is to act on what is discovered. Others who have engaged in this feedback process have successfully improved service to their customers. For example, the Fallon Clinic, a 300-member physician-group practice with a largely HMO patient population, incorporated the results of a patient-feedback process into its physician reviews. Results were shared with the doctors, and one year later, follow-up surveys showed improvement in patient ratings of participating physicians.

Such changes do not just happen by accident, however. It takes an open mind and willingness to change before the information can be utilized for improvements. With some issues and in some instances, it also requires training. For example, following the reporting of initial patient-satisfaction results at the Fallon Clinic, the OB/GYN department provided a communication skills program for its physicians, and the next survey showed improvement among the targeted doctors.[5] An appropriate conclusion is that the training helped the physicians to focus on their communication behaviors and also taught them some techniques and methods for improving this skill. If the Fallon Clinic had not engaged in an official process of inquiry, problems could not have been uncovered and documented, and improvements could not have been made.

FACTOR 4: ONLY THROUGH A STRUCTURED APPROACH TO DATA COLLECTION CAN SERVICE IMPROVEMENTS BE ACCURATELY MEASURED.

Before you can even start to improve service in your practice, you must have a benchmark, an indication at a specific moment in time of how your practice is doing in those nonclinical areas of importance to customers. Improvements can only be determined when measured against these carefully documented starting points. For example, the Fallon Clinic was able to do just that. They began by conducting patient-satisfaction surveys in one year, going over the results with physicians, and conducting a follow-up study the next year. The results indicated that the actions taken to correct service problems in the intervening 12 months had been successful because patient ratings had improved. In addition, physicians indicated that the surveys significantly improved the physician evaluation process because they had some tangible data to study and specific areas on which to concentrate.[6]

FACTOR 5: STANDARDIZED SURVEYS CANNOT AND SHOULD NOT REPLACE PRACTICE-SPECIFIC CUSTOMER RESEARCH.

Some excellent standardized patient-satisfaction surveys are available, and they are useful for comparing practices and/or physicians. However, each practice needs to measure what is important to its own customers. Thus, your practice needs to create its own vehicles for doing so. Your practice needs to talk to customers to find out what matters to them and then to construct questionnaires to determine how the practice is doing in those areas.

The first phase of this process is very important. If you begin with structuring a questionnaire based on your own perceptions of what is important to any given customer population, you will quite likely be measuring customer reactions to some irrelevant points. You may unwittingly discover that you are doing fine in areas that don't matter to your customers, while at the same time not discovering attitudes and perceptions about items that do matter to them. John Maben, in his article, "Market Research: The 90's Way to Increase Your Odds of Business Success," pointed out: "All the issues important to the customer must be included in [a] survey. Failure to do so can produce misleading results; therefore, exploratory research is often needed. A recent client provided a list of 27 issues management believed to be important; exploratory interviews with customers revealed 26 additional issues management did not think of."[7]

FACTOR 6: CUSTOMER RESPONSES TO DIRECT QUESTIONS CAN CONFIRM OR DENY THE PRACTICE'S OWN PERCEPTIONS OF ITS SERVICE.

Self evaluation is another way to frame the results of the official research in a positive way. The process works much like the breast self-examination encouraged by doctors today. Such an exam may discover some potential areas of concern that need to be officially confirmed or denied. It also may not reveal an existing problem that requires closer scrutiny. In both instances, when the absence of a problem is confirmed by self-analysis, everyone feels good. Also, when problems are discovered or confirmed by expert examination, then action can be taken to handle the situation.

From a practice standpoint, the confirmation or dis-confirmation of the self-evaluation is also an indication of just how well a practice knows its customers. If the customer research reveals that the self-assessment of service issues has been confirmed, you know that your practice is close to its customer and that's good! If the self-evaluation is not confirmed, then you know your practice needs to get closer. Prior to asking any customer population what it thinks, I urge medical practices to make their own best guesses of what those responses will be. Then, when the actual customer responses are received, they can be compared to those anticipated by the practice.

FACTOR 7: OPENNESS TO FEEDBACK REQUIRES MENTAL AND EMOTIONAL PREPARATION.

When customers are asked to offer feedback, they will respond, which will mean both good news and bad news for the practice and its personnel. The good news is that a clear and complete picture of what your customers think of your practice will emerge, and the bad news is that a clear and complete picture . . . You get the idea. When your practice begins to seek feedback, you will hear it all—

the good, the bad, and the ugly. The acceptance of such honesty without falling into those defensive behaviors discussed in Chapter 3 depends on proper mental and emotional preparation.

For the practice leaders—the physicians and managers—this preparation requires the willingness to appear fallible in the eyes of your employees. You will need to set this process in the proper framework in your own mind. Just as *nobody* is perfect, no physician nor office manager is either. The best can be improved and the worst is not without hope. I want to reassure you: Those who have already conducted this type of research report that it isn't so bad. In fact, they hasten to add that it is very helpful. Charles Gaughn, formerly the director of research for TakeCare and now for FHP Inc. in Denver, reports that after TakeCare began a carefully structured process of seeking the patients' opinions about its network physicians and their practices, the doctors responded quite favorably. "Most of our physicians now fully support the survey. In fact, to gain more insight into our patients' concerns, some physicians have requested that we survey more than the standard 20 to 30 patients from their practice each year."[8] Morris Spierer, M.D., medical director of Fallon Clinic, and his colleagues said, "Surveys of patient satisfaction provide . . . direct feedback regarding the management of [the] practice. The results . . . can be used to identify problems, set goals, and motivate staff [physicians] to focus on quality."[9]

Clinical and nonclinical staff also need to be prepared mentally and emotionally. You too will receive feedback that will reflect both the positive and negative opinions of the customers. That alone can feel threatening. Also, you carry with you the additional knowledge that you do not own the practice and are not a part of management. That ultimately means that you can be more easily replaced, or so it can seem. So, as your practice starts down this road, your leaders need to help you prepare to accept the feedback in a positive way.

Proper preparation for all practice personnel means, first, that open and honest discussions are conducted regarding the rationale for engaging in this customer-feedback process. It is also helpful to place the seeking of customer feedback in the context of the larger perspective of creating and maintaining a Total Service Medical Practice. It is critical that all practice personnel understand that this is an information-gathering process only, that jobs are not on the line. Everyone should remember that there will be some good news to celebrate, that customers can and do compliment as well as criticize! Practice leaders should commit to celebrating all successes and working toward solutions to any problems.

Even though you think you know your customers, you probably don't. You may know what is bothering some patients who will voluntarily complain. You may have an idea that certain things are important, but you have no reliable data to tell you how important. You may have some notion that a few patients really appreciate what you do, but those seem to be too few and too far between. Without reliable valid data, which are collected in a systematic way, the chances are high that you will be basing service decisions on inaccurate or, at the very least, limited information.

Now, you are ready to move on to Step 6—Get Close to Your Customers and Stay There!

END NOTES

1. Steven Brown and Teresa Swartz, "A Gap Analysis of Professional Service Quality," *Journal of Marketing* 53, no. 2 (April 1989) pp. 92–98.

2. Stephen J. O'Connor, Richard M. Shewchuk, and Lynn W. Carney, "The Great Gap: Physicians' Perceptions of Patient Service Quality Expectations Fall Short of Reality," *Journal of Health Care Marketing* 14, no. 2 (Summer 1994), pp. 32–39.

3. "Treating Patients the Way They Want to Be Is Critical to Success," *Dental Group News* 28, no. 5 (May 1994), pp. 1–2.

4. Dorothy Pennachio, "What Parents Want from Your Office," *Pediatric Management* 4, no. 11 (November 1993), p. 35.

5. Morris Spierer, et al., "Assessment of Patient Satisfaction as a Part of a Physician Performance Evaluation: The Fallon Clinic Experience," *Journal of Ambulatory Care Management* 17, no. 3 (July 1994), p. 5.

6. Ibid, p. 7.

7. John Maben, "Market Research: The 90's Way to Increase Your Odds of Business Success," *Advertising and Marketing Review* 17, no. 10 (October 1994), p. 7.

8. Charles Gaughn, "TakeCare's Patient Satisfaction Survey Gauges Quality of Physician Care in HMO Setting," *Group Practice Journal* 42, no. 6 (November/December 1993), p. 30.

9. Spierer, 1.

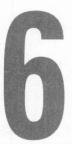

C H A P T E R

Step Six—Get Close to Your Customers and Stay There!

"It's really remarkable! When you are doing something that they don't like, it really comes through when you take the time to ask!" With these words Office Manager Marilyn Haley summarized her reaction to asking customers what they want and need. She continued, "The problem was we made an administrative decision to put a computer at our front desk, so when patients checked out we could put their numbers in right then. We could just hand them a bill at checkout and wouldn't that be wonderful! Right? Wrong! They hated it. They said, 'We come out and your head is in the computer! No one pays any attention to us.' We couldn't get rid of that computer fast enough." With this example, Ms. Haley illustrated one of the major reasons you should ask customers for feedback—you may find out that your view of service and theirs differ considerably. She also demonstrated the appropriate response to such discoveries—when you ascertain that something bothers the customers, do your best to change it!

GETTING CLOSE TO YOUR CUSTOMERS

When I use the phrase *getting close to your customers*, I am talking about a complete process of inquiry. Customers need to be *asked*

73

for their opinions and, as they answer, your practice needs to *listen*, to *empathize*, and to *respond*. The areas that are perceived by the customers as positive should be maintained; those about which there are complaints should be improved, if at all possible; and ways to exceed the customers' expectations should continue to be found. Only through this process of inquiry can your practice ensure that quality service is being provided.

Methods of Inquiry

The various tools available for getting close to your customers fall into two major categories: quantitative and qualitative. Quantitative data are obtained when something is counted. These data occur, for example, when functional performances are measured, such as the number of rings that occur before the telephone is answered. Quantitative data also occur when customers' perceptions are tabulated, such as the number of responses to items on a survey. Conclusions regarding the quality of service are usually determined by comparing these numerical outcomes against a desired standard. Theoretically, the closer the quantification comes to the standard, the better the service. When the standard is achieved or, in appropriate instances, surpassed, quality service is said to have been provided.

Qualitative data are based on *individual* perceptions, revealed through spoken and, on occasion, written comments. This perceptual base makes these data vulnerable to the criticism of being personality driven; it is easier to argue with the verbalized perceptions of someone else than with the numbers on survey results. Due to their reliance on the customers' *own words*, however, qualitative data carry their own power and cannot be underestimated.

Quantitative and qualitative methods range along a continuum from the formal to the informal. (See Figure 6–1.) All provide useful information. The more-formal methods require a carefully structured research design, while the more-informal methods do not. Those methods found along the midrange are less structured than the formal, but not so casual as the informal. All methods, regardless of their formality, are helpful tools for getting close to your customers.

FIGURE 6–1

Continuum of Research Methodologies

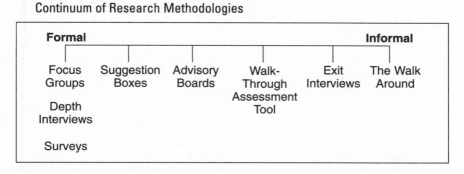

Formal Tools: Creating Your Official Customer Report Cards

The term *customer report card* is being used a lot lately with slightly different meanings. What I am referring to is the discovery of what matters to the customers of your practice and the determination of what these customers think of your practice's efforts in those areas of importance. Structuring customer report cards (there should be one for each key customer population) requires a formal process which relies on both quantitative and qualitative methodologies.

The first step in creating any report card is to ask representatives of the customer groups the following question:

What is important to you about the nonclinical aspects of your experiences with a medical practice?

In order to find the answers, begin the *formal* process of inquiry with qualitative methods.

Focus Groups

Brought into the popular vernacular by political campaigning of the 1990s, focus groups have long been a legitimate research method. Consisting of 8 to 12 customers, focus groups solicit responses from the participants to open-ended questions posed by a facilitator. Transcripts of these group interviews are analyzed later for trends in the data (sometimes called "critical incidents"): topics that are repeated by several people or that are returned to over and over again by a smaller number of participants.

Focus groups and the data they provide are valuable for several reasons:

■ *Focus groups allow customers to drive the discoveries.* Due to the open-ended nature of the questions, the responses reflect what is on the *customers'* minds. The trends in the data that emerge describe the customers' opinions and experiences, not those predetermined and imposed by the practice or the creator of a standardized survey instrument.

■ *The facilitator can probe into issues and elicit detailed information from the participants.* A skilled focus-group facilitator enters the process with a set of open-ended questions, called *protocols*, but as the participants respond, additional questions are created on the spot. This allows the facilitator to ask for clarification, examples, further explanation, and even for possible consensus among these participants.

■ *Interaction among group participants stimulates even further discussion.* While some criticize this aspect of focus groups for being a type of *group think*, I have found it to be otherwise. When participants come to a focus group, they have a general idea of the topic at hand, but they are not usually given questions in advance. Thus, they can be caught a little off guard as the actual questions are asked. The discussion serves to stimulate their thinking and helps them to recall examples of their own. Another factor that argues against the group-think criticism is that focus-group members often disagree. They seem to take the facilitator's request for their *own* opinions quite seriously.

■ *During these face-to-face interactions, the nonverbal messages can be observed and recorded.* In Chapter 7, I discuss the specifics of nonverbal communication. At this point, keep in mind that the facial expressions, the sound of the voices, the gestures and body movements (such as nodding heads)—all provide important data. These nonverbal behaviors can show the strength of an opinion, the depth of a feeling, and the power of the experience being described.

■ *The exact words of the customers can be preserved and shared with others.* As previously indicated, the power of specific quotations from customers cannot be underestimated. They can bring your practice close to the customer in a way no quantification can. While the old saying "There's strength in numbers" is true, it is also true that in customer-service research nothing can replace the impact of the customers' own words.

One question I am frequently asked is, "Can we conduct our own focus groups?" My answer to that is a qualified "yes." The caveat I offer is this: If it is at all possible, hire someone from outside the practice to conduct these groups, and if that is prohibitively expensive, then do it yourself but with caution.

Why should your practice spend money to have someone else ask perfectly simple questions? There are several reasons. First, the questions themselves are not as simple as they might appear. Trained focus-group facilitators know what the appropriate initial questions should be and have developed a skill for structuring probing follow-up queries that have to be created on the spot; this is not as easy as it may seem. Second, when the responses are not what practice personnel want to hear, a facilitator from the practice can become defensive, thus impairing his or her ability to think and to process the information. Negative responses also can stimulate the practice-facilitator to offer a verbal defense or merely an explanation, neither of which reflect the data-collection purpose of the session. In addition, practice-facilitators are often prone to simply filtering out or ignoring data that they don't want to hear. Although usually an unconscious reaction, when this filtering process occurs, important data are never reported. Finally, focus-group participants can have difficulty seeing practice personnel as researchers and not as problem solvers. Thus, they can expect explanations and even solutions to their difficulties, which shifts the entire focus away from data collection. Additionally, if the facilitator does not attempt to solve problems on the spot, then the participants can become angry, affecting the information that they provide, and, at times, creating unproductive distractions.

The advantage of having practice personnel present for the focus groups is so that they can observe and hear the participants. This advantage can easily be provided by videotaping the session or by having practice personnel observe through the one-way window that is available in most standard research centers, the best places to conduct these sessions. When I am facilitating a group, I handle the hidden presence of the observers by simply saying, "We have some guests from my client's organization here today, and because I need your complete attention on me and these questions, I've asked them to just observe quietly from behind that window there. They are very interested in what you have to say and appreciate your participation." Sometimes we even wave at the unseen observers and that seems to break the ice; to my knowledge, their presence has been accepted as *standard procedure* by the participants.

I have noticed no difference in the level of participation between those sessions that are being taped and/or observed, and those that are not. Most focus-group participants have agreed to be interviewed because they have something to say; neither a camera nor an observer appears to hamper their willingness to say it. In fact, the major inhibitor to participation seems to be face-to-face interaction with practice personnel. Reluctant to offend, customers are less likely to be open and honest in the visible presence of physicians, managers, and staff. This is yet another reason not to rely on in-house facilitation.

If, however, your practice simply does not have the resources to hire outside facilitators, then proceed on your own . . . with caution. The practice personnel who will be conducting the sessions should receive training in focus-group facilitation. They also should prepare themselves mentally and emotionally for what they may hear. The data-collection purpose of the session needs to be made clear to the participants from the first contact and reinforced by the facilitator at the beginning of the session. If necessary during the session, reminders of the fact-finding/data-collection purpose should be offered, if the participants get off track.

The following are suggestions for the effective use of the focus-group research tool:

1. Eight to 12 participants per focus group should be selected, based on such demographic data as age, sex, socioeconomic status, etc. For example, if your practice is interested in the possible varying wants and needs of the different *age* groups it serves, then it may be advisable to use age as a selection factor: one focus group of young adults with no children; one focus groups of young adults with children; two focus groups of middle-aged adults, and two of the over 65 population. This should allow some indication of possible differences based on age. It is a good idea to invite three to four more participants than you think you'll need. Attrition will take care of the extras.

2. A cash stipend, usually of $25, should be offered in advance and paid at the time of the session. Refreshments should be provided, especially if the session occurs during a meal time.

3. Participants should be contacted via telephone first, inviting them to be a part of your practice's customer service initiative. The data-collection nature of the process should be clearly explained.

4. Participants should be reminded of their oral commitment with a follow-up letter which provides directions to the location, and they also should receive a telephone call the day before the session reminding them to attend.

5. The focus groups should be held at a site away from the practice, if possible. The familiarity of the practice's location can be an inhibitor for some people and can also obscure the research function of the focus group. Most cities have marketing research firms with focus-group facilities, including videotaping and/or observation room setups. They also usually have a staff of consultants who can be hired to conduct the focus-group sessions. These facilities are usually on the pricey side, but, if the money is available, they are well worth the investment. A second facility-choice would be a conference room at a local hotel; a third would be a similar room at a hospital.

6. Trained facilitators should be used, if possible. If the budget does not allow for this cost, and in lieu of using practice personnel, another option is to check with selected graduate programs at your local or even regional colleges and universities. Many of these programs have mature graduate students who frequently are familiar with focus-group methodologies, and they would be available at little to no cost, especially if the data could be used in their theses or dissertations. The most likely departments for such folks are the departments of communication or communications studies, business administration, marketing, psychology, or sociology/anthropology. The Office of the Dean of Graduate Studies could also make recommendations.

7. The room should be set up with a conference table and comfortable chairs. If the video camera has to be visible, it should be placed in a far corner and kept as unobtrusive as possible.

8. If audio or videotaping will occur, which it should, participants should be told in advance and be reminded before the session starts. Anyone not wanting to be taped should be excused. It is probably a good idea to secure a signed permission statement from those who are taped.

9. Protocols, the open-ended questions, should be prepared in advance. (See Appendix for samples.)

10. The facilitator should be nonthreatening but able to control the group.

11. Depending on the size of the group, sessions should last between one and a half to two hours.

12. The session should be followed up with a letter and a summary of the results; participants want to know what happened to their input.

13. After the sessions are completed, analyze the data. Working from written transcripts, trends or common themes should be determined. First, similar comments from different participants that come up repeatedly should be identified. Although, in most instances, the sample size of focus groups is not large enough to consider this type of quantification statistically valid, it is sufficient to determine a trend. Also, any topic that is revisited *repeatedly* by a small number of participants or even one individual should be noted; this repetition can indicate an issue of great importance to these people, and it is worth adding to your list. Based on the trends in the data, a survey can be constructed and submitted to a larger sample for validation. The best quotations from the focus groups should be preserved for inclusion in the report that will be written at the end of the research process.

Depth Interviews

Another useful tool for collecting qualitative data is the depth interview. Similar in methodology, although different in format, depth interviews and focus groups extract the same kind of spontaneous data that will help your practice determine what is important to its customers. Usually relied on for interviewing upper management and professional personnel, this depth interview technique uses the same type of open-ended questions that are asked of focus-group participants. Rather than meeting in a group at a neutral location, however, the depth-interview participants are queried one-on-one at their own offices or locations of their choice. (I interviewed a doctor for this book at the nurses' station in a hospital, while we waited on an expectant mother to deliver!) Sometimes interviewees are offered a stipend, and other times they are not. If the offer is made, it usually is between \$50–\$100. Most professionals do not accept the stipend, and some seem offended at the offer. Others seem to appreciate, but decline. This is your call. My experience has been that most appreciate the offer, but turn it down. One physician asked me to donate his stipend to his favorite charity. Because only one person is being interviewed at a time, depth interviews usually take around 30 minutes and never over an hour. Probing questions are very important in a depth interview, because it is up to the interviewer alone to stimulate thoughts in the interviewee; there is no group to assist with this process. These interviews are usually audiotaped with permission in order to preserve the specific content. For structuring a report card, usually between 6 to 10 individuals are interviewed. The interviews are transcribed, and the trends in the data are then identified.

After the qualitative data obtained during the focus groups and depth interviews have been analyzed and after the items of importance to the customer population that is being queried have been determined, the next step is to answer the second question on the customer report card:

How is this practice doing in those areas of importance?

The best method for answering that question is to survey a representative sample of the customer group under consideration, seeking to quantify the responses.

Customer Satisfaction Surveys

In order to move the qualitative data into some measurable form, the information discovered during the focus groups and depth interviews must be transferred into a survey. By considering the list of important items, which was extracted from the qualitative data, survey items can be written. Customer-satisfaction questionnaires seek reactions to specific customer experiences. For example, if the focus groups and depth interviews revealed that a *positive staff attitude* is important to patients, then a patient-satisfaction survey should include items that will help ascertain how successfully the practice's staff performed in this area during a patient's recent visit to your practice: Was the receptionist courteous? Was the nurse helpful? Was the check-out clerk pleasant?

Each question provides the respondents with a range of options, known as *descriptors,* from which to choose. One such scale is called the Likert Scale, named after the inventor of this type of instrument. The options or descriptors from which the respondent chooses can range from "Strongly Agree" to "Strongly Disagree," from "Very Satisfied" to "Very Dissatisfied," from "Very Positive" to "Very Negative." Between the two extreme ends of each of these scales are three to five additional choices, representing degrees of reactions; the middle choice on a Likert Scale is always Neutral. The following question from a patient satisfaction survey illustrates a typical Likert Scale item:

Was the receptionist courteous?
Strongly Agree   Agree   Neutral   Disagree   Strongly Disagree

Another example looks like this:

The doctor took time with me.
Strongly Agree   Agree   Neutral   Disagree   Strongly Disagree

The respondents are instructed to circle the most appropriate response based on their recent experience with the practice.

The following example illustrates another common scale used on survey items:[1]

How would you rate each of the following, based on your satisfaction during your recent visit to our practice:

The overall visit:
Excellent   Very Good   Good   Fair   Poor   N/A

The personal manner (courtesy, respect, sensitivity, friendliness) of the provider you saw:
Excellent   Very Good   Good   Fair   Poor   N/A

The length of time you waited to get an appointment:
Excellent   Very Good   Good   Fair   Poor   N/A

Regardless of what kind of scale is used, one allowing for degrees of responses is preferable to a dichotomous, forced choice of *yes* or *no.*

Most customer-satisfaction surveys include a section for additional comments that is particularly important on the shorter forms. Sometimes each specific item has a space for a written explanation. In other instances, the comments section is included at the end of the questionnaire. Wherever these sections appear, they provide important opportunities to gather, in the customers' own words, additional insights into the specific incidents that shaped their reactions to the experience.

The following questions represent typical queries of many people regarding the use of surveys:

> Question 1: *How much does it cost to survey customers?*
> Depending on how much outside assistance your practice requires, a very simple self-conducted study might cost approximately $500. A simple study conducted by an outside vendor will probably range from $500 to $5,000. More complex studies which should probably be conducted by an outside vendor will vary from $5,000 to up to $20,000. Advanced studies will cost more. (The more complex and advanced studies usually include several customer populations).

> Question 2: *How many people should be surveyed to have a representative sample?*
> It all depends. Studies have indicated as few as 25 patients provide reliable rating information on an individual physician. Other studies indicate a need for 20 to 40. A sample of 300–400 qualified respondents can be said to represent an *entire customer* population, particularly if the majority of the respondents give similar answers.[2]

> Question 3: *What kind of response rate can we expect?*
> In the area of patient-satisfaction surveys, medical practices are lucky. Compared to the response rate for hospitals (often only 20 percent or lower)[3], medical practices frequently find a 50 percent, or better, response rate, plenty for a statistically relevant sample.[4] Part of the explanation for this high response rate has to do with the ongoing personal relationship that is established between practices and their patients, which hospitals may not have. Also, in some cases, patients may perceive that their input might well have greater impact on the usually smaller entity of a medical practice. A third reason is that, in many instances, the patients of the practice are not as ill or injured as those in a hospital, and so they actually feel more like completing a

questionnaire. Whatever the reason, you can expect a fairly high return on your patient surveys. If your practice has already distributed surveys with a low response rate, then consider the timing, the length and complexity of the questionnaire, and the ease of return. Often problems in these areas contribute to a lack of response. Suggestions for increasing your return are:

- Keep the questionnaire brief.
- Provide clear and accurate instructions.
- Deliver the questionnaire personally when possible. For example, hand the survey to the patients before they leave the practice. Consider having the physician hand the questionnaires to the patients.
- Mail questionnaires in a timely manner, if using that distribution method.
- Include a self-addressed, stamped envelope with the mail-in questionnaire.

Surveys of the secondary external customer-populations are unusual, so they may result in a low return at first. In addition to following as many of the above suggestions as possible, also follow up with reminder mailings and/or phone calls. Secondary customers can be persuaded to participate by:

- Sharing with the customers a brief statement of your practice's motivation for conducting this survey: that your practice considers its customers to be important members of a customer population, and that your desire is to serve them more effectively.
- Sharing a brief summary of the qualitative research that preceded the survey.
- Sharing the positive responses made by your practice to previous report card feedback.
- Reminding the customers of your practices' on-going efforts to stay close to its various customers.

As you can see, most of the above suggestions involve showing the customers that their input is wanted, needed, and will be responded to. Then their involvement will seem to be worth their time.

Question 4: *How long should our questionnaire be?*
There may be a tendency to want to ask every conceivable question that comes to mind. I have seen some patient satisfaction surveys that were so long and intimidating that many potential respondents probably threw them away. "Health care marketers need to weigh carefully the negative implications of lengthy questionnaires that include assessments of such things as expectations and importance against the limited contribution these data provide for decisionmaking."[5] Irwin Press, president of the well-known hospital-based Press Ganey Satisfaction Measurement indicated, "Report cards should be short . . . Twenty-five [items] is too many and two or three is too few.[6] Office manager Marilyn Haley said, "We use a one-pager."

Question 5: *What kind of results should we be satisfied with?*
Realizing that all customers cannot be satisfied and that practice personnel will make mistakes, perfection in service is not an achievable goal. The notion of Zero Defects[7] or even Zero Defections[8] fails to recognize this fact. Arguing for an error-free environment, these theories do not allow for the human aspect of service interactions and for the resulting occasional imperfections.

Having said this, I don't mean to imply that poor service can and should be tolerated. It should be the service goal of your practice to work toward providing quality service to all of its customers. Meryl Luallin, an experienced researcher in patient satisfaction, concluded the following about service standards in medical practices: "No medical practice would be satisfied with a 10 percent error rate in diagnosis or similar lack of accuracy in laboratory test procedures . . . no less should be expected in service than is demanded clinically. If you have a 90 percent (Good + Excellent Rating) that means that one in 10 [of your customers] was unsatisfied . . . ninety-three percent should be at least the norm expected."[9]

Question 6: *How often should we survey?*
As will be discussed in greater detail in Chapter 17, the process of inquiry should be conducted on an ongoing basis. Focus groups should be conducted at least once every two

years, and surveys should be conducted at least annually. In cases where trouble spots have been identified, more frequent surveys will provide current data on the effects of management's attempts to improve service and/or performance.[10]

Question 7: *What kinds of surveys should be conducted?*
So far I have been discussing paper-and-pencil surveys. While these are the most common, you can also conduct similar surveys via the telephone or, with some customers, even the Internet. Director of marketing research Charles Gaughn of FHP of Colorado and formerly of TakeCare, described the success of his telephone-survey approach: Within 60 days of a visit to a provider's office, patients were contacted by telephone and asked to respond to a short survey. Gaughn reported, "What we've found has been overwhelmingly positive. Patients appreciated the opportunity to discuss their experiences. . . In fact, we doubt that the goodwill created in conducting the survey could be duplicated. Of the more than 12,000 surveys conducted each year, only 3 percent of the members called declined to participate."[11] Given the electronic capabilities of many of your practices' secondary customer populations, it is possible to conduct a survey over the Internet. Until all potential customers in any given population have this capability, however, a limiting variable will be introduced into the study, which can impact the generalizability of the results. For now, the best methods to use are the written or telephone-survey approaches.

The following example illustrates an effective use of the survey approach: The Fallon Clinic, cited in Chapter 5 for the success of its patient-satisfaction process, designed a questionnaire to assess patients' perceptions of the quality and timeliness of care during their recent visits to the clinic. (In this instance, quality of care referred to the nonclinical or service aspects of the customers' experiences.) Patients were asked to rate a number of issues on a five-point scale from Excellent to Poor. Quality-of-care issues in the survey included response and courtesy shown by the physicians; explanations about tests, procedures, and medications; and the likelihood that the patient would recommend the physician to others. Timeliness-of-care issues included the patient's ability to reach the physician, the length of time between calling to schedule an appointment and the day of the appointment, the ability to obtain follow-up care, and time spent waiting after arriving for a visit. Other survey questions asked patients why they chose Fallon and their physicians, and how long they had been patients of Fallon and of that doctor. The patients were also asked to indicate their age and sex and to answer three questions regarding their health status.

Morris Spierer, Fallon's medical director, and his colleagues explained, "The surveys were sent out with a postage-paid return envelope and a cover letter signed by [Spierer]. The letter explained why the survey was sent, thanked the patients for their participation, and assured them that their responses would remain anonymous . . . For each full-time physician evaluated, 150 patients were randomly selected from a computer database of all patients that had seen their physicians in the previous three weeks. For some part-time physicians, names were selected from as far back as three months in order to get a sample of 150. The sample population included both fee-for-service and Fallon Clinic Health Plan members."[12] The overall response rate was a respectable 43.6 percent in the first year and 37.3 percent in the second. (See the sample patient-satisfaction questionnaire from Facey Medical Foundation in the Appendix.)

Service Quality Surveys

As discussed in Chapter 1, service quality differs from customer satisfaction in that the former focuses on long-term attitudes that are shaped by repeated experiences with your practice, while the latter seeks perceptions of specific experiences. The questions asked on a service quality survey differ from those seeking to measure customer satisfaction. Service-quality-survey items guide the respondents to consider their overall impressions of the practice. The surveys are given to people who have interacted with the practice over a longer period of time (usually a year or more) and have had several contacts during that time.

Service quality questions might look like the following:

Based on your long-term relationship with our practice, please respond to the following questions:

How would you rate the attitude of the staff with whom you've interacted?

Excellent   Very Good   Good   Fair   Poor   N/A

Explain:_____

_____

How would you rate the attitude of the physicians?

Excellent   Very Good   Good   Fair   Poor   N/A

Explain:_____

_____

How would you rate the appointment accessibility?

Excellent   Very Good   Good   Fair   Poor   N/A

Explain:_____

_____

Since respondents are asked for overall reactions, opportunities to explain are especially important on service quality surveys, allowing respondents to justify the rating in more specific terms. This measurement of long-term attitudes provides a useful comparison with the short-term reactions discerned via customer-satisfaction surveys. Transitory conditions can impact customers' perceptions of specific experiences, so it is helpful to know if the pleasure or displeasure seems to be universal and chronic.

Positive responses on the service quality instrument should not prevent the practice from being concerned about the problems brought out on customer-satisfaction instruments, however. If the problem has occurred once, it is worth examination. If it has occurred several times, it demands attention.

The distinction between customer satisfaction and service quality is a relatively new one, and standardized instruments for measuring the latter have not yet been written, nor have many organizations created their own. Thus, your practice will be more on its own when creating a service quality tool. (See the Appendix for a suggested service quality questionnaire.)

Quantification of Functional Tasks

Functional tasks refer to those tasks that are necessary for the daily operation of the office. The number of times that a telephone rings before it is answered is a typical example. Although perhaps unusual, I also have included measurements of time in this category: the number of minutes a customer must wait before being seen (in the case of a face-to-face interaction) or heard (in the case of being placed on hold during a telephone call); the number of days, weeks, or months between a request for an appointment and the appointment itself.

Counting functional tasks can be very revealing, but it can also lead to putting quantity over quality. Customer service representatives from all industries complain about the pressure to take more telephone calls, for example. Based on the often erroneous notion that *more is always better*, this approach does not allow for any appraisal of what transpires during those customer interactions. Most service personnel subjected to those quantitative measures complain that the pressure to take more calls prevents them from really listening to the customer and from taking their time to offer satisfying assistance to them. Independent physicians who are pushed by capitation to see more patients or staff doctors pressured by an organization to reduce the number of minutes per patient interview are often caught in the quantity versus quality dilemma as well.

As your practice examines these and other functional tasks, care should be taken not to consider quantification to be the absolute determinant of quality. Although it provides important and useful information, quantification of functional tasks does not present the entire picture.

Pitfalls of Measurement

Although measurement is an important part of formulating customer report cards, be aware of some its pitfalls:[13]

- Microvision: Your practice can become so caught up in measurement that the reason is forgotten. I've had receptionists tell me: "We are supposed to answer the telephone within three rings." When I have asked them the rationale for this policy, they have not been able to remember.
- Averages: When quantifying service, averages do not say very much. As we know, to arrive at a numerical average there must be figures above and below. When it comes to service, *below average* is far from acceptable. For that matter, neither is *average*.
- Counting Complaints: In Chapter 14, I discuss in greater detail how complaints can be appropriately used to assess service. For now, the point to remember is that counting complaints will not

necessarily reveal if service is good or bad. In fact, once customers discover that your practice is listening to them, the number of actual complaints will very likely increase, thus leading to the erroneous conclusion that service is getting worse, not better. By the same token, practices that have not actively sought customer input can be lulled into a false sense of security by a small number of complaints. (Remember, most customers have to be encouraged to complain.) Complaints should be used to track the trends for problems but not relied on as measures of service improvements. (For that you need to compare follow-up data with benchmark data.)

■ Random Sampling: When measuring customer satisfaction, a totally random sample will probably not sample the appropriate population. For example, customer satisfaction research wants to measure those with recent experiences; service quality is aimed at long-term perceptions. Thus, these and other variables will need to be factored into the sample taken.

A Report on Your Report Cards
If the title of this section seems redundant, I hope you'll find solace in the fact that during my academic career I once served on the Committee on Committees. At least my redundance here seems worthwhile! But I digress. Once the survey data for each customer population has been tabulated, you can shape your customer report cards and to present them in the report-card report.

The report should begin with a brief introduction, explaining the rationale for the study, who was queried, and any other relevant information. Then, the answers to the key questions posed to the customer populations should be provided, one population at a time:

> What is important to you [the customers] about the nonclinical aspects of your experiences with a medical practice?

and

> How is this practice doing in the areas of importance?

Qualitative and quantitative data should be offered to support the answers presented. Next, an analysis of the positives and the areas for improvement should be offered with recommendations for needed changes prioritized. (For a briefer, more concise version to supplement, not replace, the longer report described above, the important customer-items for each population can be listed with a brief summary of how the practice is doing following each item.) The report, then, should contain (1) an introduction, (2) the results of the answers to the two key questions for each population queried, (3) an analysis of the positives, and (4) an analysis of areas for improvement accompanied by prioritized recommendations.

The report-card report should be shared with practice personnel. Those items that have to do with the practice as a whole or with systems involved in serving the customers should be shared with the entire practice. Any personal information, especially problems, should be handled privately. As long as praise serves as a motivator for others, positive feedback for specific individuals can also be shared with the practice as whole. A summary discussion should be offered to customers who participated in the qualitative phase. If the number of survey respondents is small enough, they too should receive a similar summary. An important final note: The results of the report cards for each customer population should be compared, looking for any conflicting desires between or among customer groups that should be resolved and finding all complementary wishes that can be granted.

Midrange Methods for Getting Close to Your Customer

Although not usually included in official customer-report-card research, the midrange methods for getting close to your customer can provide important information to your practice. On the methodology continuum, these methods fall between the formal and the informal. The two most often used in medical practices are suggestion boxes and advisory boards.

Suggestion Boxes

Falling midway on the continuum between formal and informal methods is the ever-popular suggestion box. Usually the place you will find people registering complaints, this tool can provide an opportunity for quick responses to the question of "How are we doing?" The following suggestions will help institute a successful suggestion-box system:

- Place the box in a visible location. Don't hide it away in a corner as though you are afraid of the feedback. Put a sign nearby that says: "Please tell us what we're doing right and what we can do better."

■ Make the box big enough to encourage participation. Little boxes don't convey an eagerness for feedback. However, a huge box can indicate you expect lots of problems.

■ Keep cards and sharpened pencils handy! Be certain that a suggestion-box form is readily available and that the respondents have a writing utensil. I recommend a pencil because it allows respondents to make changes, it is not expensive, and it won't be removed from the practice as readily as a pen.

■ Have an assigned member of the practice manage and monitor the suggestion box. Someone needs to be in charge. The above-mentioned supplies must be provided, and the contents of the box must be collected and analyzed. At the Sansum Clinic in Santa Barbara, an employee group evaluates and makes recommendations on patient suggestions.[14]

■ Act on the suggestions! I cannot stress this enough. If your practice wants people to participate in a suggestion-box system, they must see a willingness to implement their suggestions. They will stop completing the forms if they don't see results.

■ Respond personally to anyone who has signed a suggestion form. Place an optional section on the form that requests the name, address, and phone number of the respondents, should they want to provide this information. Even if a little research is needed to find the address or phone number, do it. That personal response will earn many jewels in your crown not to mention points with the customers.

Advisory Boards
The most frequently used advisory boards deal with patient issues and are composed of active patients of the practice. Daniel Gottovi, M.D., described the following suggestions for establishing a patient-advisory board:[15]

■ Announce in billing notices and notices in the office. Dr. Gottovi's advisory board received coverage in the local newspaper, which resulted in great public relations for the practice, the story also brought phone calls from additional volunteers.

■ Screen applicants for a representative mix on the following demographics: age, sex, ethnic background, or other pertinent factors.

- Keep membership at a manageable number. Dr. Gottovi wanted 15 members; but after attempting to eliminate some, he decided to keep all 19 applicants. Although that may seem like a large number, it also allows for the inevitable absences that will occur with such voluntary groups.

- Set a regular, but not too frequent, meeting schedule. Again, Dr. Gottovi recommends monthly meetings. His patient advisory board meets the second Tuesday of each month at 5:30 P.M.

I will add my own suggestions to those of Dr. Gottovi:

- Be certain that the mission and purpose of the advisory board is clearly explained at the first meeting. At the initial meeting, take the time to explain why this board was created and what the practice hopes to gain from it.

- Allow the advisory board to establish its own guidelines for operation. Once the members have been informed about the board's purpose, practice personnel should step aside and let the members themselves decide about such issues as absences, meeting length, even date and hour. (To be effective, patient advisory boards should meet once a month; other customer boards may not need to meet as frequently.)

- Coordinate the agenda with the board's representatives. Usually the office manager acts as the liaison to the board. Usually, but not always, the board chairperson acts as the liaison from the board to the practice. Regardless of whom is performing that role, prior to each meeting these two people should meet to set the agenda, which can then be sent in advance to the board members. Each meeting should allow issues to be brought from both the board, as the patients' representatives, and from the practice.

- Be certain to respond to the suggestions made by the advisory board. As with the suggestion-box system, nothing will deflate the respondents' enthusiasm more quickly than feeling as though their ideas have disappeared into a black hole. If at all possible, implement their suggestions. If not, explain clearly and patiently why it can't be done. Then, try to find an alternative that will please them.

Dr. Gottovi's practice received and implemented many suggestions made by the advisory board:

- Expanded hours for walk-ins.
- Changes in fee structure.
- Consistency in payment policies.
- Direct patient refunds.
- More parking for the physically challenged.
- Creation of a practice newsletter.
- Improved doctor/patient communication.
- Clarified points of contact for patients.
- Added patient education staff (teaching nurses in gastroenterology, cardiology, and pulmonary disease, as well as a dietitian.)
- Improved pharmaceutical counseling (special room for pharmacists to counsel patients).
- Expanded range of medical services (added dermatologist, pediatrician, and ambulatory surgery).[16]

Advisory boards take time to coordinate effectively, and they take a real commitment to listen to what your customers have to say. But, as you can see, many important improvements can be made in your practice via this more informal, but useful, contact.

Informal Tools for Getting Close to Your Customers.

Although the most reliable data are obtained through more formal research methods, other less carefully structured but equally revealing methods will help your practice get close to your customers. Often called point-of-contact methods, they are relied on to drop in on the customers' experiences spontaneously.

The Walk-Through Patient-Focus Assessment Tool (WTPFAT)

Intended to supplement traditional methods of collecting patient-satisfaction data, "the WTPFAT is an instrument that has been developed for use by healthcare workers, managers, and professionals in order to examine their environment from the patient-focus point of view."[17] I am reminded of an old M*A*S*H* episode which was filmed entirely from the perspective of the young man in the post-op ward. The sight lines were only those he could have had; the conversations were only those he could have heard. This perceptual point of view reinforced for me the importance of seeing the world through the customers' eyes. It may look quite different to them than it does to you. The application of this *through the patients' eyes* technique grew from the experiences of physicians who became ill and found that the medical scene looked quite different to them from the vantage point of a patient. "Placing oneself in a patient's shoes and understanding what the experience is like in a personal manner can cause a fundamental change in the way that one approaches patients and medicine in general. [In fact], several medical schools have begun to have physicians-in-training spend time as patients to sensitize them to the patient's experience.[18]

You can design the WTPFAT to fit your practice. Still relying on the items of importance discovered in the focus group and depth interview data, a simple checklist can be designed that will allow practice personnel to view the practice through their customers' eyes. Keeping in mind that although patients are the primary customers of your practice they are not the only customers, this same experience should be accorded to all staff, and separate checklists should be designed for each of your critical customer populations.

The Exit Interview
Another informal method for obtaining feedback is to conduct exit interviews with customers who leave. Marc Lato, M.D., a family physician in Phoenix, Arizona, contacts patients who have asked that their records be transferred, asking them to call if there has been a problem. This tactic has led to changes in office policies and has occasionally retrieved an unhappy, departing patient.[19]

The Walk Around
An even less formal method was described by an office manager in one of my workshops: "Once a month I take some time and I walk through the office and talk to people. I talk to patients. I talk to staff. I also talk to the physicians. I find out 'how things are going.' Those walks have provided some of the most important insights I've had about this practice and what it takes to bring

satisfaction to people." Although this approach should not replace the formal creation of the customer report card, it will bring you up close and personal to the people both inside and outside the practice in a special way.

Another suggestion I have is to assign a staff member to go through the practice from the patient's point of view, from scheduling an appointment through leaving the practice or even after receiving the bill. Then, that person can share his or her experiences at a staff meeting. By rotating this opportunity on a regular basis, your practice can begin to see the world through the patient's eyes. The same approach can be used with other customer populations as well.

Although not usually statistically valid, these informal approaches to getting close to your customers can reveal many interesting and important insights into your practice.

CUSTOMER REPORT CARDS REVISITED

In Chapter 4, I identified patients as the primary external customers of your practice. I also identified a ring of secondary customers whom your practice needs in order to provide quality care and quality service to the patients: family members of patients, other physicians, insurance carriers, and hospitals. Although your practice may identify different secondary customers, the patients are at the heart of the enterprise.

Earlier in this chapter I recommended that your practice conduct its own qualitative research to discover what is important to each of the external key customer populations it serves (and to the internal customers, for that matter). Although this section should not replace that process, I would like to share the results of my own attempt to discover what matters to the five external customer populations identified in Chapter 4. Through focus groups, interviews, literature review, and more casual interactions with workshop participants, I have formulated the following lists of items important to these customer populations. *Let them serve only as a comparison for what you find in your own qualitative research.*

As you read the lists below, understand that any relationship is a two-way street; your customers have their own responsibilities to uphold. Bear in mind, however, that if your practice is paying attention to these areas or to those discovered through its own qualitative research, the chances are much higher that the practice/customer relationships will be positive and that the interactions will run much more smoothly.

Patients

The following are items of importance to patients, not listed in any particular order:

- Attitude of physicians: Courtesy, respect, communication.
- Attitude of staff: Courtesy, respect, friendliness, communication.
- Immediate acknowledgement: wanting to be acknowledged when entering reception area.
- Waiting time: After arriving at the practice for a visit and in the examination room.
- Ease of appointment scheduling: Actual process used and length of time before being seen.
- Office hours: Usually wanting expanded hours to cover early morning, evening, and in some instances, weekends.
- Telephone Communication: Responsiveness, voice mail, being on hold, pleasantness and helpfulness of staff.
- Cleanliness of facility: Neat and unsoiled.
- Parking: Ease of parking, availability of spaces, and, in some instances, cost.
- Patient Education Efforts: Availability of written and even video materials; availability of teaching nursing staff.
- Payment Policies: Cost, billing procedure and forms, co-pay policies and implementation thereof, assistance with insurance companies.
- Referrals: Ease of process, quality of specialists, location of specialists, attitude of specialists and their staffs, availability for appointments.

Family Members of Patients

Family members of patients have indicated the following items are important to them:

- Honesty: Sensitivity of approach, truthfulness of what is told.
- Information: Amount, clarity, lay language.
- Answers to questions: Willingness to provide; encouragement to ask; detail, clarity, and understandability of response.
- Recognition: Seen and treated as an individual, not just the patient's relative; involvement in discussions with patients.
- Treatment of patient: Involvement of patient if he or she is capable; courtesy, respect, and caring accorded to patient.
- Treatment of family members: Courtesy, respect, understanding, empathy.
- Involvement in patient care: Extent to which they are allowed to assist in providing care.

Other Physicians' Practices

In order to be able to help each other provide quality care for the patients, physicians' practices request the following from their colleagues.

Primary Care Physicians' Requests of Specialists:

- Insurance knowledge: Is the specialist's practice in the plan? What is the plan's referral process?
- Referrals: Cooperative development of a successful practice/practice system.
- Treatment of referred patients: Treating the patient *right*—courtesy, kindness, friendliness, speed of appointment.
- Information regarding referred patient treatment: Complete and timely updating.
- Empathy: Understanding of the differences in volume of patients, differing stresses in PCP practices.
- Telephone accessibility: Physicians are directly and immediately accessible by phone.

Specialists' Requests of Primary Care Physicians:

- Referrals: Smoothness of the procedure, cooperative attitude.
- Clarity of Game Plan: Knowledge of what the PCP doctor does not want to deal with, communication of this knowledge to specialists' practices.
- Empathy: In some instances, an understanding of the acuity of the patients' situations and the accompanying impact on specialists' practices.
- Attitude of PCP physicians and staffs: Cooperative, understanding, courteous.

Insurance Companies

Insurance carriers have indicated that the following items are important in establishing a positive working relationship with them:

- Insurance knowledge: Understanding of how insurance works in general—including fee-for-service and managed care; willingness to become informed on specific plans.
- Familiarity with representatives: Availability to positively interact with insurance representatives (medical directors, provider relations staff, case management staff, etc.), regularity of the contact.
- Role in insurance company: Staff and physician willingness and activity (in advisory committees) to evaluate policies and procedures.
- Orientation toward difficulties: Willingness and ability to work toward solving problems.
- Shared commitment: Sharing of commitment to and understanding of the importance of patient satisfaction and service quality issues.
- Self knowledge: Practice's awareness of its standing in the network; practice's knowledge of its strengths and weaknesses.
- Improvement: Demonstration of efforts to improve in problem areas.
- Attitude of physicians and staff: Pleasant, courteous, cooperative, although not necessarily compliant.[20]

Hospitals

Hospital administrators and staff have indicated that the following are important to them as secondary customers of medical practices:

- Understanding: Awareness of issues that hospitals must manage, patience with slower processes, limitations placed on resources.
- Shared commitment: Shared mission regarding patient care; shared commitment to service.
- Attitude of physicians: Positiveness, cooperative (although not necessarily compliant), courteous.
- Attitude of staff: Friendly, courteous, cooperative, helpful.
- Scheduling: Adherence to promised schedule.
- Communication: Openness; ongoing nature; spoken, not just written; respectful.
- Cooperation: Willingness to work with, not against; adherence to admitting procedures.
- Empathy: Understanding of the frustrations of hospital staffs.
- Availability of medical personnel: Ease of access, on-call availability, office hours access.
- Information: Clarity of instructions, availability of information, timeliness of information, thoroughness.
- Insurance issues: Accurate, timely, and cooperative handling of practice's responsibilities in this process.

STAYING CLOSE TO YOUR CUSTOMERS

Getting close to your customer is only part of your job; the next part is staying there. Karl Albrecht reported an important lesson of service when he said, "The longer you are in a service business, the greater the odds you don't know your customers."[21] There are several reasons for this, as discussed in Chapter 3, and one of the most important is that customers change. The truth is that even your satisfied customers of today probably will not be satisfied tomorrow. This phenomenon has nothing to do with your practice; it occurs because customers are in a constant process of change. "When their expectations are understood at any given moment in time and the organization meets or even exceeds those expectations, customers don't say, 'Oh, thank you so much. That will be all.' Instead, they continue to develop new expectations because the old ones are now accepted as Standard Operating Procedures (SOP)."[22]

Also, customers themselves change. Age, life events, even something as simple as a mood on any given day can impact how easily they will be satisfied.[23] This situational nature of customer satisfaction is particularly important when thinking of patients. For example, studies indicate that there is a correlation between the health of the patient and his or her satisfaction with the care. Healthy people tend to register a higher level of satisfaction than ill ones. Thus, if asked on a day when they are not feeling well, your patients may record dissatisfaction in areas that would be less important or even nonexistent on days when they are well.[24] Also, patients who have received an unpopular recommendation from a physician, such as smoking cessation or weight reduction, may well be less satisfied than those who hear what they want to hear.[25] Given the transitory nature of perceptions of satisfaction (reactions to specific incidents or experiences with the practice), it is important to keep asking the questions and comparing the results. It also is important to measure service quality (long-term impressions of the service aspects of your practice over time). Karl Albrecht's lesson about service need not become a truism, and it won't be if your practice engages in the ongoing process of inquiry described in this chapter.

END NOTES

1. Haya Rubin, M.D., et al., "Patients' Ratings of Outpatient Visits in Different Practice Settings," *Journal of the American Medical Association* 20, no. 7 (August 18, 1993), p. 836.

2. Meryl D. Luallin, "Surveys Lead to Service Improvement," *Marketers Guideposts* 2, no. 1 (Summer 1991), pp. 1, 4–5.

3. John Burns, "Hospitals Use Patient Surveys to Meet Consumers' Needs, Get Edge in Negotiations," *Modern Healthcare* 23, no. 15 (April 12, 1993), pp. 56, 58.

4. Anne-Marie Nelson and Stephen W. Brown, "Do You Know What Your Patients Expect?" *Family Practice Management* 2, no. 5 (May 1994), p. 54.

5. James McAlexander, Dennis Kaldenberg, and Harold Koenig, "Service Quality Measurement," *Journal of Health Care Marketing* 14, no. 3 (Fall 1994), p. 35.

6. "Providers Refine Satisfaction Surveys as Weapons in Fight for Capitated Contracts," *Capitation Management Report* 1, no. 4 (September 1994), pp. 66–70.

7. Mary Walton, *The Deming Management Method*, (New York: The Putnam Publishing Group, 1986).

8. Joan Koob Cannie, "Turning Customers into Gold . . . the Art of Achieving Zero-Defections," (New York: AMACOM, American Management Association, 1994).

9. Luallin, 4.

10. Ibid.

11. Charles Gaughn, "TakeCare's Patient Satisfaction Survey Gauges Quality of Physician Care in HMO Setting," *Group Practice Journal* 42, no. 6 (November/December 1993), p. 30.

12. Morris Spierer, et al., "Assessment of Patient Satisfaction as a Part of a Physician Performance Appraisal," *Journal of Ambulatory Care Management* 17, no. 3 (July 1994), 3.

13. William H. Davidson and Bro Uttal, *Total Customer Service: The Ultimate Weapon*, (New York: First HarperPerennial, 1990) pp. 197–202.

14. Nelson and Brown, p. 56.

15. Many of these suggestions are based on the following article: Daniel Gottovi, M.D., "The Best Experts of All Help Run Our Practice," *Medical Economics* 68, no. 9 (May 6, 1991), pp. 56–57; 61–63.

16. Ibid., p. 62–63.

17. David J. Shukin and Jeffrey Otten, "The Walk-Through Patient-Focus Assessment: Preliminary Results in Augmenting Patient Satisfaction Data," *Consumer Satisfaction* 8, no. 2 (Summer 1993), p. 68.

18. Ibid., p. 70.

19. Nelson and Brown, p. 56.

20. Many ideas for this section were provided by Sue Phillips, Director of Provider Relations, Capital Community Health Plan, Washington D.C.

21. Karl Albrecht, *At America's Service* (Homewood, Illinois: Dow Jones–Irwin, 1988), p. 3.

22. Vicky Bradford, "The Voyage to Total Quality: Time to Course Correct," *Medical Interface* 8, no. 11 (December 1995), pp. 85–89

23. Ibid.

24. Judith Hall, Michael Milburn, and Arnold Epstein, "A Causal Model of Health Status and Satisfaction With Medical Care," *Medical Care* 31, no. 1 (January 1993), pp. 84–94.

25. Spierer, p. 6.

PART THREE

FOCUS ON THE PEOPLE

Service is a very human activity. It takes customers to receive it and practice personnel to provide it. Just as careful attention is paid to the former in a Total Service Medical Practice, equal time must also be devoted to the latter. The commitment, cooperation, and participation of all practice personnel to the process of creating and maintaining a Total Service Medical Practice is essential to the successful implementation of the steps described in this book.

The chapters in Part III focus on the people, the providers of the service. Beginning with a topic of importance to all practice personnel, Chapter 7 concentrates on methods of effective communication, the most essential ingredient for service success. Then, the next three chapters focus separately on the roles and responsibilities of the Physician (Chapter 8), the Office Manager/Administrator (Chapter 9), and the Staff (Chapter 10) in the Total Service Medical Practice. Returning to a broader perspective, Chapter 11 offers suggestions for creating an effective practice team.

7

CHAPTER

Step Seven—Master the Communication Process

I would be willing to bet that medical practice personnel are not unlike most other people when it comes to communication. Although we do it every day and quite likely could not survive without it, we spend very little time thinking about it. So, in this chapter we are going to do just that—think about communication. You see, all practice personnel, from the physicians to the managers to the staff, must be effective communicators if quality service is going to be provided. In fact, effective communication is the cornerstone of the Total Service Medical Practice.

COMMUNICATION IS COMPLEX

Imagine my surprise when the professor of my first doctoral class in the Department of Communication at the University of Colorado made what seemed to me to be a rather easy assignment: we were to write and explain a definition of communication. "Everyone knows what communication is!" I thought as I dashed off what I was soon to realize was a very simplistic response. My surprise was intensified when at the next class meeting I heard an amazingly wide variety of responses to the assignment. It seemed that even we graduate students in the field did not have a common understanding of the very subject we were in school to study. This experience underscored for me, very dramatically, the complexity of the communication process. It also helped me to shape the following definition of communication, which I still find useful today:

Communication occurs when behavior is perceived and meaning is attached to it.

A few key words contained in this definition are important to understanding what happens in the communication process.

■ Behavior—When most people consider communication behavior they think primarily of verbal messages, and certainly words are important tools for conveying meaning from one person to another. However, nonverbal tools also send powerful messages. In fact, when verbal and nonverbal messages are in conflict, such as the frowning receptionist saying "It's good to see you," the person receiving the conflicting messages almost always believes the nonverbal one.[1] So, any study of communication must include focus on both verbal and nonverbal tools.

■ Perceived—Each person has his or her own unique filters, such as attitudes, beliefs, values, experiences, emotions, and senses through which messages must flow. These filters influence perceptions, and thus the shaping and the interpreting of messages.

■ Meaning—As the above explanation implies, meaning is not an absolute fact. Remember the old communication adage that I cited in Chapter 1? "Meanings are not in words, they are in people." Because of each person's perceptual filters, the recipient of the message may interpret a very different meaning than was intended by the sender. For example, one doctor told of his surprise when he recommended that his patient go to the hospital for tests and observations, only to have the patient respond with an absolute and firm "No." What was occurring was a difference in the interpretation of the word *hospital*. To the doctor, it represented the most technically advanced, and thus, the best, location for providing what he believed the patient's condition required. The patient, on the other hand, interpreted the word *hospital* as a *place to go to die.* Unknown to the doctor, the patient had lost several family members during the previous two years—all of whom died while in the hospital. These differing interpretations of one simple word caused a major communication breakdown.[2]

■ Attached—This word implies a very important fact about communication that many people do not realize: communication can be unintentional. As long as one individual perceives a message, intended or not, and attaches meaning to it, communication has occurred. In other words, we can convey messages that we are not even aware we are sending. For example, even physical appearance can communicate a message to others. One patient reported during a focus group discussion: "I don't want to see people working in a doctor's office who are pierced all over. If they will do that to their own bodies, what will they do to my own!" (Later in this chapter, nonverbal communication is covered in much greater detail).

As the above discussion indicates, when closely examined, this simple definition captures the complexity of the communication process.

COMMUNICATION IS A SKILL

Even with its inherent complexity, there is no magic to being an effective communicator. It requires conscious effort and a willingness to learn new behaviors and refine old ones. Some people appear to be born communicators and seem to have a natural talent for conveying information, converting ideas into words, conveying interpersonal warmth, and so forth. While some people may be more extroverted and thus find the process of communication to be more comfortable for them, no one was born with the polished skills necessary to be effective. Whether it is through the carefully structured process of study or through learning by life experiences, these so-called born communicators have actually worked hard to turn their ease with people into a refined skill.

By the same token, those people who claim to be naturally shy can learn to be effective communicators too. I interviewed Neil Sullivan, M.D., my own primary care physician, for this book, mainly because he is such an effective communicator. When I asked him if he had any training in these skills, he smiled and said, "Yes. I'm naturally a shy person and I wanted to get better at this part of my job." He went on to explain that such training was unavailable to him until he was in his residency, and since that time he has actively sought out other opportunities, such as volunteering as a subject in a study of physician communication behaviors during patient interviews. I can report that his efforts have not been in vain and I applaud him for his proactive steps toward improvement. As Dr. Sullivan stated, "Even if it is not your favorite part of being a doctor, effective communication is becoming more and more a part of the job description."

Effective communication is at least an implied part of the job description for any individual working in a medical practice. As Dr. Sullivan exemplifies, everyone can learn to refine communication skills, and he reminds us that it can and should be done.

COMMUNICATION IS A PROCESS

As a process, communication is dynamic and difficult to analyze without employing the same freeze-frame approach I used in Chapter 3 when visualizing the model of the Total Service Medical Practice. So let's apply that method again here as a tool for understanding the way the communication process actually works. Figure 7–1 illustrates a freeze-frame image for us to study.

At any given moment in the process, there is a sender and a receiver of a message. The message can be sent through both verbal and nonverbal channels, and is received through the receiver's senses. Both the sender and the receiver bring their own perceptual filters to the communication situation. The message sent must travel through these filters, affecting both the clarity of the expressed message and the interpretation of its meaning. Communication noise, mentioned in Chapter 2, is defined as environmental, physiological, or emotional disturbances that can interfere with both the sending and receiving of the messages, usually resulting in distortion or even obliteration. The receiver responds to the sender's message through both verbal and nonverbal feedback.

Let's see how this model works by applying it to a typical daily interaction in a medical practice. In this freeze frame, the receptionist is the sender of the message and the patient is the receiver. The message being communicated concerns scheduling the patient's next appointment to see the doctor. Using words and nonverbal signs such as gestures and facial expressions, the

FIGURE 7–1

The Communication Process

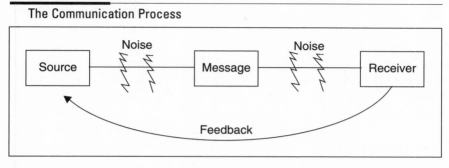

receptionist explains the time options available to the patient. The patient is watching and listening, but he is also experiencing some physical noise due to his fever, throat pain, and overall body aches. The receptionist's experience with patients in this condition, as well as this particular patient's pained and distracted facial expression, tells her that he may not be comprehending her instructions. To verify that the patient has in fact understood the message, the receptionist asks, "Were those options clear to you?" Now the patient responds, providing specific verbal feedback to the receptionist. At the moment when he begins to send a message, the roles in the communication situation have changed, making the patient the sender and the receptionist the receiver. As this everyday scenario demonstrates, the communication process is not as simple as it might seem. By understanding how it works, however, you will be able to analyze any communication situation, and by applying the model in Figure 7–1, you will gain greater understanding of what has occurred.

COMMUNICATION USES A VARIETY OF TOOLS

As communicators, we have many tools open to us for sending our messages. These tools fall under two general categories: nonverbal and verbal.

Nonverbal Tools

One entire area of the field of communication study focuses on the elements of nonverbal communication. When you consider that researchers have estimated that in face-to-face communication as much as 90 percent of the social meaning may be carried in the nonverbal messages, such specific emphasis is obviously warranted.[3] Thus, to be an effective communicator you must learn to manage your nonverbal messages. I say *manage*, because while verbal behavior is almost always under your voluntary control, nonverbal behaviors are not. A conscious focus is required if you are to be alert to what is being sent to others via your nonverbal channels.

Defined as messages without words, nonverbal communication takes the following forms:

Kinesics—body movements and facial expressions.

Proxemics—physical distance between the communicators.

Personal Style—clothing, treatment of time.

Physical Environment—fixed space such as office floor plan, parking, appearance of the building; semi-fixed space such as furniture placement and appearance, temperature, lighting, and color.

Paralanguage—pitch, rate, and volume of voice.

When these forms are applied to the messages conveyed in the medical practice, their importance becomes clear.

Kinesics
Facial Expressions Practice personnel need to examine how they express themselves kinetically, especially their facial expressions. A smile on your face and in your eyes can go a long way toward calming frightened or upset patients. Looks of genuine concern can increase trust and confidence. A friendly demeanor toward each other can also make any stressful day go more smoothly.

Eye Contact The old saying, "The eyes are the windows to the soul," is certainly true when it comes to nonverbal messages; they will give away your emotions almost every single time. Thus, be certain that you truly feel caring for your patients and for each other. Because your eyes will say whether you really do or not.

From a patient's point of view (pardon the pun), direct eye contact is important. For example, the patient wants the doctor to look him or her in the eye as much as possible, and wants even a busy receptionist to visually acknowledge his or her presence when entering the office. (A smile is appreciated at these moments as well.)

Body Movements All practice personnel, perhaps most especially doctors, need to understand the importance of one simple yet very important kinetic posture: sitting. All people like the feeling that practice personnel have time for them. Simply sitting, when possible, conveys that impression. In fact, Carol Mullinax, an associate executive director of the Ohio State Medical Association, pointed out that doctors who sit when talking with their patients are perceived to have spent more time than they actually have.[4]

Patients have reported very positive impressions of the service in the office when other personnel also sit when discussing their case with them. Again, that perception of *time available for me* was stressed when patients explained the impact of such simple behavior. One woman told me, "I don't know what kind of training they had at my new doctor's office, but it's great! On my first visit the nurse *sat down with me* and talked about the way things are done there. I've never had that happen before and I liked it."

Proxemics Edward T. Hall, in his landmark research on proxemics, identified four distinct physical distances that exist in face-to-face human interactions: *Intimate distance,* up to about 18 inches, is considered appropriate for private, intimate conversation with close friends, parents, and younger children; *personal,* 18 inches to 4 feet, is appropriate for casual conversation; *social,* 4 to 12 feet, is used for impersonal business such as a job interview; and *public,* more than 12 feet, is used for most public presentations. These four distances were determined by Hall after his intense scrutiny and observation of human behaviors in the Anglo-American culture.[5]

In a medical practice, a great deal of patient communication is conducted within intimate space. Because intimate space is protected by many people and is only open to those who are near and dear, entry into this space by practice personnel may create anxiety in the patient. By the very nature of the physical examinations necessary in providing medical care, this space is entered frequently by medical personnel. Kindness, gentleness, and interpersonal warmth can make this experience less stressful for the patient.

Colleagues who are cramped into small office space may also find themselves invading each other's intimate and personal space out of necessity. You need to be aware of these distances and respect them as much as possible. The forced close proximity that comes with limited space can create tensions and anxieties for workers.

Individuals vary and problems can occur when communicators have, for one reason or another, developed even slightly different standards of acceptance for entry into their intimate space. For example, some people come from very demonstrative families, where hugs and affection are given with ease. These folks are less intimidated or uncomfortable when their intimate space is entered than are those from less demonstrative backgrounds. Sadly, when people come from violent situations, entry into their intimate space often results in pain and fear, making them reluctant to having that space violated even for medical reasons. Differences in cultural norms can also impact an individual's comfort with entry into his or her intimate space. For example, in some Far Eastern cultures, normal casual conversation is often conducted close enough for the communicators to bathe in each other's breath. Knowing your customers, whether internal or external, as people will help you know how comfortable they are with entry into their intimate space and will help you know how to handle those situations when that entry is necessary.

Personal Style

Clothing Patients report that one way they determine the professionalism of the medical practice personnel is through the clothing that is worn. They like to see uniforms of some type, even if it's only a smock cover-up. One patient told me, "I don't think that doctor knew what he was doing." When pushed to provide the basis for this conclusion, she responded "Well, he didn't look like a doctor! He didn't even have on a uniform." The *uniform* she sought was nothing more than a white lab coat, but its absence mattered to this patient. I have also had office managers express their concern about what certain staff members were wearing to work. Skirts that were too short or other clothes that were too casual were conveying usually unintentional negative messages to patients about these staff members.

Time   Time is a powerful nonverbal tool and one of the most difficult to manage in a medical practice. Regardless of whether you are dealing with an internal customer or an external one, people in the Anglo-American culture tend to attach meaning to time. Most want prompt attention to their needs, whatever they might be, and find that anything less is a negative. Given the power of this nonverbal message, medical practices must work doubly hard to manage the timing problems they inevitably face.

Being on schedule is a constant source of stress for all medical practice personnel. Because patients can become unpleasant and angry if they are kept waiting too long, it often becomes a source of major practice concern. (In Chapter 12 I offer some specific suggestions for improving the timing problems in the medical practice.)

Paralanguage
Referring to how something is said rather than to the actual content, paralanguage is a most powerful tool. Listening to the sound of your voice—its pitch, pace, and volume—is a useful exercise, especially to those who do a lot of telephone work. Also, people who ask routine questions, such as doctors or scheduling clerks, need to be aware that asking repetitive questions can result in a monotone pitch, and this is often interpreted as boredom. All practice personnel should make their voices sound interesting and interested.

Fixed and Semifixed Space
Although we know from patient satisfaction research that it is not the most important item on most patients' lists, the physical environment of the medical practice does matter to them. The floor plan of some offices, for example, has been criticized soundly by some patients. One woman commented about the large clinic that had a payment window set up outside of the waiting room and had notices that patients should make their co-payment before they even entered the office. "They are just interested in money! That's what that says!" she stated angrily. Another patient had the reverse experience, stating, "When I left the examination room and

started out, I couldn't find the checkout counter. I knew I owed a co-payment, but I couldn't find out where to pay it! It was almost like they were embarrassed or afraid to ask!"

Customers also report that the inconvenience of parking is a negative for them. Patients in particular often state that searching for a parking space worsens their already negative moods. In addition, the practice's location communicates to the customers as well. One asthma specialist's practice has set up seven sites around the Denver area, for example, to meet their patients' need for convenience. According to the patient satisfaction surveys conducted by this practice, patients report appreciating these location choices, and they cited this as an example of how much the practice cares about them. Even the appearance of the building in which your practice is housed can communicate a message to people. For example, a large medical building can be intimidating to some patients, while others find it reassuringly professional.

Since often the fixed space may be beyond your control, paying attention to the semifixed space becomes doubly important. Arrangement of furniture, for example, communicates messages to people and is well within your power to manipulate. One patient reported finding the new clinic where her doctor had moved to be "cold and impersonal." When asked why, she said,"There's all these rows of chairs all lined up like in Canon City [the state prison in Colorado]." While serviceable straight-backed chairs are probably the most useful and perhaps cost-effective furnishings, they are now available with padding and colorful upholstery. See what you can do to personalize the waiting areas. Little things such as lamps, flowers, plants, pictures, play corners, etc., will communicate a more inviting message to your customers. Also, groupings of furniture convey a more relaxed environment than rigid rows of chairs.

While you are checking your decor, take a look at your examination rooms. Patients report spending a lot of time in those rooms and they find them to be too cold and too sterile for comfort. In a patient focus group, one participant suggested piping soft music into the examination rooms. He thought it might have a calming effect on him while he waited. Another wanted to know if there could be some pictures other than drawings of the human body with the skin "scraped away." One patient described the comfortable dressing area in her gynecologist's examination room, complete with a small, soft settee; a lamp; and a table with magazines on it for her enjoyment. She reported that this provided a very pleasant environment in which to wait and she didn't mind doing so under these circumstances. She said, "If they went to this trouble to provide a nice space, then they must care that I am waiting and want to make it as pleasant as possible." Patients also report that the temperature in examination rooms is too cold, especially when they have to spend a long time waiting in those "funny little gowns."

Even the colors of the rooms in your practice will communicate messages. Communication professors Rudolph and Kathleen Verdeber explained, "People react predictably to various colors: red as exciting and stimulating; blue as comfortable, soothing, calming, peaceful; yellow as cheerful, jovial." They also indicated that much of our reaction to color comes from expectation. When a color does not meet expectations, reactions are unpredictable. "Mashed potatoes tinted green in honor of Saint Patrick's Day may nauseate diners who are not color blind, even before they attempt to eat."[6]

As I suggested in Chapter 6, take a few moments to really see your office as your patients do. I remember my own gratitude to some thoughtful hospital worker who had placed a smiling happy face on the ceiling in the waiting area outside the X-ray lab and to the gynecologist who had decorated his ceiling with an interesting paisley pattern! Both incidents showed me that someone had cared enough to see the space as the patient sees it and had acted accordingly.

Nonverbal messages, then, cover a wide range. We need to be aware of what we look like when we communicate, as well as what we sound like. We need to be tuned in to the fixed and semifixed space that surrounds us. The personal style we each have will convey messages that we may not even realize we are sending.

The secret to effective nonverbal communication begins with awareness. Because nonverbal tools become so automatic for us and are such integral parts of who we are as well as of the environments in which we communicate, we can and do become oblivious to them. By being aware, we can discover the areas we would like to change, and reinforce those we would like to retain.

Verbal Tools

Verbal tools consist of the words that you use to convey messages, which are organized into specific identifiable structures. The two most important structures found in verbal messages in the medical practice are explanations and questions.

Explanations

Offered when providing initial information or responding to inquiries, this structure is very important to effective communication in the practice. Regardless of to whom the explanation is directed, there are some important tips for providing clear explanations.

Tip 1: Make the technical content of the explanation appropriate for the receiver. Two types of terms can make explanations problematic: technical/medical terms and professional jargon. Patients are the most obvious nonmedical receivers of messages in a medical practice. As such, both types of terms probably contain little if any meaning for them. Even those patients who think they know a lot about their condition will need some guidance if they are to completely understand either type of language. So, when speaking to people outside the field, such as patients, speak plainly and simply. I don't mean talk down to your patients, but rather speak in terms they can understand. When you need to rely on medical terminology, provide adequate definitions. Double check to be certain that your message has been understood. Jargon, defined as a slang or short-cut language, is hardly ever appropriate for messages to the patient. On the occasions when it might be, take care to define its meaning for the patients so that they will understand.

Although it may be surprising, many practice personnel also report that they too have difficulty with highly technical messages. People working in nonclinical areas report needing help in learning the important medical terminology required to perform their jobs. Even clinical personnel indicate that many medical terms are used differently from practice to practice and that they too need definitions to establish the meaning in a given office setting. Also, managers and administrators should keep in mind that most doctors and nurses are not familiar with business terminology, and such words undefined will carry little or no meaning for them.

Tip 2: Check with the receiver to determine that your intended message is being received. Even when using words with which you expect your receiver to be familiar, you cannot always be certain that is the case. Therefore, it is helpful to stop periodically in any message to double check. Simply seeking feedback by saying, "Have I been clear so far?" opens up the opportunity to correct misinter-pretations as you go. Waiting until the end of the explanation to ask, "Do you have any questions?" may well be too late. When receivers of a communication message encounter terms and phrases that they do not understand, they tend to stop listening. Providing the opportunity for their expressions of confusion as you go will save time in the long run and make certain that your intended message is getting through.

Tip 3: Don't be afraid of softer words that show emotion. Words such as "I'm sorry," "I understand," or "I care" are just as important as the technical language needed to explain. Explanations that are dotted with such softer words are very effective. When receivers believe their emotional state is being understood or that someone really cares about them, then they are more receptive to the technical explanations so often needed in a medical practice.

Tip 4: Answer questions effectively. Not only do personnel in the medical practice volunteer information, but they find themselves answering questions as well. These responses constitute a form of explanation that can be enhanced by using the following format:

- Be certain you understand the question.
- Clarify if you do not.
- If the question has been long and rambling, paraphrase it to focus your answer.
- Offer a one-line, direct response such as "Yes, you should expect some side effects."
- Elaborate on the one-line response such as: "They will be . . ."
- Ask if you have answered the question.

By practicing this format at every opportunity, you will soon become quite comfortable with it. You will also offer well-organized explanations that will not only fulfill the receiver's needs for information, but also will require less time.

Questions

The process of inquiry is important in a medical practice. From the general routine questions to those that are person-specific, questions elicit vital information. Patients report that they wish doctors would ask more questions. Many doctors fear that in so doing they will lose control of the interview. More than merely a *control* issue, their fear is connected to the expectation that if asked questions, patients will ramble on when answering. Though understandable, that fear is usually unfounded. Studies show that patients who are allowed to describe their problem or complaint without interruption take an average of just two minutes to answer; often they take even less.[7]

In addition, all practice personnel with similar fears should remember that well-placed questions can be your friends! They can move patients along in their stories, thus reducing rather than expanding the time taken. Questions such as "What happened next?" or "And that's when you started feeling this pain?" will refocus them on the physical complaint if they wander too far afield.

Patients indicate that practice personnel tend to ask rote, repetitive questions. One very simple suggestion will help soften this impression: explain why you are asking the question. Patients report that merely being told "I need to ask a few questions so that the doctor will have an idea of where to start," or "I need to ask a few questions so I can locate your file in the computer," softens and personalizes this process.

All questions should be asked with interest. This can be a challenge if it's the tenth or fiftieth time you've asked that question in a given day . . . or hour. It also is hard to remember to do this when you are asking for simple demographic information such as, "What is your street address?" However, try! Remind yourself that although you've asked the question many times before, it is probably the first time that day that it has been asked of this respondent. Also, for the patient who has undergone hours of inquiry, your interested attitude will be appreciated. In addition, remember that even the most basic information is important.

Perhaps making a game of it can make even the most repetitive task interesting! I'm reminded of the ticket taker at a theater in Denver whose job it was to stand in one place and receive the tickets from the patrons as we entered. This particular young man surprised me by taking my ticket with a smile and a look of sincere interest on his face. "I was wrong!" he said with a laugh. "About what?" I asked. "Oh. I thought you'd be going to see *Nixon*!" He explained that he enlivened this very routine task by trying to guess what movie his customers were going to see. With just a little imagination, you too can find a reason to be interested in the answers to the routine questions you have to ask.

What kinds of questions should you be asking? It all depends; you have many choices. Let's apply the various types to a doctor / patient interview situation.

Closed Questions   A closed question is one that takes only a "yes" or "no" answer or limits the respondent to a set answer. These help obtain a specific response to a specific query and are especially useful to double-check symptoms: "So, these headaches started last Saturday?"

Open Questions   Open questions allow the respondent more latitude in answering and encourage explanation. They are especially useful at the beginning of the patient interview: "What can I do for you today?"

Direct Questions   Direct questions guide the respondent toward a specific topic, as do closed questions, yet they allow a greater breadth of response than yes or no: "How much time do you spend exercising?"

Indirect Questions   Indirect questions set a general topic area, making them more structured than an open question, yet still allow a great deal of room for the respondent to answer: "Tell me about your fitness regimen."

Empathetic or "Putting the Shoe on the Other Foot" Questions   Empathetic questions express understanding and can be especially helpful when trying to defuse a hostile situation or get patients to discuss a difficult topic: "Do you find getting exercise every day as difficult as I do?"

"Why" Questions Why questions seek rationale for a certain act, behavior, or method. Although troublesome for most people to answer because they can put the respondent on guard, they can be very effective in getting to the root of problems. When asking these questions, soften their impact in some way: "I wonder if you could help me understand why this keeps happening to you?"

Awareness is the key to improving both the verbal and nonverbal communication; your practice needs to take stock of both types of messages that are being sent to its customers. Then, action should be taken to correct any problem areas.

THREE KEY COMMUNICATION SKILLS

Now that you have an understanding of the communication process and the tools available to you for sending and receiving messages, I would like to spend the remainder of this chapter talking about three specific communication skills: empathy, listening, and managing conflict. These skills, when mastered, will lift you above others in your ability to communicate. When left unattended, they can quickly become major sources of communication problems.

Empathy

The word *empathy* conjures up different images for different people. There are those who see it as some magical process by which one person is transported into the emotional web of another and is thus able to feel *exactly* what the other is feeling. There are others who subscribe to a definition similar to that offered by Jack Platt, M.D.: "[Empathy is] a cognitive skill . . . [an] intellectual process that requires understanding of feelings. It uses our sensory observations, what we see and hear, but then processes those observations mentally to come to a true understanding of . . . feelings."[8]

Actually, empathy is a term coined around 1910 by E. B. Titchener to apply to aesthetics, and then adapted by psychologist Theodore Lipps to refer to the common feeling between patient and therapist.[9] From a layperson's point of view, it is perhaps best defined by the little plaque that hung in my high school principal's office more years ago than I care to admit. "Never criticize a man unless you've walked a mile in his moccasins." Empathy is the ability to walk a mile in someone else's shoes. In a more clinical sense, empathy becomes a bit more involved. Grattan and Eslinger distinguish between affectively based empathy and cognitively based empathy. The former is defined as "an ability to construct for oneself another's emotional experience; a sort of vicarious arousal." The latter is explained as "an ability to take another's viewpoint, infer his feeling, and put yourself in his shoes."[10] Although for some people it seems to come more easily than for others, I believe empathizing can be learned, and thus the latter definition works best for me, and it is the one I'll be referring to throughout this book.

Sometimes people confuse sympathy with empathy. The confusion is understandable because the two reactions look very much the same at the beginning: They both involve the observation of the sensory data sent by someone else and even go as far as identifying or labeling the feelings being experienced by the other. However, that is where the similarity stops. While empathy evolves into the internalization of the named emotion and the search for and ultimate location of similar feelings in yourself, sympathy takes a detour. Sympathy results in feeling sorry for the other person. "I sympathize" implies "I am so sorry for you." "I empathize" means "I understand." Although most people probably appreciate your efforts, few of them really want your pity. What means the most to someone experiencing an emotion is "I understand," and that comes from empathy.

In fact, in a recent experience of my own, I heard *understanding* beautifully turned into a statement of action that left me feeling reassured and at peace. I was having difficulties regarding a claim that had been filed with my insurance carrier. The woman I spoke with at the managed care company was wonderful. As I told her about my concerns, I also said, "You understand how I feel about this, don't you?" Her response was perfect: "I certainly do. I would be frustrated and angry too and I wouldn't want this to happen to my claim! I promise you I'll treat this situation as if it were my own." That is the best articulation of the desired result of empathy that I have ever heard.

The following steps for achieving empathy are adapted from those offered by Frederic Platt, M.D., in his book *Conversation Repair*:

1. *Determine the emotional content of the message.* Pause a moment and consider what emotion you are observing the other person display. A simple rule to go by is that most people experience some variation of the following four basic emotions: Mad, sad, glad, or scared. If you can identify the emotional state as one of the above or a version thereof, you will have accomplished the first step toward empathy. A note of caution: What appears to be anger is often a mask for some other more personal emotion, usually fear or sadness. Especially when dealing with patients, you will need to look behind the anger to determine what it is most likely masking.

2. *Remember how such emotions feel.* Reflect on your own life experiences. Has anything similar happened to you? Have you felt that emotion yourself on some occasion? It is helpful if you can recall a specific situation from your past, because the details will intensify your recollections and help you access how such emotions feel. A favorite saying of mine explains what can occur in this moment: "Same context, different content." You need not experience exactly the same situation or event to be able to understand the context of what the other person is facing.

3. *Pause if necessary to access these emotions.* Don't be afraid of the pause. That silence can be as powerful as any words you might say. If you need to, say, "I need just a moment here. I want to try to really understand what you are feeling." That honesty will show your desire to empathize and it will be honored and appreciated by the person with whom you are communicating.

4. *Ask if you can't identify the emotion.* Dr. Platt put it this way: "When in doubt, be curious. It is perfectly correct to ask, 'DR: I can tell that you feel strongly about this. PT: Yes. DR: But I am not sure I understand exactly HOW you feel. Could you tell me?'" Dr. Platt also encourages people to ask about the reasons behind an emotion if they are not clear.

5. *Acknowledge the emotional impact.* Don't tell the person that you understand by saying, "I know how you feel." With all due respect, you probably don't know exactly how anyone else feels, because each person is unique. The preferable expression is "You must be feeling _____ about this," or "You seem to feel _____ about this." By labeling the emotion, you place your empathy in a descriptive, not an experiential mode, which is more acceptable to the other person. It also helps the other person to identify the emotion for himself or herself. He or she may well disagree with you by saying, "Well, it isn't so much sad as it is depressed." Or the person can agree with your description, and you are able to move to the next step.

6. *Allow the person to be in the emotion.* You don't even have to say another word for a while. Just sit there and allow the emotion to run its course, within reason. People cannot be rushed out of their emotional states, nor would you want them to be. A short-circuited emotional reaction will eventually surface at some other time. People also appreciate having someone who understands with whom to share these moments.

At this point you are ready to move the conversation on. Asking a more factual question, for example, will help refocus the other person on the topic at hand.

Some practice personnel are reluctant to show empathy, fearing it will violate some artificial standard of professional demeanor, or because they have trouble accessing their own emotions and find it embarrassing to try to access those of others. To these people, I would like to say, please confront your fears and your discomfort. Showing empathy is one of the most precious gifts you can give to others. Your expression of it will only heighten their impressions of you. In showing empathy, you are honoring their emotional processes rather than hiding from them, hoping they will do likewise. Also, a side benefit of showing empathy to others is that it makes you more open to your own feelings, and there is nothing more human than that.

The subject of empathy appears often in this book. Customers, internal and external, ask for it and need it. An additional side benefit of empathy is that when you show your willingness to empathize with someone else, that person is much more willing to empathize with you. Just imagine how effective your customer interactions would be if both you and the customer were able to walk a mile in each other's moccasins!

Listening

Some people are surprised to find this topic included in a discussion of communication. However, just as often as you are a sender of messages, you will find yourself the receiver of them. In fact, most patients report that they wish all practice personnel could do a better job of really listening to them. Research shows that they are probably right. Studies indicate that on average, after asking a question, doctors interrupt their patients only eighteen seconds into the answer.[11] Other practice personnel, who find themselves hearing the same story over and over from the same or different patients, report that they, too, tend to cut off the sender before he or she has actually finished. The following tips for active listening will help you become an effective listener.

Tip 1: Get ready to listen. This means both mentally and physically you should make the shift from the speaker to the receiver in the communication process. Stop thinking about the many other pressing issues that are on you mind. Don't start forming your answer before the question is complete. For the period of time it takes to ask the question, even if it's only for a brief instant, give your undivided attention to this sender. An Arizona computer operator described the feelings he had when his doctor demonstrated these behaviors: "He gives you the feeling that you're his only patient."[12]

Tip 2: Have a sincere desire to listen. Sincerity cannot be faked, because your eyes will give you away. So, it is essential that you focus on *this* sender. Then you can sincerely care about this person and sincerely want to hear what he or she has to say.

Tip 3: Show an interest in what is being said. Don't just sit by passively. Look and act interested. Nod your head once in a while. Smile or frown where appropriate. Even a few "um hums" now and then would be nice. In short, demonstrate to the sender that you are listening.

Tip 4: Pay attention to both verbal and nonverbal messages. Most people think of listening as only a verbal exercise, and in the literal sense it is. However, to be an effective receiver of any communication messages, you need to be certain that all available channels for receiving the message are being used. Listen for the verbal content; it *usually* will tell you the *facts* that you need to know. Watch for nonverbal cues, especially the paralanguage and facial expressions; they will usually tell you the *emotional* message.

Tip 5: Control your emotional hot buttons. You are a human being, not a cold, emotionless machine. As such, you too have feelings and your emotional hot buttons can get pushed, especially when dealing with an angry customer. Thus, be aware when that happens. You will feel yourself wanting to interrupt in order to defend yourself. Your nonverbal behaviors will give you away also, unless they are monitored. The reason you need to control your emotional responses is that when these feelings are running through your mind and especially your body, you can't think about what is actually being communicated. These emotions function as the *communication noise* we have discussed before.

Tip 6: Avoid mental detours. While listening, our minds will want to wander from the topic under discussion, especially if the communication flow has been one-way for even a brief period of time. The reason for this is that the human mind can process information much faster than speakers can speak it. In fact, although we are capable of understanding speech at rates up to six hundred words per minute, the average person speaks between one hundred to four hundred words per minute.[13] Thus, you have plenty of time to take mental detours such as day dreaming and debating the speaker. Again, these prevent you from listening effectively.

Tip 7: Concentrate. Active listening is hard work! At the end of a day of listening, I know that the participants in my workshops are going to be tired. If they really want to receive the message I am sending, they will be exerting a great deal of effort, and most of that effort will come in the form of concentration. Many thoughts will compete for my message in the minds of even the most motivated listeners. It takes conscious, concentrated effort to focus attention and to attend to what is being communicated. One workshop participant said jokingly, "I think I'll just call Dr. Braden and tell him I can't come back this afternoon! I'm just too worn out from listening!" Although everyone laughed, including me, she probably was feeling the result of concentrating on my message for an entire morning.

Tip 8: Avoid negative, personal judgements. Sometimes what you hear in a medical practice can be shocking or even disgusting. These reactions can lead to a judging process that can block your reception of the message. If you are evaluating the personhood or value of the individual, you may well miss a critical piece of information. You do not have to like or even respect every individual with whom you must communicate, but the use of judgmental labels can and does interfere with your effectiveness as a listener. It can prevent you from following all of the above tips, and thus can short-circuit the communication process.

CONFLICT MANAGEMENT

In the complexity and unpredictability of human interactions, there is one constant: Every human relationship experiences conflict. Any relationship that is perceived as conflict free only appears that way because the conflict is unexpressed. The successful management of conflict on an office team is essential to its successful functioning. If these issues are allowed to remain unexpressed they will build up until there is an explosion. Sometimes called *gunnysacking*, this process of collecting and then dumping unexpressed conflict issues is a very unproductive way of handling such situations and usually does not result in an effective resolution.

If conflict is a normal part of every relationship, why then do we feel so uncomfortable when it arises? There are several reasons. First, we react as we do toward conflict because we don't understand it, and as human beings we tend to fear things we don't understand. The first way to combat your negative reaction to conflict is to learn about it. Later in this section I will discuss the five different options you have for engaging in conflict and you'll find a specific process for handling conflict in a productive, proactive manner included in the appendix.

A second reason we tend to fear conflict is because we have been hurt in conflict situations in the past. Usually, these hurt feelings are the result of engaging in a conflict with someone who was out to win no matter what. The win-at-any-cost mentality causes attacks on not just the ideas but also on the person of the other. In order to get beyond this kind of past hurt, take charge of your own behaviors. Remembering that not all conflict has to be handled in that fashion is reassuring.

Thirdly, we tend to be uncomfortable with conflict because it is hard work. It is difficult to sit down with another person and confront a difficult issue that has been bothering you. This kind of conversation is usually made more difficult because the individuals involved have not established a method by which they intend to handle conflict when it arises. Because we don't want to acknowledge conflict, we tend not to prepare for it in advance. Thus, when conflicts occur, and they always do, we don't know how to handle them effectively. This leads to blundering, stumbling, and fumbling your way through. If your office team has an agreement that acknowledges the normal, natural existence of conflict and also describes how you will handle it when it does arise, you can help remove some of the unnecessary stress. It still isn't easy, but the rewards will be great.

You have five different options from which to choose when it comes to engaging in conflict. If you are using an unproductive style, and know that other options do exist, then you can choose to change your style. The Thomas-Kilmann Conflict Mode Instrument[14] is based on the notion that most people tend to have a favored approach to conflict. This instrument helps you to determine what your preferred style might be, and offers you the range of choices open to you when facing conflict situations. The five styles are:

> *Competing:* An individual pursues his or her own concerns at the expense of the other person's concerns. This is a power-oriented mode, in which one uses whatever power seems appropriate to win one's own position—one's ability to argue, one's rank, economic sanctions. Competing might mean standing up for your rights, defending a position which you believe is correct, or simply trying to win. Such conflicts end with one party giving in to the other, with a third-party arbitrator rendering a decision, or with a stalemate in which no decision is reached. On occasion, both parties decide to "give a little," and a compromise results.

Accommodating: The opposite of competing, an individual accommodates by neglecting his or her own concerns to satisfy the concerns of the other person. There is an element of self-sacrifice in this mode. Accommodating might take the form of selfless generosity or charity, obeying another person's order when one would prefer not to, or yielding to another's point of view. When one party accommodates, the conflict usually ends rather quickly because the other party is achieving his or her goals.

Avoiding: Individuals who are avoiding do not immediately pursue their own concerns or those of the other person. They do not address the conflict. Avoiding might take the form of diplomatically sidestepping an issue, postponing an issue until a better time, or simply withdrawing from a threatening situation. When one party avoids, the conflict is not fully addressed.

Collaborating: The opposite of avoiding, collaborating involves an attempt to work with the other person to find some solution which fully satisfies the concerns of both persons. It means digging into an issue to identify the underlying concerns of the two individuals and to find an alternative which meets both sets of concerns. Collaborating between two persons might take the form of exploring a disagreement to learn from each other's insights, concluding to resolve some condition which would otherwise have them competing for resources, or confronting and trying to find a creative solution to an interpersonal problem. Clearly, collaboration involves both parties and will require a great deal of time. It involves discovering a solution in which both parties are completely satisfied.

Compromising: The objective of compromise is to find some expedient, mutually acceptable solution which partially satisfies both parties. It falls on a middle ground between competing and accommodating. Compromising gives up more than competing, but less than accommodating. Likewise, it addresses an issue more directly than avoiding, but doesn't explore it in as much depth as collaborating. Compromising might mean splitting the difference, exchanging concessions, or seeking a quick middle-ground position.

It is interesting to think about the range of conflict modes available to you. No one has to use any one style in all conflict situations, and it is completely permissible to use any of the styles above at any appropriate time. Care should be taken with the Competitive mode, however, that you do not resort to the win-at-any-cost approach; that will destroy any relationship more quickly than you can imagine.

Before you and another person address a conflict, it is helpful to have a predetermined, agreed-on methodology. The same process can be used with people who are not familiar with it, but you should be aware that they will not know the rules. Thus, they may not respond in the same way as your colleagues who do share your knowledge of this process. When your entire practice knows the Steps for Productive Conflict Management and uses them, fearing conflict can become a thing of the past. (See Appendix for the Steps for Productive Conflict Management.)

Medical practice personnel are in far more than a clinical/technical business. You are in the most highly developed people-centered profession in the world. You must see and hear the whole person in order to do your jobs effectively. As such, you must understand and appreciate the complex process of communication. You also must have a sincere desire to improve and hone that skill. Then you will be able to treat each other, your patients, and all those with whom you come into contact in the most positive and effective way. Dare I say, the way you would like to be treated yourself.

END NOTES

1. Rudolph Verdeber and Kathleen Verdeber, *Interact: Using Interpersonal Communication Skills*, 3d ed. (Belmont, Calif.: Wadsworth Publishing, 1983), p. 88.

2. This example is based on the case discussed by Frederic W. Platt, M.D., *Conversation Repair* (Boston: Little, Brown and Company, 1995), pp. 4–9.

3. Albert Mehrabian, *Silent Messages*, 2d ed., (Belmont, Calif.: Wadsworth Publishing, 1981), p. 76.

4. Carol Mullinax, "Can the Luster Be Restored?" *The Internist* 35, no. 1 (January 1994), p. 12.

5. Edward T. Hall, *The Silent Language* (Garden City, New York: Doubleday, 1959), pp. 164–165.

6. Verdeber and Verdeber, pp. 94–95.

7. Anne-Marie Nelson and Stephen W. Brown, "Do You Know What Your Patients Expect?" *Family Practice Management* 2, no. 5 (May 1994), p. 50.

8. Platt, pp. 30–31.

9. Leslie Brothers, "A Biological Perspective on Empathy," *American Journal of Psychiatry* 146, no. 1 (January 1989), pp. 10–19.

10. L. M. Grattan and P. J. Eslinger, "Empiric Study of Empathy," *American Journal of Psychiatry* 146, no. 11 (November 1989), pp. 1521–2.

11. Ken Terry, "Telling Patients More Will Save Your Time," *Medical Economics* 71, no. 14 (July 25, 1994), p. 52.

12. Howard Eisenberg, "You're Doing Something Right," *Medical Economics* 67, no. 8 (April 23, 1990), p. 50.

13. Ron Adler and Neil Towne, *Looking Out/Looking In*, 3d ed. (New York: Holt, Rinehart, and Winston, 1988), p. 218.

14. Kenneth W. Thomas and Ralph H. Kilmann, *Thomas-Kilmann Conflict Mode Instrument* (Tuxedo, New York: Xicom, 1974).

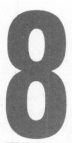

CHAPTER

Step Eight—Embrace the Physician's Role

I am not a medical doctor. I have never actually looked into the eyes of another human being, realizing that a life was now resting in my hands. I cannot express strongly enough the deep respect I have for those of you who have made this professional choice. As I have interviewed physicians in a variety of research contexts over the years I have found the reasons for this choice to be fascinating. They range all the way from "I was intrigued with the intricacies of the human body" to "I watched Ben Casey and Dr. Kildare on TV and I wanted to be like them!" to "I wanted to have a secure and comfortable lifestyle." But one constant theme emerges in some form in our conversations: "I wanted to help people. I wanted to give something back to life." As I have watched physicians rushing through their hectic daily routines, as I sat in the early morning dawn interviewing a doctor for this book, as I observed the gentleness with which my own physician patted my arm in comfort when I was injured; I have become convinced that it is the latter reason that keeps you answering the bell. No other motivation could compel you to endure the stresses and strains, the early morning hours and the late night calls, the frustration and pain you feel when a patient goes bad. It takes that kind of inner commitment to something bigger than science or heroes or dollars and cents. It takes a person with a desire to serve others. So, in this chapter, I feel as though at some level I am preaching to the choir.

Prior to my opening comments at a workshop that served as a forerunner for this chapter, one elderly doctor thumbed through the handouts and motioned me over to his table. He said with a smile but wanting to make a point: "What makes you think we aren't already doing these things?" I paused and pondered my response. Why *was* I going to talk about these things with this audience? What *had* motivated me to put this program and later this chapter together? And then I had my answer.

First, this doctor's implication is correct: As I talk with office managers and staff around the country, I am aware of how many doctors are already implementing the suggestions in this chapter. Yet, I am also aware of how easily these ideas can become pushed to the background as the pressures of daily life in a medical practice close in. So, part of the motivation is to provide reminders—to help you become refocused on these things you may already know but have perhaps forgotten to apply. I also am aware that some doctors appear to pay little attention to the nonclinical side of their practices, focusing all of their energy on the clinical processes and outcomes. However, I am convinced that most of these doctors are not aware of the negative impact that such exclusive focus can have, and thus, another motivation for this chapter is to try to fill in that gap in awareness. I always begin my workshop, *Effective Communication Skills for Physicians*, with the question: "What expectations do you have for our time together?" Invariably the most universally agreed-on goal is for me to tell them what other people are saying. One doctor reflected the physicians' feedback void I referred to in Chapter 6, when she said, "I'm hoping you will tell us what other people are saying about us. You're out there talking to them and they won't usually talk to us." By relying on original research and on research by others, I will report what the office managers, staff, and, when appropriate, patients say they want and need from the physicians.

As you read this chapter you may become somewhat overwhelmed by the lists of suggestions I have to offer. Let me explain a few things about this approach that may help you avoid that reaction. First, I chose the use of lists because they are quickly

FIGURE 8–1
Traditional Organizational Chart

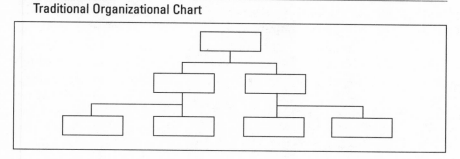

read and referenced, and I am aware of the demands on your time. Second, if you examine the lists closely, you will notice that most of the suggestions are focused on *ways of being*, not more *things for you to do*. Also, in several instances, I am suggesting actions that will actually remove burdens from your shoulders and place them on others. So, with that in mind, let's begin our discussion of your role, the role of the physician in the Total Service Medical Practice.

THE HEART OF THE PRACTICE

You are probably familiar with the traditional organizational charts, those collections of rectangles that place the CEO or the president in the top box with the remaining executives, managers and frontline employees marching downward in a rigid, inflexible order. (Figure 8–1.) Based on the military and its need for a specific, unwavering chain of command, this model has been used by a wide variety of organizations since the post-World War II period to reflect the internal structure and flow of official decision-making and responsibility.

Total Service Medical Practices do not and should not function like the military, however. Thus, a different model must be used, one that does not isolate the physician at the top, but rather places you where you belong, at the heart of your organization (Figure 8–2.) This model provides such a visualization, symbolizing the physician's influence and impact on all segments of the practice. This representation is intended to reflect the fact that physicians are not and cannot be isolated. Just as the human heart pumps the lifeblood to all vital organs and

FIGURE 8-2

The Organizational Chart of Total Service Medical Practice

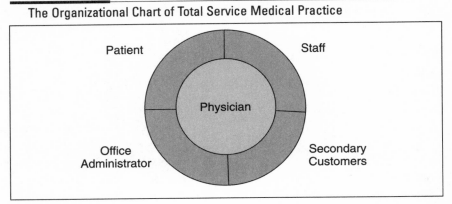

extremities of the body, so do the physicians provide the vital substance that maintains the life of your practice. As one office manager explained when asked what drove her particular practice to achieve its high patient-satisfaction ratings: "It all starts with our doctors."

In Lesson 1, I stated that service has to begin with the practice leaders. In the eyes of all concerned, physicians epitomize that role, and a unique role it is. In most other organizations, the further up the traditional organizational chart a person moves, the less contact he or she has with the frontline employees and external customers. This is not the case in the medical practice. You, as a physician, are in daily, even hourly contact with all types of customers who look at you not only as the organizational boss but also as the provider of the technical expertise on which the entire organization depends. That is a very special role and one that few if any CEOs in any other field can claim to have. Your organizational and medical images merge together to place very important and unique demands on you.

THE THREE Cs OF PHYSICIAN SERVICE RESPONSIBILITY

Of course, as a physician, you provide the technical care that drives the daily functions of the practice. In the Total Service Medical Practice, you have additional nonclinical responsibilities as well. These nonclinical aspects of the doctor's role can be classified under the *The Three Cs of Physician Service Responsibility:* Commitment, Caring, and Communication.

Commitment

Whether you are aware of it or not, as a physician you are looked to to set the example for your practice. You are depended on not just to handle the clinical duties, as important and even vital as they are. Your office personnel also rely on you to show them, through your own behavior, that you consider the service aspects of the practice to be important too. In other words, as I mentioned in Lesson 1, you are expected to walk the walk of service.

Before your commitment to service can be demonstrated, however, you first must actually make one. That is often the stumbling block for many organizational leaders. They know they should be committed to service, they may even want to be, but they don't really go through the process, inside themselves, to actually become so. Such surface buy-ins result in inconsistent or even nonexistent decisions that contradict or deny a personal commitment to service as a way of life. In addition, making the kind of service commitment to which I refer may be uncomfortable for you because it is not a totally linear nor scientific process. This means that at some point the truly committed leader will say, "I am willing to make the leap. I will do whatever it takes." When you can say that and mean it, then you have reached commitment.

Once you have made your own personal journey to service commitment, your next task is to demonstrate it and in so doing take significant steps in your walk of service. How is this accomplished? The following suggestions came from office managers and staff members who have been participants in my workshops or who were interviewed for this book. I offer them to you as a means of stimulating your own thinking.

The Steps in the Walk of Service:
■ *Model service-behaviors for your staff.* Office personnel look to you, as the physician, to set the example. How you interact with people, including them, shows your manager and staff how you want them to behave. Patients notice this connection between you and your employees, as was indicated by the following comment

from a focus group participant: "You can tell how the doctor relates to people by watching how the employees behave."

■ *Make service-oriented decisions.* Another way to demonstrate your commitment is through the decisions that you make for the practice. During my interactions with a wide variety of healthcare organizations including medical practices, I have heard the following complaint coming from frontline employees: "Our leaders tell us to provide quality service, but then they do not make decisions that put service first." This is disheartening to even the most motivated employees. I realize that outside entities are increasingly dictating certain decisions for your practice, which means that you will need to search even harder for the areas that you can and do still control. By making certain that these areas reflect the service perspective you want for your practice, you will also be providing viable indications of your commitment to service.

■ *Celebrate the service successes.* When employees believe that you place a high value on service, they will also believe in your commitment to it. Chapter 16 deals with official rewards and celebrations in greater detail. However, there are many things you can do personally to show your appreciation to practice personnel when they serve internal and external customers well. One of the simplest and yet most important is a sincere "Thank you for doing a good job."

■ *Allow your employees to make their own service-oriented decisions.* As an entrepreneur and quite possibly a partner or owner of the practice, it may be difficult for you to let go of some of your decision-making authority. However, doing so will result in three very distinct advantages. First, by empowering employees to make decisions, you can give yourself more time to practice medicine. Second, it will make employees feel valued and trusted, which is essential to keeping a satisfied work force. Finally, and very importantly, it says to all concerned that you want service to pervade your practice. Of course, clinical decisions should be made by medical personnel, but not all require a doctor's input. Nurses, nurse practitioners, physicians' assistants, and midwives can assume responsibility for many such decisions. Nonclinical issues can be handled by office managers and their nonmedical staff as well.

■ *Honor your commitments.* When you do what you say you will do, you demonstrate your commitment to service. Making promised phones calls, being on time for appointments, keeping your word about salaries and vacations—these and other similar actions indicate that you mean what you say. If patients, employees, and other practice customers are to believe in your commitment to service, then they must see that your words can be trusted. Each time your deeds match your words, you build on that belief.

Caring

Did you ever stop to ponder why the word *healthcare* is used to describe the medical field? While *care* can refer to clinical treatment, it also refers to something else: a personal, humanistic response from one human being to another. The actual demonstration of *caring* depends on individual personal style.   When I asked patients to describe what their doctors did to demonstrate their caring, here is what they told me:

> "He treats me with respect. He doesn't talk down to me. It's like I matter to him as a person."

> "My doctor really listens to me. That makes me feel he really cares."

> "She is honest with me. I hate to be lied to. She cares enough to tell me the truth."

> "My doctor spends time with me. I don't how she does it, because I know her schedule is full, but she makes me feel that we have all the time in the world. It really shows she cares."

> "He answers all my questions fully and clearly. I know some of them may seem simple to him, but he doesn't seem to mind. I think that shows he cares."

A caring attitude is important to staff members, too. They want to feel cared about as human beings and want to feel that their feelings and opinions matter. Office personnel have shared with me some of their descriptions of physicians who care about them as employees. As I have listened, I have noticed some definite trends in the data. The first and perhaps most interesting trend involves the use of the possessive pronouns. If the employees felt cared about, I heard frequent references to *"my* doctor" or "*our* doctors." If there was strain in the relationship, I heard "*the* doctor" or "*those* doctors."

When asked to be specific as to the ways their doctors demonstrated *employee* caring, some common themes emerged from the staff members' comments. According to practice personnel, the doctors who care do the following:

> "He makes me feel as though I am a valued, contributing member of the practice."
>
> "She makes me feel like she's glad I work here."
>
> "He makes me feel trusted."

One of the biggest obstacles physicians face to the demonstration of their caring attitudes is also one of the most difficult to remove: time problems. I know that this is a sensitive topic for most, if not all, physicians, and I am certainly aware that many external demands on your time are outside of your control. However, it is possible that you might fall into the group of doctors described by Eric Anderson, M.D., when he wrote, "Doctors get into the habit of not bothering to be punctual. We turn up late for meetings, events, and parties with no excuse except 'we're always late.'"[1] Robert Taylor, M.D., stated it quite bluntly: "Physicians who receive complaints about waiting time should examine their personal sense of promptness and correct any deficiencies."[2] So, I ask you to stop a moment and consider the question, "Can I more effectively manage my time?" If the answer is "yes," then act accordingly.

All of the behaviors desired by patients and practice personnel are visible, tangible indications of a caring attitude, but they will only be surface tricks if they are performed without one critical ingredient—sincerity. Caring has to come from the heart. As you can see from the above descriptions, the manner in which it is shown can and does vary from person to person. It doesn't matter how you show it; it only matters that you do.

Communication

Effective communication is the means through which, among other things, caring and commitment are conveyed. Yet, as important as it is, communication is an area that is seldom covered in medical school. The future doesn't look appreciably brighter for official training in this skill. In fact, current efforts in graduate education reform seem to be focused on many other aspects of practice development , but there is little indication that training in communication skills will be added also.

Yet, the physician's communication skills are important, because problems in that area are directly connected to the patient-retention rate. Remember, the survey conducted by the Miles Institute of Health Care Communication revealed that 1 in 4 of the 1,000 participants switched physicians at some time because of communication problems.[3] In addition, as was discussed in Chapter 2, communication problems lead many patients to do more than merely take their business elsewhere; these difficulties also are traced to patients' decisions to file malpractice suits. In fact, Robert E. Taylor, M.D., the medical director of Northwest Physicians Mutual Insurance Company in Salem, Oregon, indicated that about 70 percent of malpractice suits have at least a relationship to poor doctor/patient or staff/patient communica-tion.[4] Northwest believes in this connection so strongly that it grants physicians a 7.5 percent discount on their liability premiums if doctors receive training in physician/patient communication.[5]

On a brighter note, we also know that the more effective the physician's communication, the better the patient's compre-hension of questions asked during the diagnostic phase, retention of information about their condition and therapeutic regimen, and compliance with treatment. Thus, effective communication is of clinical importance as well.

As the leaders at the heart of the medical practice, physicians are called on to communicate with a wide range of populations in addition to patients. Clearly, effective communication skills applied internally will enhance those intraoffice relationships that will be more thoroughly discussed in the next section of this chapter. Also, being able to express themselves clearly will help the doctors effectively present their opinions in external settings as well.

To begin working on your communication skills, review Chapter 7, and focus carefully on the twelve steps of an effective patient interview in Chapter 13. As you study the suggestions offered in these chapters, find the ones that make sense to you and start implementing them. Also, avail yourself of workshops and seminars, or volunteer to be a subject in a physician communication study. Actively seek feedback either from taping yourself and listening with a critical ear or soliciting input from those with whom you interact. By making improvements in your communication a priority, you can and will sharpen this most essential skill. You also will be fulfilling one of the three most important service responsibilities you have as a physician in a Total Service Medical Practice.

THE PHYSICIAN'S ROLE IN EFFECTIVE INTRAOFFICE RELATIONSHIPS

Quality service starts from within! In the Total Service Medical Practice, the relationships among all personnel, including those involving the physicians, are key to creating the kind of environment in which both internal and external service can flourish. As a physician, an essential part of your role is to manage your intraoffice relationships effectively. Of course, others must do their share, but how you relate to the manager, the staff, and other physicians will set the tone for everyone else.

Doctor–Manager Relationships

In every smoothly running practice, the doctors and the office manager work well together. They have a relationship that is based on mutual respect, trust, and clearly defined roles. Both parties are responding to the needs of the other. In Chapter 9, I will talk to office managers about your needs, but now I would like to tell you about theirs. Based on the interviews I have done with office managers, comments from participants in my workshops, and a survey conducted by the Professional Association of Health Care Office Managers (PAHCOM), I have designed several suggestions for you to consider in your relationship with your office manager.

1. *Ensure that you and your office manager agree on the manager's role.* Sometimes there is simply a mismatch in this area. In fact, I would say that an incompatible agenda is the cause of most

FIGURE 8–3

Doctor–Manager Business Decision-Making Continuum

Doctors Make All Decisions/ Manager Implements	Doctors Seek Input Before Making Decisions/ Manager Implements	Doctors Offer Vision While Manager Makes Daily Decisions	Manager Makes All Decisions/ Doctors Approve	Manager Makes Decisions/ Doctors Informed	Manager Makes Decisions/ Doctors Not Involved

problems between office managers and physicians. These difficulties can be corrected if you will consciously determine the kind of responsibilities you want to have as well as those you are willing to relinquish, and then find an office manager who is comfortable with that. As you make these determinations, consider the continuum of practice business decision making offered in Figure 8–3.

Darlene Wojciechowski, CMM, office manager of a specialty group in Springfield, New Jersey, operationalized the optimum situation when she advised that physicians make clear to the office manager the goals of a practice and then give the manager the authority to work toward those goals.[6] This will allow the physician(s) to guide the practice from a philosophical position and yet allow the managers to do what most of them believe they were hired to do: manage.

One note of caution: Stay involved. Even though office managers want to be free to do their jobs, they also still want and need your participation and interest. Meeting with your manager on a regular basis and showing a willingness to discuss practice issues and problems will provide the kind of continuing support he or she needs. As your practice grows, you may even need to head and/or participate on some business-related committees. Be willing to do whatever your practice administrator needs you to do without micromanaging his or her job.

2.*Avoid reversing your manager's decisions.* Decision reversals tend to come most often when dealing with people issues. More than one participant in my office managers' workshops has echoed the following words: "It is frustrating when I have made a decision only to have the staff member run to the doctor and have him side with the employee." Others report another common area of decision-reversal involves billing issues. As one manager in a seminar stated it: "When a patient goes to the doctor and complains about a decision I have made regarding a bill, the doctor almost always reverses me. That makes it hard for me to maintain credibility with the patients, and it makes me feel unempowered." As difficult as it may be, and recognizing that on occasion a manager might make a poor decision, this kind of intervention should be kept to a bare minimum and should always be discussed with the manager first. Also, when both the office manager and the doctors are in agreement regarding the manager's decision-making role as discussed above, then the need for reversals will be almost, if not totally, eliminated.

3. *Stick to your decisions.* When doctors do make decisions, office managers report that they have a tendency to reverse themselves. In a PAHCOM survey of three hundred office managers, one of the most frequently voiced complaints concerned doctors who contradict their own rules, especially on billing.[7] Imagine the office manager's confusion when she thinks she knows the practice's policies and attempts to implement them, only to have the doctors apply them inconsistently. This is not to say that rules should never be broken. However, what this complaint reflects are those times when the doctor does it without consulting the office manager or without explaining the rationale.

4. *Understand the role of the office manager.* Everyone likes to feel that they are understood, and office managers are no exception. They often report the feeling that no one truly grasps the range and number of demands that are made on them. When you show your understanding as a physician you will greatly enhance your doctor/manager relationship.

The first step toward such understanding is education. Doctors should exert the effort to find out, not just the content of the office manager's job description, but how it plays out on any given day. One physician in one of my workshops told of his annual day to walk in his manager's shoes. Once a year he spends the day shadowing his office manager. He does not interfere nor does he allow others to turn to him instead of the manager. Rather, he merely observes. At the end of the day, the doctor and manager sit together and discuss what has occurred, what were the most stressful parts for the manager, what questions the doctor has about any particular event of the day. It is important that any doctor who might engage in this shadowing activity create the appropriate rationale for it. Office managers should not feel that they will be second-guessed or corrected. The purpose of this day is to gain understanding.

Another, less dramatic, way for gaining this insight and conveying an interest in what the manager does is merely to ask and then really listen to the response. This inquiry can be accomplished with a casual but sincere question, or in a more structured way during those regularly scheduled meetings I referred to earlier. Office Manager Arlene Stolte told me about the arrangement she has with her physicians: "We meet every two weeks. I can talk to my doctors about the progress we have made as well as any problems we might encounter, such as staff, patient, or contract problems."

5. *Show appreciation for the office manager.* Closely tied to understanding the office manager's role is the physician's appreciation of it. The first and most obvious place to look is at the pay scale. How well compensated *is* this valuable individual? Recognizing that most medical practice personnel do not choose this field for the money, paying them a competitive salary is still money well spent.

Appreciation is not shown through dollars and cents alone, however. Some of the most unhappy employees of any organization are those who are paid well but who are not told in softer currencies that they are appreciated. These currencies will be discussed in detail in Chapter 16. I can't resist sharing one with you now, though. As mentioned earlier, office managers express their desire for an easily supplied indication of physician appreciation: a simple and sincere "thank you."

6. *Show respect for the office manager's professionalism.* Closely aligned with understanding and appreciating the office manager's role is showing your respect for it. Not only will it please office managers that physicians understand their jobs, but it will delight them that they also consider the office manager as a professional colleague. The PAHCOM survey contained some rather blunt criticism indicating that such respect is not always accorded. One manager wrote, "The doctor does not see clerical or office managers as professionals—only the RNs." A manager in a cardiologist's group stated that her doctors could show "more respect toward me as a professional specializing in medical management." One manager of a small OBG group wanted her boss "to stop asking me to do his personal business."[8]

What the office managers seek is recognition by physicians that they are healthcare professionals too. One sure-fire way for doctors to demonstrate this acknowledgement is through the tangible support of professional development activities for their office mangers, such as time off to attend workshops or seminars. Of equal importance are practice-funded memberships in the Medical Group Management Association and/or PAHCOM, and practice funded trips to the state and national conventions sponsored by these organizations.

7. *Be open to feedback and suggestions.* As I have discussed, physicians often exist in a vacuum. Patients and even staff members are reluctant to share any feedback with the doctor, whether it be good or bad news. The person they usually turn to is the office manager. So, frequently office managers have obtained important and useful information which they would be happy to share if they felt that their doctors were open to receiving it. I urge you to reread Chapter 5 on preparing for receiving feedback, focusing especially on Factor 7, and then tell your office manager you would like to know what he or she has to share! You must create a safe, nonthreatening environment for these feedback sessions and sincerely *want* to find ways in which you can improve.

8. *Be time-conscious.* Earlier in this chapter I discussed the importance of physicians' time-consciousness. This is especially important to office managers, because they are usually the ones who must explain your tardiness. Thus, do what you can to stay on schedule. It will be greatly appreciated.

The PAHCOM survey revealed three more important time-related areas for your consideration. Office managers expressed their appreciation for the doctors who honored the commitment to meet with them on a regular basis. In addition, managers found it was much easier to perform their jobs when their doctors' paid prompt attention to paperwork. They also appreciated the physicians' consideration of the demands placed on other employees' time too.[9]

One final thought: lest you think that the office managers only complain about their doctors, let me assure you that this is not the case. The PAHCOM survey is replete with positive examples and the overall ratings were high. The vast majority of the office managers in my workshops speak of their doctors with the warmest regard and pride. All of the office managers interviewed for this book were highly positive about the doctors for whom they worked. I conclude, then, that many physicians have already built and are actively maintaining positive relationships with their office managers. My hope is that the above suggestions will offer some new ideas that will make this important relationship even stronger.

Doctor–Staff Relationships

Your practice needs competent, motivated, satisfied, challenged, self-actualized employees. Not only do the clinical and nonclinical staff have extensive interactions with patients, but they can affect the patients' perceptions of their entire healthcare experience. Terry Sullivan of Sullivan, Hall, Boot, and Smith, an Atlanta, Georgia, law firm that defends physicians in negligence and insurance cases, points out that staff reinforce the impressions—positive or negative—that patients form about their doctors. "When you have a patient in the 'gray zone' who is doubting the quality of care, staff certainly aggravate or improve the situation.[10]

Where do staff members get their role models? Earlier in this chapter I discussed the importance of focusing on your own behaviors as a doctor, because your staff will be looking to you as an example of how to act and interact. Also, whether you realize it or not, you are an influential person in their lives. They want to admire you and respect you and, as I indicated earlier, they want to believe that you care about them. Unfortunately, in too many cases, this does not occur. In my conversations with staff members in medical practices, I have heard the following comments:

"I have to walk on tippy toes sometimes!"

"Some days it's like walking on eggshells."

"I wish he'd at least talk to me."

"I wish he'd talk to me as though I'm human."

"I wish he'd ask me how I felt or what I thought, and mean it."

And this one from an office manager:

"I only wish the doctors would realize how much a kind word and a smile would mean to my staff."

It isn't always this way, however! Lisa McCollum, now director of certification for the American Association of Medical Assistants, recalls the days when she worked for Dr. Robert Bright. She says he acknowledged the value of his assistants by paying for their association fees and continuing education and giving time off for them to take classes. As a result, the staff took a personal interest in patients and talked with them. Assistants attached notes to patient files, alerting the doctor to patients' personal problems or mentioning upcoming anniversaries he might bring up when talking with patients. "We were an extra set of eyes and ears for him, not just an extra set of hands." At the end of each day, the staff would meet briefly with the doctor to discuss how things had gone and to make future plans. McCollum says the resulting team feeling helps Dr. Bright keep a low turnover rate among his workers, and a high referral rate among his patients.[11]

There are several suggestions for building the kind of positive doctor/staff relationship that will reap the type of results Ms. McCollum describes.

1. *Share your mission and expectations.* Staff members need to understand the physician's philosophy of patient care and the practice's mission. When prospective employees are being interviewed is an ideal time to introduce them to these key areas. It is also important to be clear about your expectations of your staff. Sometimes physicians feel frustrated and don't understand why they aren't getting what they want from their staff, and they assume that the staff just doesn't care about doing a good job. While on occasion that may be true, in most instances the problem

is not a lack of caring but rather a lack of clarity about expectations.

2. *Empower staff to make decisions.* How can a doctor make sure that staff members are doing their jobs? Ownership. By not only allowing the office manager to make certain policy decisions but also empowering staff to make specified on-the-spot decisions as well, you can instill a sense of ownership that is so important to staff longevity and effective external and internal practice communication.

3. *Be open to staff input.* Staff members are on the front line daily. They are in a position to observe a lot and can be gold mine of information and ideas. In the PAHCOM study, 68 percent of the surveyed practices have made at least one improvement as a result of staff suggestions. They included adding a silent alarm in a psychiatry practice to alert police if an employee is confronted by a psychotic patient; sending patients thank-you notes for referrals; setting policy on forwarding messages to doctors; and sending a map, parking instructions, and brochures to new patients before the first visit. A cardiologist's staff now uses color-coded flags to identify what procedures the patient in each exam room needs while a urology group manager reports "improved decorum" as the result of staff suggestions.[12]

Not only do new ideas for implementation come from the staff members, but their input can prevent some erroneous decisions. For example, one practice manager described what happened when the physicians decided to change the telephone system without seeking input from the people at the front desk. Without advice from those in the best position to offer it, the doctors' decision created more problems than it solved. Moreover, the staff members felt left out of the loop and were angry that their opinions had not been solicited.

Staff members are also in a position to learn a great deal about the patients, bits of information that are important but may not be shared with the doctors. Collectively, staff members spend more time with the patients than the doctors do, so it's important to keep them informed and to seek their insights. In Dr. Bright's end-of-the-day discussions with his staff, they cover potentially difficult interactions and anticipate the expectations and special needs of patients.[13]

4. *Appreciate what the staff does, and show it!* In practices where the physicians and their staff enjoy positive relationships, the doctors understand the importance of the contribution made by each staff member. For example, one of the most hectic, vital, and frequently unappreciated positions in the practice is that of the receptionist. An article in *The Physician's Advisory*, entitled "Help Your Receptionist Deal With Patients" made this appeal: "Your receptionist has the thankless job of discussing a number of delicate matters with your patients. How would you, the physician, like to pin down a patient to say exactly when or how she will pay her overdue bill? Or tell a patient he can no longer expect to be seen by the senior doctor— despite his preference for that doctor—but that your new associate will see him from now on? And how would you tell the new patient to be prepared to make payment over the counter on the uncovered part of your fee when she comes for her first visit to your office? Consider also saying these things while two telephone lines are ringing, one or two patients are checking in, and someone else is checking out."[14] Just as your office managers appreciate being appreciated, so do all members of your staff.

The same methods that work for managers also can apply to staff members. The one that costs the least and yet means more than you can possibly imagine is the doctor's personal expression of thanks and interest. Take the time to stop for a quick "good morning" to the records clerk, express your appreciation for the juggling act performed by the receptionist, compliment your nurse on her skill with a patient: it will work wonders for office morale and will provide the cement for your positive doctor/staff relationship.

5. *Communicate effectively.* It is understandable why all of the focus on physician communication seems to be between the doctor and the patient. However, it is equally important to demonstrate effective communication skills when interacting with your staff as well. PAHCOM found that the most common complaints are summed up by a plastic surgeon's manager who wishes the boss would be "a better listener, a little less opinionated, and more patient."[15]

There is a practical reason for effective communication with your staff. It can avoid mistakes. For example, consider the surgeons in a multidoctor practice who switched their rotation schedule without informing the staff, figuring it did not matter as long as they were all doing the same procedure. What they did not realize was that the staff had been preparing the instruments and positioning the patients differently for each doctor, according to each physician's habits. Once they'd entered the new rotation pattern, the doctors' needs were not being met by the staff. The physicians became short-tempered and angry, while the staff became sullen and difficult. All of this could have been avoided if the channels of communication between the doctors and their staff had been kept open.

6. *Be available.* Although the responsibility and authority for the daily management of personnel should appropriately be in the hands of the office manager, the physician needs to be available to staff members who would seek his or her advice or perspective. Office manager Debra Goodyear explained, "My staff knows they can talk to the doctor about any decisions that are made. Our Fearless Leader . . . has an open-door policy and he wants them to come to him if they feel they need to." For this kind of open-door policy to work effectively without undercutting the office manager, however, it should be thoroughly discussed with and agreed to by the manager.

Sometimes a staff member would merely like to discuss other issues with the physician, such as career path or personal problems. How much of this kind of interaction you engage in is really up to you, but it is important that the staff knows that either they or the office manager can gain direct access to you for such input.

7. *Don't be intimidating.* Believe it or not! You can be an intimidating presence. Sometimes it is the result of an angry tone of voice or the way your sentences are worded and sometimes it is in the very aura surrounding your image as a physician. By being friendly, respectful, and courteous you can reverse this impression.

On occasion, intimidation can turn to abuse. William Rock, M.D., Vice President of Medical Affairs at Dean Medical Center S.C. in Madison, Wisconsin, explained what happens when physicians become abusive to their staff.

> "In the past when one of our colleagues displayed an outburst of temper . . . there was often a tolerance for the offense . . . One frequently hears the comment, 'You know what a short temper Dr. So & So has when he is really busy and pressed; he can be a bear.' Unfortunately, employees, technicians, nurses, clerks, or students are often the targets of such rude behavior and one's colleagues

may only be vaguely aware that it occurs . . . In today's workplace, such disruptive behavior cannot be tolerated. In addition to the need of asserting common courtesy, decency, and/or responsible professional decorum, there is now the very real threat of lawsuits and/or action by the Equal Opportunities Commission. No longer can medical organizations overlook such activities."[16]

While you probably do not engage in any of the behaviors described above, I suggest you open yourself to feedback. As Dr. Rock pointed out, in many instances the doctors themselves are not aware of the impact of their behavior. Self examination and an open, honest discussion with your office manager can help you determine if you are perceived as intimidating or abusive. Then, you can take action to correct these behaviors before they destroy any hope for effective doctor/staff relationships.

Doctor/Doctor Relationships

How well physicians communicate and relate to each other is important to the success of the practice. Some suggestions for building positive doctor/doctor relationships are:

1. *Select a medical director based on his or her ability to bring people together.* Feuding doctors can lead to major problems in a medical practice. Selecting a medical director who knows how to capitalize on the strengths of each individual and can assist people in managing their conflicts will help build positive professional relationships.

2. *Be willing to work together.* A medical director cannot provide the entire answer. As a member physician of the practice you must also be willing to learn how, if you don't already know, to resolve conflict productively and without personal affront.

In a very real sense, the physicians in the practice represent the executive team of your organization. You need to learn how to function as a team and not as independent entities. Read the section on team-building in Chapter 11 and apply it to your group.

3. *As a group of physicians, define your vision for the practice.* Issues such as ethics, management responsibilities, patient loads, and compensation can be addressed much more easily when all doctors are on the same page. If they are not, then conflict almost inevitably will result. Also, office managers and staff need to be informed of this vision in order to function appropriately in the practice. Thus, taking the time to create a physician team's vision for the practice will reap important benefits down the line.

4. *Express appreciation for each other's differences.* Differences can tear a group apart or can lift it to a higher level of creativity and accomplishment. Rather than resenting competing ideas of how things should be done, showing appreciation for the variety will build positive doctor/doctor relationships. How boring it would be if all of you thought alike, talked alike, and even practiced medicine alike.

5. *Make the effort to communicate effectively with each other.* Just as with any person you encounter during your day, your professional colleagues deserve your attention to the ways in which you communicate with them. Being aware of your nonverbal and verbal messages will help you be sure to practice effective skills. Listening to each other, really listening, can go a long way to erasing conflict. Also, if anyone in the practice can understand a doctor's life and problems, it should be another doctor; extend empathetic understanding to each other on a daily basis.

7. *Do not contradict each other in public.* Although doctors often can and do provide needed consultation for each other, any disagreements should be discussed privately. Nothing is more upsetting to a patient than to hear his or her doctor's assessment of the situation contradicted by another physician. Also, it is a matter of professional courtesy. No one wants to be challenged in public.

When I interviewed my primary care physician for this book, I asked him what brought a smile to his face during any given day in his practice. Without hesitation he said, "The interactions I have with my colleagues in the practice. I believe I have learned more about practicing medicine from them than anyplace else in my career." That is the way it can be, should be, and hopefully is in your practice. If not, then as doctors you and your colleagues need to take the steps necessary to make it happen.

As a physician, then, you are the heart of your medical practice. As such, you must never underestimate your importance to all aspects of it. Your demonstrated commitment, sincere caring, and effective communication will help ensure that your practice remains a healthy one. If you build and maintain effective relationships with all those with whom you work, you will find that you actually have more time to do what you want most to do: practice medicine.

END NOTES

1. Eric Anderson, "The One-Minute Office Call," *Physician's Management* 30, no. 9 (September 1990), p. 78.
2. Robert Taylor, "What Do Patient's Look For in Their Physicians," *Physician's Management* 31, no. 10 (October 1991), p. 56.
3. J. Gregory Carroll and Robert Engle, "Communication Techniques for HMO Physicians," *HMO Practice* 7, no. 1 (March 1993), p. 40.
4. Flora Johnson Skelly, "Communicate . . . or Litigate," *AMNews* 35, no. 25 (June 29, 1992), p. 41.
5. Ibid.
6. "Office Managers Offer Tips on Running Practice," *Physicians Marketing and Management* 7, no. 2 (February 1994), p. 16.
7. Lauren M. Walker, "How Do You Rate with Your Office Manager?" *Medical Economics* 69, no. 22 (November 16, 1992), p. 96.
8. Ibid., p. 98.
9. Ibid., p. 96.
10. "Don't Let Staff Push Patients into Malpractice Suits," *Medical Office Manager* 7, no. 1 (January 1993), p. 1.
11. Robert McCoppin, "Service Is the Key to a Healthy Practice," *American Medical News* 34, no. 11 (March 18, 1991), p. 15.
12. Walker, p. 100.
13. McCoppin, p. 15.
14. "Help Your Receptionist Deal with Patients," *The Physician's Advisory* 44, no. 6 (June 1994), p. 7. (To subscribe, call 888-941-4488.)
15. Walker, p. 96.
16. William Rock, "The Disruptive Physician," *Group Practice Journal* 43, no. 5 (September/October 1994), p. 38.

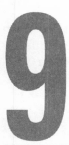

CHAPTER

Step Nine—Embrace the Medical Practice Administrators Role

LEADERS OF THE PARADE!

I will never forget my first day as the drum major of my high school band. As I stood in front of the school and looked down the street at my 125 classmates, all looking to me for leadership, I was almost overwhelmed by the responsibility. Whatever direction I led, they were to follow. Whatever tempo I set, they were supposed to keep pace. I hoped that I was up to the task. As the year began, I made my beginner's mistakes: Turning the wrong direction on the midway at the Kansas State Fair or marching so far ahead of the band in the homecoming parade that the announcer thought I was my own entry—"Ladies and Gentlemen, the Fredonia High School Marching . . . Drum Major?" But, things got better. I developed my own style and soon made the role my own. By the end of the season, I was acclaimed one of the best drum majors our high school had ever had.

When I think of your role as the administrator of a medical practice, I envision the leader of a very special parade. The doctors have entrusted its successful operation to you. Your staff members look to you for direction and tempo and much, much more. When you first began in your job (or if you are just starting now), you may have had your own versions of beginning drum-major blunders. However, as you continue to live with this role, you are no doubt making it your own. The suggestions I offer in this chapter are to help you on your way. The band has gathered behind you. The job is officially yours! "Forward! March!"

THE WOWS OF BEING A PRACTICE ADMINISTRATOR

At first blush, you may not think of your job and say, "WOW!" but I do! When I think of the responsibilities you have in the practice, it produces in me that expression of amazement and appreciation. More than that, however, this simple word represents the key responsibilities of your job!

Work with your doctors and staff
Organize Your Office
Welcome Your Patients

Let's look at each of these now.

Work With Your Doctors and Staff

Later in this chapter I will discuss, in detail, some specific suggestions for establishing effective relationships with the doctors and with your staff. At this point, I want to examine some important responsibilities that you have in working with both groups.

Help Doctors and Staff Stay Informed
About Changes in Healthcare

Before you can help anyone else, you must first become and stay current. To stay up to speed on the cutting-edge trends in healthcare and on their impact on medical practices, you need not stand alone. You can join professional group practice organizations, such as the Medical Group Management Association (MGMA) (for practices of all sizes) or the Professional Association of Health Care Office Managers (PAHCOM) (for smaller practices). These organizations have publications, conferences, library support, and research facilities that can help you stay up to date.

Next, you should keep your doctors and your staff informed as well. Your professionalism will provide a key resource to them as they adjust to the changes in healthcare. Doctors need to know how these changes are going to impact them and their practice of medicine. Staff members need to know how they will be affected in the performance of their jobs. This information can be conveyed in meetings, in-house newsletters, and posting of important items on office bulletin boards.

Help the Practice Personnel Handle the Change Process.

People seem to vary in the time it takes them to adjust to change. What seems to be common among us, however, is the process itself. Those who have studied human reactions during periods of transition have discovered specific phases of the change process.

Based on Elizabeth Kubler Ross's phases of death and dying, these phases are:[1]

Denial: "Change isn't going to come."

People in denial continue to behave under the old paradigm, which only leads to their continued frustration.

Anger: "How dare they change things like that!"

As I have traveled the country conducting my workshops for those in the healthcare field, I have discovered many angry people. Since so many of the changes impacting the medical practice are coming from external sources, the anger arises primarily from a sense of losing control of professional lives.

Bargaining: "Maybe we won't have to do it that way. Maybe this will work just as well!"

At this stage, people realize that they will in fact have to change if they are going to remain in their current jobs. Thus, they begin to offer some other kind of alternative, assuming anything will be better than the change that is in the offing.

Depression: "I feel so sad about this. Things just aren't like they used to be."

People in this phase have realized that change is here. It does no good to rant and rave about it. There is really no chance of any other option: this is the change and there's no alternative. So, they feel helpless, unhappy, victimized. Some people never move beyond this phase. It keeps them trapped in negativity. They may change their behaviors, but their hearts are stuck in the old system.

Acceptance: "Well, I guess if this is the way things have to be, I'll go along."

Although not the same as agreement, the people in this phase are willing to accept the change without being negative. They do their jobs, but with little if any enthusiasm.

Reconstruction: "Hey! This new way of doing things works pretty well!"

During this phase, the people have begun to actually see the value of the change. They can even get excited about it. They are well on the way to the essential buy-in that will lead to the next step.

Commitment: "This is the way we do things here!"

These people have moved through the process. They are now able to embrace the changes and have incorporated them into their lives. What was a change has now become status quo.

As the office manager, you will have experienced or will be experiencing these phases yourself. Yet, it is your responsibility to handle your own process as well as lead the doctors and the staff through their own. Helping them understand what is happening by sharing and discussing the change process will assist all of you in adjusting to the changes that are occurring.

A specific kind of change that is impacting many medical practices today is sudden and rapid growth. As I mentioned previously, doctors are finding many advantages to joining together, and often this takes the form of a larger group practice. Nancy Miller, the manager of OB & GYN Specialists in Winter Park, Florida, found herself administering a practice that leapt from two doctors to 11, with four midlevel practitioners, 80 staff, and three offices. Between 1995 and 1996, the practice added three physicians, expanded its second office from 2,300 to 7,800 square feet, and opened its third location. What suggestions does she have for handling such spurts of rapid growth? The creation of a successful management team and physician management committees.

The management team at Ms. Miller's practice meets monthly and is composed of the office managers from each of the three locations and the department supervisors who report to them. She said, "I try to give them as much autonomy as possible so that I don't have to micromanage." The supervisors' roles differ somewhat from location to location, but all are responsible for managing their departments, setting schedules, handling patient complaints in their areas, and doing staff reviews. Ms. Miller added "We all are working managers," which means that if a staff member is out for some reason, the supervisor may fill in for that person. Similarly, the three managers fill in for the supervisors when needed.

The five physician committees were established as a direct result of the growth in the practice, and cover all aspects of the practice operation: managed care, facility management, staff management, computers, and education. Ms. Miller meets once a month with all 11 physicians, plus the nurses and physician assistants. At that meeting, the doctors report on their committee meetings and go over their schedules and hospital coverage. She also has a monthly financial meeting with the shareholders.

To the managers of practices that are growing fast, Ms. Miller has four specific pieces of advice: delegate, gain the physicians participation, hold effective meetings, and establish on-site management for each location. The most difficult of the four was the solicitation of the physicians' participation in the business of the practice. Although it took a while, Ms. Miller reported that the doctors eventually came around. After a long time, she said, "it becomes a mutual admiration society. The doctors are proud of me, and I am proud of them."[2]

Change and growth is almost a constant in medical practices today. Understanding the process and seeking advice from others who have been there will help you help your staff and your physicians.

Generate a Sense of Community

In Chapter 11, I talk specifically about how to create an effective practice team and, as the office manager, you will be an important part of that effort. What I am referring to here, however, is the development of your own sense of ownership and belonging, and the sharing of that feeling. As the office manager, others will look to you for your example, even your physicians. If you show your commitment and express your belief in the greater good this practice has to serve, then you will move others to feel pride in that as well. The result will be a sense of community, where people can be accepted for themselves and for the strengths they bring. David Bowen, a dedicated office manager for 36 years, posted the

following poem in his practice, noting that it was this kind of
environment which he hoped to create for everyone who worked
there.

Where Can I Go?

If this is not a place where tears are understood,
Where do I go to cry?

If this is not a place where my spirits can take wing,
Where do I go to fly?

If this is not a place where my questions can be asked,
Where do I go to speak?

If this is not a place where you'll accept me as I am,
Where can I go to be?

If this is not a place where I can try, and learn and grow,
Where do I just be me?

If this is not a place where tears are understood,
Where do I go to cry?

Poem by Ken Medina,
modified by Bill Crockett[3]

How do you, the office manager, help create such a space?
The suggestions offered in this chapter will give you practical
ideas for helping people feel this kind of belonging. More than
that, however, you must actually feel it in your heart and soul
yourself: This is where you want to be. This is where you want to
work. No place else will do. As one office manager described her
feelings to me: "I love the medical field. I've loved every doctor
I've ever worked for. I love this office. It's like my home." Of
course, I don't mean that you should lose yourself and your own
identity in any profession or job. But the kind of dedication and
commitment expressed by this woman is the kind of enthusiasm
that is catching. Others in her practice will feel the same. That is
what I mean by a *sense of community.*

Organize Your Office

From the paper to the people, a medical practice needs to be
organized, and the responsibility for creating that structure falls on
the shoulders of the office administrator.

Develop Efficient and Customer-Friendly Processes

When a practice is engaged in an internal process, you can be sure of one thing: A customer, either internal or external, is waiting on the results. You can also be certain that the longer they wait, the angrier they will become. Thus, as the office manager, you need to lead an evaluation of the processes in your practice. A specific model for doing this is offered in Chapter 12. The important point here is to realize that the initiation of this analysis is up to you. One process to study carefully is that of billing and collections. Probably the most troublesome internal process, even it can be made efficient and customer-friendly. (See Chapter 14 for a thorough discussion of this process based on suggestions provided by well-known medical practice consultant, Diane Palmer.)

Keep Files Organized and Up to Date

Workshop participants have told me about the black hole that swallows medical charts and files and holds them forever. While at times you may well wonder if that has happened in your practice, a carefully organized filing system can help eliminate it. Of course, computerization has helped tremendously in accomplishing this task. Regardless of how it is done, though, you must develop a system for reviewing, updating, and organizing all patient charts and business files. All appropriate employees should be instructed in how to maintain these systems as well.

Organize Your Staff

The easiest method of keeping people on task and away from unnecessary repetition is the creation and use of a practice employee handbook. One of the best I have seen was created for an opthalmologist's office.[4] The general categories include: introduction, orientation of new employees, financial policies, job descriptions, office procedures, staff policies, employee benefits, inventory, and phone directory. (This book is available on diskette from the publisher. Similar publications pertaining to other specialties, such as Family Practice and General Surgery, are also available.) If everyone in the practice, including the doctors, has a copy of this handbook, and you have discussed the elements during the training period, your staff members will know where to look for answers to many of their questions. Also, they will clearly see what is expected of them if they are to be a part of this practice.

Organize the physicians

One of the most important contributions you can make to the smooth operation of your office is to keep your physicians informed about their schedules. Office manager Arlene Stolte described it this way: "I make sure they know what their schedules are for the next day. [She faxes the next day's schedule to each of the doctors.] I make their lives as stress-free as possible by helping them stay organized." She added, "My responsibility is to keep the physicians informed about where they are to be and when."

Welcome the patients

No, you will not be sitting by the front door with a box of candy, like a greeter at Wal-Mart. However, you may have direct contact with many patients later in their visits, and your influence will be felt vicariously when your well-trained staff makes each patient feel welcome. How can you ensure that this will happen? The warmth of the office decor, especially in the waiting areas, helps. Hot coffee or hot water for soothing herbal teas creates a very gracious feeling, as is in evidence at the mammography clinic where I go for my annual exam. As we know, though, physical facilities are only a small part of the message patients find important. The personal contact with practice personnel is what makes the difference. It is up to you to see that your staff receives training in how to manage these moments effectively. The patient's first personal contact is with the receptionist. We know already that patients want to have a pleasant smile of acknowledgement on their entry into the office, and they want to be greeted verbally when the receptionist is not on the telephone. One office manager I interviewed pointed out the absence of any computers in her office. All billing, insurance filing, etc. is handled in another location, away from the patient's eyesight. She believes that these machines create a distancing effect between her staff and her patients, and she is probably right.

Many times when office managers speak directly to the patients, it is to resolve problems that have arisen. It is at these moments that you must work doubly hard to stay pleasant, and yet sometimes firm, as well as showing empathy for the patient's predicament. One office manager told of her interaction with a patient who was very upset about his bill. Even after she had clearly and carefully addressed the patient's confusion, he was not satisfied. He finally blurted out loudly and angrily, "Well obviously you don't want to help me. I want to speak to someone who can! Who has the final say around here?" She smiled and said, politely, "That would be me, sir. I'm as high as you can go." The man paused and then laughed. They resolved the situation and he went away feeling satisfied at being heard by the highest possible authority in that practice.

Clearly, several things were going on in that situation. The office manager was able to say with confidence, "The buck stops here," because she and her doctors had clarified what her decision-making function was to be. She also knew that her decisions, whatever they were, would not be reversed by the physicians. Also, she maintained her poise, did not allow herself to become pulled into the customer's anger, and was able to remain courteous, polite, and even friendly.

So, WOW! Office managers have a lot to do. You must work with physicians and staff, helping them through changing times as well as keeping them informed. You must organize the business and the people of the practice. You must establish the kind of situation in which employees feel a sense of belonging and patients will feel welcome. These are but a few of the responsibilities that you must uphold in your role as the administrator of the medical practice.

BUILDING POSITIVE RELATIONSHIPS WITH THE PHYSICIANS

In your role as a practice administrator, you have to balance many relationships. None must be given more careful attention than the one you have with your doctors. In chapter 11, I will talk further about the doctor/administrator team, but for now I want to offer some suggestions to you for upholding your share of the creation and maintenance of an effective doctor/administrator relationship.

Understand Your Doctors

The times, they are a-changing! And for no one more than for physicians in healthcare today. You will be better able to relate to your physicians if you pause a moment to realize how many changes they are facing.

In fact, Barbara J. Linney, the director of career development for the American College of Physician Executives in Tampa, Florida, conducted a study to determine the specific areas in which physicians perceive major changes. She concluded, "Four changes were discussed by everybody: lowered income, brought about mostly by Medicare; loss of control over the provision of patient care; the constant threat of malpractice litigation hanging over their heads, and actual lawsuits in some cases; and mountains of paperwork for third-party payers, requiring additional staff to manage." Quoted by Ms. Linney, Tully Blalock, M.D., an internist in Winter Park, Florida, described the impact of these changes: "We have a dreadful period to go through . . . There is so much more stress. We work longer hours and harder and make less money for the same amount of work. There are not many happy people practicing medicine." Ending on a positive note, however, he concluded, "I think things will work out."[5]

Given all of these changes, when doctors may seem a little out of sorts or unwilling to give up any more of their autonomy, try a little understanding. They are caught in a constant process of change, never quite completing all seven phases of the process before a new wave overtakes them, plummeting them back to denial and anger. The changes you want your doctors to make will be for the good of the practice in the long run, but you will need to be patient, present your case well (to be discussed later in this chapter), and be willing to give the doctors some time.

Understanding your physicians also means you need to understand their limitations. We all can fall into the trap of expecting a doctor to be perfect. We expect them to make accurate diagnoses and prescribe the best treatment for our illnesses. Even people like you, who work around them every day, can begin to expect physicians to be infallible in all dimensions of their lives. The truth is that they are not. Doctors have, as was pointed out in Chapters 2 and 8, received very little if any training in effective communication skills, for example. Not only does this impact their patient interactions, but it also affects how they communicate with you, the staff, and each other. In addition, in medical school they were trained to forge a tough independence and decisiveness. In fact, "these are assets in their arsenal of survival skills."[6] Finally, a physician's medical school and residency training typically does not further his or her managerial skills. In fact, according to Mark Shields, M.D., the medical director of the Dreyer Clinic in Aurora, Illinois, many aspects of this training make it more difficult for the physician to be a successful manager. The emphasis on the "captain of the ship" mentality for the clinical responsibilities makes it difficult for the physician manager to delegate responsibility or accept the give and take of a management team.[7]

Understanding your doctors also means getting to know each of them individually, because in spite of their shared state of constant change, each doctor is different. Richard Thompson, M.D., a former private pediatrician and then hospital-based chair of pediatrics of a 500-bed medical center, offers the following rather amusing but accurate descriptions of the differing attitudes doctors may have:

> There is no such thing as a single approach to a group of physicians. Rather, any approach must reflect the unique characteristics of several subgroups . . . Dr. Wonderful: clinical skills, cooperative attitude, sense of responsibility, and sense of humor make this physician a delightful working companion. Dr. Today: Reluctant to change (who isn't?), but willing to change if convinced by persuasive arguments that change is necessary. Dr. Yesterday: Has the Gloria Patri mentality: As it was in the beginning, is now, and ever shall be. Dr. Tomorrow: The physician's vision matches that of healthcare executives. Dr. Entrepreneur: May be a subspecialist in a highly technical but revenue-producing clinical area; may be an economic partner of the healthcare organization in some joint venture. Dr. Trouble: Usually has excellent oratorical skills. Urges colleagues not to 'collaborate with the enemy.' The Warrior: May be working on, or have obtained, a law degree. Begins most sentences, 'On the advice of legal counsel . . .'—handle with care.[8]

Sometimes these differences among physicians make reaching decisions difficult. Office Manager Marilyn Haley told me, "Consensus-building in a medical practice is almost impossible. They will never all have the same opinion to start with." Another office manager provided her solution to this problem: "I have assigned each doctor to a specific area, after consultation with them, of course. Then when I need a decision regarding equipment, I can go to Doctor X. When I need one regarding personnel, I go to Dr. Y., and so forth. It cuts down on everyone's time, and I don't have to solicit five responses from five very different doctors." Long-time office manager David Bowen offered this suggestion for dealing with the differences among doctors: "All physicians are not alike. An effective manager will study the personality and idiosyncrasies of each physician and develop a rapport with each one."[9]

Understanding your physicians does not mean that you should pity them—they don't want that; nor should you cave in to them—you don't want that. It does mean that you should help them gain insight into the changes in healthcare, be patient as you work to establish your positive relationship with them, and get to know them each as individuals if at all possible. (Specific suggestions for presenting your ideas to physicians will be discussed in the last section of this chapter.)

Build a Trusting Relationship with Your Physicians

The first step to a trusting relationship is the demonstration of your loyalty. In a time when doctors are doubting the loyalty of the very people they are trying to help (the patients), it is doubly important that they sense yours. A difficult word to define, I asked an office manager what she meant when she talked about loyalty. She answered: "It means that you don't talk about your doctors behind their backs. You don't run them down to other doctors inside or outside the practice. You don't criticize them in front of the staff. Slowly, over time, you build up their knowledge that they can rely on you. That you can be trusted." Loyalty does not need to be blind allegiance, however. Sometimes it means being candid in your assessment of a situation. Most doctors will appreciate and value that honesty.

Another way to build a trusting relationship with the doctor is to show professional competence. You can be honest and reliable, but if you do not have the skill levels necessary to do your job, complete trust will not result. Going to classes and workshops, reading, attending professional conferences, and simply asking good questions of those who have good answers—all will help you hone your skills.

A final way to build trust is to be sure you are giving the most accurate response possible to physician inquiry. Don't be afraid to say, "I don't know," but follow up quickly with "I'll find out and get back to you by [specify a time and/or a date]." Then, of course, do so, even if it is to say that you still don't know the answer.[10] That kind of concern for accuracy will build the physician's respect and trust.

Support Your Doctors

I've already talked about the kind of support that comes through loyalty and positive feedback, and, in an odd way, through honesty. However, now I am talking about a different kind of support. As you know, probably better than anyone other than the doctors themselves, their lives are hectic, stress-laden, and emotionally as well as physically draining. There are times when these strains can create seemingly insurmountable obstacles. At these moments, doctors need your support most of all. Build in a mechanism for dealing with physicians' emotional problems, alcoholism, or other addictions, promptly and sympathetically, in an orderly, established manner.

Support doesn't always have to look so serious, however. Often, all your doctors need is the sense that they aren't in this by themselves. I'm reminded of the story of the physician who was running late . . . again. As he dashed in the back door of the office looking harried and hurried and tired, he was met by his office manager. Instead of scowling and growling at him about being late and ruining her schedule, she smiled and handed him a milk shake and a sandwich. "You sit down a minute, Doctor, and eat this. Then we'll take care of those patients." This too is support. Pay attention to the little things.

Clarify Your Decision-Making Authority

If you are a new office manager, then make certain, during the hiring process if possible, what role you are supposed to play in making practice decisions. The continuum offered in Chapter 8 Figure 8–3, will give you a useful tool for charting the doctors' desire for your involvement and the level of participation you would prefer. You should be at or very near the same place on this continuum or your relationship is doomed to having difficulty. You can accept a position in which you think you will be allowed to grow into more responsibility, but you will have to do it slowly over time. When doctors see that they can trust you, they will usually give you more and more authority.

If you are already in an office manager's position, then you need to clarify that position now. One office manager told me about the day that she had to face her physicians with an uncomfortable fact—she was not happy with her decision-making role. Rather than blaming the doctors, however, this manager said, "I think you need a different type of administrator, because I can't do it this way." She confided that her doctors had no idea that she was unhappy or that they had been undercutting her authority. Together they reached an agreement concerning who would do what, and she reported that everything had been worked out satisfactorily.

Meet with the Physicians on a Regular Basis

Many doctors do not consider meetings to be an important part of their jobs. Others regard them as a necessary evil. But very few, if any, actually look forward to sitting down in a meeting with anybody. They would much rather be providing direct patient care. Because of this attitude, you need to use the following suggestions for scheduling meetings:

- Find a convenient time.
- Keep the time and place consistent.
- Anticipate monthly meetings, at which corporate, philosophical, visionary issues will be discussed, to last one to two hours.
- Send a written reminder a day or two before each month's meeting.
- Keep staff informed in case they need to help prepare materials.

■ Hold interim shorter meetings weekly or biweekly to discuss hot-spot items that come up.

In addition to scheduling the meetings, you must also be certain that the time in them is well spent. By following these steps to holding an effective meeting, you can make certain that you do just that.

■ Plan a specific agenda and distribute it in advance.

■ Be certain that topics are of general interest and not something that can be worked out with individuals.

■ On topics that will probably bring about a lot of discussion, institute what is called a "timed discussion." Each person is allowed a specified number of minutes to present his or her point of view. Your group should decide in advance that it will be using timed discussions, and under what conditions. Thus, no one will feel cut off or unvalued when this technique is applied.

■ Attempt to get opinions of all participants by soliciting input when it is appropriate.

■ Have someone take careful notes of the meeting so that you will be able to record these for future reference.

Not all useful dialogue between the office manager and the physicians occurs in formal meetings, however. Office manager Bowen recommended that you go into the doctor's area on a spontaneous, unobtrusive, but frequent basis. Making regular visits to each physician in his or her practice area (consultation room) affords an opportunity for both you and the doctor to express concerns about problems and to discuss opportunities. Bowen cautioned that you should make sure that these visits do not unduly interrupt the physician's schedule,[11] and I would add that you should cease immediately if a doctor asks you to.

In return for the freedom to wander into the doctor's area, you must also make the doctor feel free to wander into yours. Whenever a physician shows up in your office, you can bet there is an important reason. Therefore, take the time to see a physician who stops by. If you have another appointment or an urgent

matter demanding prompt attention, explain the situation and
suggest that you resume the discussion later. Be sure to follow up.

Provide Opportunities for Feedback to the Physicians

Finding ways for the physicians to monitor their own work, and thus
determine their own feedback, produces the best results in behavior
changes. The least effective results come about when others correct
them. So, for example, the installation of a tape recorder to record
their patient interviews (with the patient's permission, of course) will
allow the doctors to hear, and if videotaped, view their own work.
When showing physicians the results of patient surveys, allow them
to draw their own conclusions as much as possible; it will help them
to self-determine areas for improvement. Also, offer positive
feedback to the physicians, but be sure that it is tactful and sincere.
Remember, doctors are just like other people. They need to know that
they are valued and appreciated. They are like others in another way
as well; some of the most difficult are the ones who need positive
feedback the very most.

Be Time-Conscious Yourself

If, in fact, you expect physicians to be aware of time commitments,
you need to do the same. Carry out your own tasks in a timely
manner. Have materials ready for the physician when he or she
asks for them . . . or before! Don't waste the physician's time with
piddly little items that you can handle. Don't allow the staff to do
so either. (Actually, these problems will be all but eliminated by a
clearly defined chart of who decides what and when.) When I
asked one office manager to give me her best advice for building
relationships with doctors, she responded by saying, "Doctors
don't want to hear the whiny, petty things. They just want to
practice medicine. They really don't want to be bothered with, 'She
said that I said, but I didn't.'"

Manage Your Staff Effectively

Doctors do not usually want to be involved in the daily
management of personnel. In fact, most report that this is not

something they enjoy and that they expect their office managers to "handle things." One practice administrator described it this way: "My job is to keep the office running smoothly, to keep the staff motivated and productive, and to allow my doctors to do what they love the most—practice medicine." Another said, "I tell my girls that our jobs are to keep our doctors happy. We are to do whatever it takes to let them concentrate on what only they can provide—effective patient care." If you are leading this parade in the right direction, the physicians should be able to do just that.

Take Care of Yourself!

What does this have to do with building effective relationships with physicians? It's simple. If you are relaxed, in good health, and in a good mood, you will be better able to do all of the above. So, find a hobby. Get adequate exercise. Spend time with your family. Take your vacations and get out of town. Your physicians need you in your top form to help them see that this practice is a successful one.

BUILDING POSITIVE MANAGER/STAFF RELATIONSHIPS

Keeping good staff members is important to your practice. When I was researching this book, I interviewed the office managers of medical practices that were rated high on patient-satisfaction surveys. My assumption was that these people already knew a great deal about service, and I was curious as to what was working for them. The most constant trend in the data, which did not vary across all types of practices, was the longevity of the staff. Employees who are knowledgeable about the practice, both from a business standpoint as well as from a clinical standpoint, are better able to respond to the patients' needs and will make fewer errors. In addition to enhancing the actual performance of service responsibilities, the mere fact that a patient sees familiar faces or that referring doctors can talk to the same nurses creates the impression of stability. High turnover in staff makes people wonder what is wrong. Also, it is costly to hire and train new people, so it is cost effective to keep employees as long as possible. Marriott International estimates that it costs as much as $1,100 to recruit and train each replacement.[12] Your practice doesn't want to face too many of those costs each year.

In a field where the pay is usually low and the stressors are usually high, what keeps staff members motivated, happy, and fulfilled? In other words, what makes them stay? There are many answers to that question, most of which will be discussed in this section. Although the effectiveness of the doctor/staff relationship is a contributing factor in staff longevity, probably the most important is the way the employees are managed, and that is the responsibility of the practice administrator, and in larger clinics also of the supervisors. So, in this section, I will offer some specific suggestions for providing the kind of environment in which your employees will want to stay for years.

Be an Effective Role Model

As I mentioned in Chapter 3, the first lesson of service is that it must begin with the leaders of the practice. Carol H. Jones, RN, president of Health Care Excellence, a healthcare marketing firm recommended, "Treat staff the way you want them to treat patients. A manager who doesn't smile, doesn't make eye contact, doesn't listen, can't expect staff to do the same."[13] I would go even further and say that your role modeling should go deeper than smiles and pleasantries, although those are certainly important. Modeling more subtle behaviors such as initiative, organization, creativity, dedication, and pride in work well done are equally important. The bottom line is that you should be the kind of employee you want your staff to be. They will notice and most will respond in kind.

Hire Well in the First Place

To secure effective employees for your practice, you should be clear as to the attributes you want them to have.

I asked office managers what they looked for in candidates for employment in their practices. Here is what they told me:

"I look for a candidate that demonstrates a *concern for people*."

"I look for a *caring person*."

"I want someone who shows *initiative* and *spunk*."

"There should be indications that the person is a *team player*."

"Friendliness and *courtesy* are top on my list."

Office manager Deborah Goodyear explained a sixth and difficult-to-define element: a gut feeling that the candidate belongs in your practice. She also believes that most employees will determine their own level of comfort and will know quickly whether they belong or not. She has actually paid prospective employees to come in for four hours to see if they would be comfortable in her practice. Ms. Goodyear explained, "After their four hours, we sit down and talk about it. This method has worked out well. Sometimes they say, 'No thank you. That's not for me.' Others say, 'This is exactly what I want!' Then we both have a better idea of whether this will work out or not."

One additional and essential way to discover whether potential employees fit in your practice is to tell the finalists exactly what your practice culture is like. Is yours an informal environment or one of more formality? Do employees have the authority to make certain decisions, and if so what? Is there extensive interaction among all practice personnel or not? For example, in one practice, everyone has the right to question everyone else. Nurses can and do question doctors, staff members can question the manager, and so on. These are not challenges, but queries to provide a double check to reduce errors. Prospective employees would need to know that this kind of behavior is the norm, and should be allowed to decide if it would be a comfortable situation for them. The office manager in that practice described a new physician they had just hired from a large staff-model HMO where no one questioned anyone. She smiled and said, "He's had a little trouble at first getting used to it, but now he values these opportunities to double-check his work."

Two last pieces of advice on hiring:

Take your time. If you can't find someone right away, fill in with temporary employees or pay regular employees overtime until you can search again. It is much easier to handle this temporary upheaval than to deal with the long-term pain of making the wrong hire.

Be willing to pay competitive salaries. If you pay slightly higher than the average you will have a larger pool of qualified candidates from which to choose. If at all possible, offer a salary at least 10 percent above the going rate for that job in your geographical area.[14]

Train the Employees

Office manager Marilyn Haley described her practice's realization that training was the key to creating and keeping good employees. She said, "About three years ago we had a terrible, terrible turnover problem. The management team sat down and said, 'We bring staff members in here, give them about two days of training, and then throw them in the water and see if they can sink or swim.' And they were sinking." Ms. Haley then described a very proactive and effective new employee training program that has worked wonders in helping her employees adapt to the practice and remain involved with it. Their turnover rate was drastically reduced as a result. "We developed an in-house training program, hands-on, every day for two full weeks throughout the practice, and for four weeks in their own area."

This kind of new employee orientation is very important. It gives new employees some structure and some support during their transition into the practice as well as providing an excellent opportunity for clarification of expectations. It also allows office personnel to help incorporate the new member into the practice team. Finally, new-employee orientation provides useful information to the employees and gives an overall impression of how the practice operates. (See the Appendix for an outline of a new-employee orientation plan.)

Training can't stop with orientation, however. It must continue as long as the employee is with your practice. One office manger pointed out that most of the staff members in medical practices are young and need ongoing development and training. Ms. Haley described how her practice continues to invest in its employees on a long-term basis as well. She offers two types of ongoing staff development programs: mini brown bags held once a month and conducted by practice personnel on specific practice-related topics, and Saturday morning workshops held quarterly and usually conducted by people from outside the practice on more general business topics, such as service. Employees are told when they are hired that they are expected to attend a specified number of each of these sessions per calendar year and are allowed to choose the ones they will attend.

I asked Ms. Haley how the staff had responded to this training, and she said, "Very well. We have many people who attend many more sessions than are required. I think that's a sign that they like the opportunity for continuing education." In that regard, Ms. Haley has made those CEUs (Continuing Education Units) official by getting her practice certified through the Colorado Nurses Association to offer CEUs to any appropriate staff who attend. Practice employees report that when they are informed right up front that this ongoing training is a part of their job expectations, when they are given some leeway in choosing the specific training sessions, and when it is paid for by the practice, they are ready and willing to attend. In fact, they are quick to recognize it as an indication of their value to the practice—and an affirmation of them as professionals.

Don't Be Afraid to Terminate Those Employees Who Do Not Work Out

I realize that I just made a serious appeal for keeping employees, but there are times, unfortunately, when the match between your practice, the job, and the employee is not a good one. It is never easy to let someone go. It hurts you and it certainly hurts the employee, at least temporarily. It may also hurt those within the practice with whom the employee has bonded. However, I have seen practices torn apart by one individual who simply did not fit. I have also seen these same individuals suffer endless pain at being forced into a job that was wrong for them. The discomfort these people feel becomes reflected in negative, angry behaviors that can be a disruptive, if not devastating, influence.

The three keys to addressing problematic employee behavior are describe, discuss, and document. You must describe the behaviors and their impact; discuss the situation with the employee on more than one occasion, to either praise or begin the warning process; and document *everything*. Using the following Progressive Discipline Process provides the opportunity for employees to change their problem behavior and provides legal protection for your practice.

When an employee displays problematic behavior, do the following:

Bring the problem to the employee's attention:

- Document the problem when it first comes to your attention.
- Describe what you have observed. Be specific.
- Describe the impact of the behavior on the organization; either on internal or external service or both, on the work flow, and so forth.
- Allow the employee to respond.
- Advise the employee on how the behavior should be changed.
- Express your support and willingness to be of assistance.
- Schedule another meeting to review the situation.
- Document the details of the conference after it is over.

Follow up:

- Coach and encourage the employee as he or she is making the change.
- Document any interactions regarding this issue.
- Warn the employee if there appears to be no change.
  - Informal, oral warning—document!
  - Two written warnings.
  - A final warning, leading to termination.

Terminate (when necessary):

- Check the federal guidelines regarding illegal reasons for dismissal, such as race, religion, and sexual preference.
- Check your state regulations regarding termination and follow them!
- Explain the behavior expectations that were not met and the inappropriate "fit" that seems to exist between the employee and these expectations.
- Give the employee a reasonable time frame for dismissal, usually one to two weeks. (In extreme cases a shorter time frame may be necessary.)

- Document! Document! Document!
- Wish him or her well!

As you can see, the above process involves several face-to-face conferences with the employee. Take care to prepare yourself adequately and keep the following tips in mind during these interactions: (1) Ask yourself "What's my 50 percent? How am I part of the problem?" (2) Whenever possible use "and" versus "but." (3) Be brief and concise. (4) Stay focused on your purpose: to bring about a change in behavior. (5) Separate the behavior from the person: "You are a good person. It's your behavior that is the problem." (6) Address one issue at a time; if more than one, look for a trend or a common thread. (7) Be open to exploring solutions with the employee.

Terminating employees is probably the most difficult part of being a manager. With adequate counseling and coaching, most problematic behaviors can be corrected. However, in those rare but difficult situations when termination is warranted, do it with kindness yet firmness, and make a plan to take care of yourself afterwards. Remember, ultimately, the act of termination was necessary for the overall good of the practice and of the employee involved.

Be Visible and Available

Just as I suggested to the doctors in Chapter 8, you too, as the practice administrator, must be approachable. Your staff needs to know that they can talk to you. One way to ensure that is to maintain an open-door policy. You should never be too busy to listen to your staff. They look to you to be their leader and often their mentor. If you are administering a large practice with supervisors, then, by all means, the employees should be encouraged to work out any problems they might have at the supervisory level. But, just as the physicians should be available to listen to the staff at certain times, you too should be available. No physician wants to hear that the staff member was unable to get at least a hearing from you.

Another good technique is that of managing by walking around. You should never be too busy to say "Hello" to staff and to patients. Try sitting for five minutes in the waiting room, and talk to people. Walk into the back office to see how things are going. Don't disappear into your office, only to be bothered when trouble erupts.

Employees appreciate it when you are present for their events as well. When staff members host a birthday party for a billing clerk or when they have a shower for the receptionist's new baby, it means a lot if you are there too. (Often you will have planned these celebrations yourself.) Develop a sincere interest in your employees and let it show.

Handle the Tough Customer Situations

You should be the troubleshooter in the office. If the practice personnel, including the doctors, all know who is the final authority on what issues, then your staff will know that while they have authority to solve many customer situations, they do not have to deal with the problem cases. Office manager Stolte put it this way: "No one will get along with everybody. I tell my staff, if they have a problem or a difficult situation, 'Don't get upset. Call me and I will help you handle it.'" Another office manager said it clearly: "My staff knows they can count on me to be there when they need me."

Show Appreciation to the Staff

Rewards and recognition will be discussed in detail in Chapter 16. However, as is the case with the physicians, I want to remind you of how important your personal appreciation is to the staff. They need to be told when they are doing a good job and need to be reassured of their value to the successful operation of the practice. "Thank you" costs so little and yet means so much.

Empower Staff to Make Decisions and Solve Problems

Ownership of decisions is enhanced through staff involvement. Clearly, there are medical decisions that no one but the nursing staff, physician's assistant, or the physician can make. However, nonclinical staff should be clearly accorded areas of authority in which they can make decisions. These decisions can cover both customer issues as well as office policies. One office manager explained, "I just tell the staff, 'This is what I need done, now help me figure out a way to do it.' They come back to me with their ideas and often that is what we do."

Help Staff Feel Good about Themselves

This advice came up over and over again in my research for this chapter. How do you do this? By practicing all of the things I've just mentioned. Top on the list is showing your appreciation for their hard work and allowing them to make their own decisions and to solve practice problems. Office manager Brenda Becker of Endocrine Associates in St. Louis said, "People feel good about themselves if you give them a certain amount of authority and let them know you respect their ability to do things on their own."[15]

Keep the staff informed

The best way to accomplish this goal is through regular staff meetings, usually at least once a month. In practices where supervisors are used, the office manager should also hold regular supervisory meetings. The topics at staff meetings are varied, and should include: policy decisions, problem solving, and of course service issues.

The question always comes up, "Should physicians attend staff meetings?" The answers seem to vary. My response is that it probably depends on your practice and on the relationship that exists between your physicians and the staff. Regardless of the physicians' participation, however, the administrator and the staff should meet together on a regular basis. That is the best way to make certain that all are informed.

Other methods for informing the staff exist, of course, and include: memorandums, bulletin board postings, and newsletters. These written forms of communication cannot replace the impact of face-to-face interactions, however.

Be Creative. Be Flexible.

Employees appreciate your understanding of the unique situations that can occur in their lives. You are probably managing a primarily female and primarily youthful work force. The biggest issues facing

most of those young people are school demands and child care.
Thus, if you can consider some creative scheduling ideas, you can
accommodate the needs that accompany these demands.

Job sharing, two employees dividing one full-time position, is
one idea that has worked well for many practices. According to the
April 1995 *Information Exchange* conducted by the MGMA library,
280 responding practices used some form of job sharing, and 217
did not. When asked, "What effect has the job sharing had on
morale?" 112 indicated it was positive, 56 said it had no effect, and
only 4 registered a negative impact. When asked "Has this policy
affected turnover in a positive way?" 103 said "yes," while 43 said
"no."[16]

Some of the comments offered by office managers regarding
job sharing were:

"At present it's been good. Two excellent former full-timers
now work evenings or days."

"We were able to utilize special skills by several employees
in a single position."

"Allowed us to retain female internists during early family
years."

"We have two nursing positions in which long-term
employees wanted to job share. We advertised for the other
half of both positions and the result has been positive for
the four employees involved."

"Three happy people."

"Just knowing that it is available has helped!"

The reactions have not all been positive, however. One
administrator said:

"People don't seem to be able to take their part-time job
seriously; we get a lot of calling in sick, etc."

"It will not work for a part-time student to job share."

"We have done this in the past and found lack of continuity
was a problem; will probably not do it again."

Before starting this approach, I would recommend that you
contact the MGMA library for information on how to make this

plan work successfully. Obviously, for many practices it does.

Flexible scheduling is another creative idea and is offered as an alternative to the regular 8–5 work day. Of those responding to the December 1994 *Information Exchange* by the MGMA, 552 groups said they did use flexible scheduling, and 389 did not. The options used included: eight-hour days within varying blocks of time (e.g., 7:30–4:30; 9:00–6:00)—290 practices; 10-hour days, 4 days a week—230 practices; 9.5-hour days, 4.5 days a week—126 practices.

Managers responded with the following comments regarding flexible scheduling:

"Helps eliminate overtime, accommodates late doctors and patients."

"Each department must vote on flexible option, otherwise only standard eight-hour days allowed."

"Depending on department need, 'creativity' in scheduling is allowed."

"Excellent for retention of working mothers."

"Assured office hours are covered with appropriate staff."

"We feel that flex hours/scheduling is beneficial to company."

As these comments reflect, flexible scheduling is an option that is not necessarily followed by every employee and department in these practices. It seems to be decided on a person-to-person basis and department by department.[17]

One practice administrator described the positive impact on staff loyalty of these creative and flexible approaches: "I believe in working with my staff and I try to accommodate their needs. In return, when I need them, my staff is there for me. If I need someone to stay late or do extra duty, I know I can count on them to help me out."

Keep Employees Up to Date on Their Progress

One of the most difficult and controversial methods of management, the performance appraisal, if handled well, is an important component for helping employees know what is expected of them and how they are progressing as a staff member in your practice.

The reason these appraisals can be hard is that they mean a face-to-face conversation about areas for improvement, which is not always received in the most positive manner.

Practices that use performance appraisals give them mixed reviews. One manager said, "They are helpful in letting good employees know they are doing a good job" while another believes that they "were not always productive—employees may consider them of little value." Still a third commented, "Employees and doctors dislike these immensely."

So, why should you engage in this practice, if it is controversial? There are several reasons. One, as the above office manager stated, it is a very helpful tool in reinforcing positive behaviors in good employees. Two, it provides a structured way to give constructive criticism. No employee is perfect, and we all need to know where and how to improve. It is part of your job as the manager to provide this kind of corrective feedback to your employees. Three, motivated employees do not like to work in a vacuum and actually want feedback, even if it points out a problem. As one such staff member in a high-trauma practice explained, "I know in the crush of each day, I overlook things. I appreciate someone pointing them out to me, because I care about doing a good job." Four, in the unfortunate situation in which an employee should be terminated, the performance appraisal provides a documented record of your attempts to correct the deficient behaviors.

Since these are important reasons for conducting performance appraisals, how can you do it as painlessly as possible? I do have a few suggestions:

■ Keep the forms user-friendly for both the employee and the manager. I have seen some forms that are so complicated that the content of the feedback becomes secondary to merely understanding the forms. I've also seen some that are so lengthy that the individual becomes overwhelmed in feedback, not knowing which is the most important nor where to start first in processing it.

■ Make the forms easy to read. This means they should be printed clearly and legibly. Again, I have seen some forms so faded and difficult to read that the entire exercise was diminished in importance.

■ Terms should be clearly and simply defined. Employees need to know exactly on what they are being evaluated. Since, as we know, meanings vary from person to person, terms should be defined. Punctuality, for example, needs to be defined as "arriving at work at a specified time."

■ Allow for positives as well as areas for improvement. Just as no one is perfect, neither is any employee all bad. So, be certain that the form and that the discussion of the appraisal with the employee contains positive feedback.

■ The form should include a *Comments* section, and it should be completed. Most people prefer to have more than a check mark in an appropriate box. Rather, they like to hear and read the words of the person performing the appraisal.

■ The form should include a section for an *Action Plan* in which you specify actions you'd like to see the employee take before the next appraisal. Most employees will attempt to do what you ask of them, if they know what that is. Your performance appraisal should reflect specific steps or actions you want the employee to take.

■ When giving feedback during the appraisal session, start with some positives and then move to the areas for improvement. Most people want to know that they are not total disasters. Of course, few are, but when their performance appraisals begin with the negatives, they can quickly conclude that this is the case. The positive comments will help make the receivers of the feedback more receptive to the suggestions for improvement.

■ Inform employees about the performance appraisals. These events should not be a surprise. Employees need to know the purpose of the appraisals, the approach used, the frequency (usually every six months or annually), and even be allowed to have a copy of the form to be used.

■ When introducing the performance appraisal in a practice where one has not has existed before, allow the employees to participate in the creation of the form. Again, ownership of the process will help to minimize its threat. As they participate in structuring the form, employees can begin to see the value of the appraisal.

■ Make certain that the performance appraisal occurs as scheduled. Employees need to know that these appraisals are important. By following a regular schedule, such as every

December, you will let the employees know when to expect them and that you consider them important.

■ Have employees conduct a self-appraisal. This not only helps the employees to pause for careful self-examination but also helps them to understand that these processes are not so easily done. When you and the employee differ, then discuss the difference. Most employees will rate themselves lower than you will. It is a fact of human nature, I believe, that we tend to be harder on ourselves.

■ Consider having employees conduct appraisals of their supervisors and/or of you. This idea is even more controversial than the employee performance appraisals. Office managers comment that most employees don't know how to do this and that their responses become opportunities for getting back at someone who had to discipline them. On the other hand, if you and your staff have the kind of relationship that you are hoping to create by following the steps in this chapter, then you shouldn't have anything to fear. It seems only fair that if you are going to give feedback to your employees that they should be able to do the same for you. Besides, they constitute a part of your internal customer population, and you need to know how to serve them most effectively. (Contact the MGMA Library for samples of: performance appraisals, employee surveys, and physicians' surveys. Phone: (303) 397-7887; (303) 799-1111.)

So, the office administrator has a huge job when it comes to managing the staff. Staff employees are important contributors to the success of your practice. Building and maintaining positive relationships with them is your responsibility, yet it need not be a chore. The above steps will help you in making your association with your employees happy, pleasant, and productive for all concerned.

COMMUNICATING WITH YOUR DOCTORS

Probably the most frequently asked question in my workshops for office managers is, "How can I get my ideas across to my doctors?" So, let's pause here a moment to discuss the Ten Commandments for conveying your ideas to your physicians.

1. *Thou shalt have done thy homework!* Before even starting to structure a message to your doctors, make the following considerations:

    a. Why should these physicians, this group, accept or implement this change?

    b Why might they resist?

    c. Is this change or its ramifications an inevitable reality for this group?

2. *Thou shalt be brief!* As one office manager put it, "Each doctor is different from the other, that's for sure. But one thing they all have in common is that they are busy." Understanding this fact should give you some instant ideas in how to reach them: Be brief. Be concise. Get to the point.

3. *Thou shalt offer proof and documentation.* Doctors are trained in the scientific process, which means that they value data. Don't come to them with intuitive notions. Doctors usually are not swayed by that kind of thinking. They want to see the proof. By the same token, doctors also know the limitations of data. They need to know the strengths and weaknesses of the information. One office manager said, "I use the patient satisfaction surveys as an administrative tool. When I go in to talk to my doctors and say, 'You know, I don't think the patients are going to like this,' they tend to ignore me. But when I have the results of the surveys, I can document my claims. The docs listen to that."

4. *Thou shalt be organized!* Doctors are accustomed to a structured, usually sequential-thinking process. Thus, present your ideas in a coherent, organized format. Most of your messages seek a decision, so you are trying to persuade the physicians to your way of thinking. Give them reasons for doing so.

5. *Thou shalt use the most relevant arguments.* Doctors are trained to think about patient care first. Thus, arguments that show them how a certain action will impact the quality of that care will be persuasive to them. Also, they are concerned about the two most precious resources in any medical practice: income and time. If you can show ways to increase the former and maximize the latter and not negatively impact patient care, you will have their attention. For example, in addition to discussing the price of surgical equipment, the manager could also represent the ways that the equipment will save time and be advantageous to the patient. In a session I conducted at the 1996 national PAHCOM conference, two more relevant arguments were suggested: impact on staff and improving the quality of the physician's life, usually how he or she can carve out more time.

6. *Thou shalt use both verbal and visual means for communicating.* Interpersonal, face-to-face interaction is important when communicating with doctors because it allows for an exchange of ideas, which they like. Also, these dialogues should be accompanied by visual reinforcements such as written outlines, slides, overheads, or written materials to clarify your position.

7. *Thou shalt allow doctors to exert as high a degree of autonomy as possible.* When providing performance feedback to doctors, for example, allow them to choose their own method for improvement. Professionals are much happier when they can correct their own performance. When problem solving, also allow the physicians as much autonomy in the solution as possible. Lay out the goals of the office, explain the expectations and why they are needed, and then work with the physicians on improving the situation. This may mean that you will need to try things their way for a while. One office manager described the process she uses this way: "Sometimes the doctors need to see if their ideas will work or not. So, I'll do what they say for a while, gather my data, and then go back. 'We tried it your way and here are the results. Now let's do it my way a while.' We usually end up putting my ideas in place."

8. *Thou shalt use comparative data.* Doctors are interested in how they and their practices compare to others. So, using data that will provide comparison to peers or a generally accepted norm is particularly effective. Graphs are especially useful visualizations of comparative data.

9. *Thou shalt not speak "managerialese."* Remember that while their vocabulary regarding medical terminology is especially impressive to the lay person's ear, most doctors are not familiar with the language of business and management. Thus, use simple, everyday language and invite questions.

10. *Thou shalt look the part!* When communicating with your doctors, be certain that you dress professionally, that you look and sound confident, and that you avoid excessive gesturing. If you

have to err, err on the side of conservatism. Appearance extends to the visual presentation of your ideas as well. Any written materials, charts, graphs, or overheads should be neat and professional looking.

By the time your practice's parade reaches the end of its daily route, no wonder you are exhausted. But if you have led your practice in the right direction, kept up a lively, consistent tempo, and provided encouragement to even the most awkward of marchers, then you can rest assured that your efforts have been worthwhile. I will always remember the look in the eyes of one office manager who had just recounted her numerous daily responsibilities. Instead of weariness I saw pride. When she said, "Vicky, I LOVE it!" I knew that it was true.

END NOTES

1. Elizabeth Kubler Ross, *On Death and Dying*, (NY: Macmillan Publishing Co., 1969), pp. 38–157.

2. "Florida Manager Carries a Two Physician Practice to 10 Doctors and 80 Staff," *Medical Office Management* 9, no. 3 (May/June 1996), pp. 6–7.

3. David Bowen, Jr., "A Matter of Tenure," *Medical Group Management* 32, no. 6 (November/December 1985), p. 21. Reprinted with permission of the Medical Group Management Association, 104 Inverness Terrace East, Englewood, CO 80112-5306; (303) 799-1111. Copyright 1985.

4. Frank J. Weinstock, *The Ophthalmology Office Manual* (Columbus, Ohio: Anadem Publishing, 1993). © Anadem Publishing , Inc. (800) 633-0055.

5. Barbara Linney, "Changes in the Practice of Medicine," *Physician EXECUTIVE* 19, no. 6 (November/December 1993), pp. 59, 63.

6. Janet Reich, "Recognizing and Overcoming Barriers: Physician/Hospital Relationship Building," *MGM Journal* 38, no. 4 (July/August 1991), p. 71.

7. Mark Shields, M.D., "The Physician/Administrator Team Revisited," *MGM Journal* 41, no. 5 (September/October 1994), p. 10.

8. Richard Thompson, *Keys to Winning Physician Support: A Guide for Executives and Managers* (Tampa, Florida: The American College of Physician Executives, 1991), p. 19.

9. Bowen, p. 21.

10. Ibid.

11. Ibid.

12. Ronald Henkoff, "Finding, Training, Keeping the Best Service Workers," *Fortune* 130, no. 9 (October 3, 1994), p. 114.

13. "Guidelines to Follow for Better Patient Satisfaction," *Medical Office Manager* 5, no. 4 (April 1991), p. 5.

14. Steven Wood, "Your Office Staff: First Market for Group Practice," *Group Practice Journal* 39, no. 2 (March/April 1990), pp. 54–55.

15. "Office Manager Tips on Running the Practice," *Physician's Marketing & Management* 7, no. 2 (February 1994), p. 17.

16. "Work Schedules/Job Sharing," *MGMA Information Exchange*, #4762 (April 1995).

17. "Work Schedules/Flexible Schedules," *MGMA Information Exchange*, #4698 (December 1994).

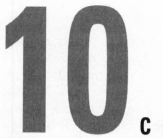

CHAPTER

Step Ten—Embrace the Role of the Staff

A TRIBUTE TO MRS. FARWELL

Grace Farwell was her name. She was the receptionist in my childhood family physician's office and I vividly remember her to this day. I can still see her long gray hair bound neatly into what we now call a french twist, and her capable, efficient stride as she disappeared into the back office to see if Dr. Bayles was ready for me. The most vivid recollection I have of her, however, is of her special way of making me feel that I mattered. The attention she paid to me, the way she looked directly into my eyes when we talked, her sincere and quiet smile—all of these things told me that she cared. I have long since moved from that Kansas town where I was raised and I have no idea what has happened to Mrs. Farwell in the following years. I hope somehow that she knows that she is remembered and that once on a time she made a difference. Going to the doctor when you are a child, and even when you aren't, can be a frightening experience. I'd like her to know that she made me feel safe.

THE STAFF CAN MAKE THE DIFFERENCE

Perhaps in the hustle and bustle of healthcare today, you may not believe that the staff in a medical practice can impact anyone's life in any significant way. Yet, staff can and most certainly do. The clinical and nonclinical staff are essential to the successful operation of any medical practice. I can offer more than my anecdotal story of Mrs. Farwell to support this claim. Patient satisfaction surveys are structured not only to measure reactions to the physicians, but also to the staff. Items such as "Telephone courtesy," "attitude of staff," "friendliness of receptionist," are commonly found on these instruments and are of considerable interest when the complete patient experience is being evaluated. In addition, as I indicated in Chapter 2, staff members can have an impact on a patient's decision to sue. This was laid out quite clearly in an article entitled, "Don't Let Staff Push Patients into Malpractice Suits:" "Office staff play a significant role in today's malpractice picture. While it's rare that an office employee singlehandedly causes a malpractice suit, staff can and do tip many a litigious patient over the edge. Conversely, it's also staff who keep a good number of lawsuits from happening."[1] So, from the patients' points of view, you have a direct impact on their satisfaction and even on their decisions to file a lawsuit.

Even more important, you can play an interesting role in patient recovery and compliance with treatment. Whether you are aware of it or not, many patients report feeling a special connection with their physicians' practices and all who work there. In the vulnerability of illness or injury, they often want to bond with you, and they will work hard to hear your praise. One woman reported, "The staff at my doctor's office was great! They encouraged me every step of the way. I wanted to do all that I could so that I would have a good report the next time I went in." Whether you have the opportunity to develop an ongoing relationship or not, your very presence on any given visit can soothe an aching back or calm a frightened soul.

From the physician's point of view, you are important as well. Perhaps the doctors in your practice don't tell you very often, but they tell me. In Chapter 8, I have encouraged your physicians to leave out the middleman (or woman in this case) and convey their appreciation directly to you. In the meantime, however, let me share what some doctors have told me about the value of their staff:

"I have an efficient and caring staff."

"I don't know what I'd do without them. They keep me going."

"I appreciate what they do for me and for the patients."

Doctors and patients aren't the only ones who speak of your value. Practice administrators also are aware that they need motivated, efficient, friendly staff. Perhaps these words from an office manager I interviewed will sum up this point most clearly: "I don't know what I would do without my people. They bolster me when I'm down, carry on when I can't, and could make this practice run even if I weren't here."

In fact, although perhaps you aren't aware of it because most people don't tell you, everyone who comes into contact with your office measures it in large part based on their interactions with you. From the front office to the back, from the face-to-face interactions to those on the telephone, patients and their families, insurance company representatives, hospital nurses and admitting clerks, managers, doctors and staff from other practices—all interact with you and your colleagues more than anyone else in your office. Their impressions of you, in many cases, are their only impressions of the practice. You matter. Believe me. You matter a great deal.

BUILDING POSITIVE PATIENT/STAFF RELATIONSHIPS

Since staff members in a physician's office often are the primary contacts for the patients, the kind of relationship you can build with this customer population is important. In preparation for writing this chapter, I interviewed both clinical and nonclinical personnel as well as patients. The following suggestions are based on what these people told me regarding the patient/staff relationship:

Be Nice

I heard this descriptor over and over. When asked to define the word *nice*, here is what some staff members told me:

"What it all boils down to is this: people just want to be treated with respect and kindness."

"Be kind. I have no tolerance for rudeness to patients."

"Friendly. I think patients appreciate a smile, even and maybe especially when they are sick."

Patients also had descriptors of *nice*:

"Pleasant."
"Friendly. Welcoming."
"Smiling."
"Gentle."
"Attentive."

Be careful of being too cheery, however. John Edgarton, M.D., a family practice physician, in Friendswood, Texas, told about one very bubbly receptionist who teasingly said to a patient: "So, are you going to live?" The patient responded, choking back the tears, "The doctor thinks I might have cancer."[2]

Perhaps my niece, who is a nurse, summed it up best when she said, "I just try to treat them the way I would want to be treated." Sounds a little like the Golden Rule, doesn't it: "Do unto others as you would have them do unto you." Not bad advice for staff interactions with patients.

Don't Get Mad at Your Patients, Even If It's Tempting to Do So

When it comes to the word *patient*, perhaps it is best applied to what staff members have to be. Remember that you are often dealing with mad, sad, or scared individuals. When people are angry, unhappy, or frightened, they are not usually at their best. Often they will strike out at the nearest perceived source of their trouble. Although you are not responsible for their illnesses, nor are you usually the one who makes final decisions about issues of cost and payment, you are often the most available individual on whom the patients can unload their emotions. I don't mean that you should endure untoward patient abuse. No one should be expected to do that. What I do mean is that you must be able to distance yourself from angry responses and see them for what they are.

One of the most effective methods for accomplishing this is called the Wall Technique, and it is best used to avoid catching the full force of someone else's anger. I have used it myself and can vouch for its effectiveness. As is the case with many such techniques, it requires self-talk. You merely tell yourself, "I am not going to let that anger in," and envision a strong brick wall rising up to protect you. The wall comes only chest high, however, because you need to be able to see the person on the other side. When I used this technique, I was amazed at how clearly I could see what was really happening. I felt incredibly safe in my own knowledge that this was not about me but was merely a reflection of the other person's pain.

Another visualization technique is one I call the Dodge. Basically, it also gives you a way to prevent the anger from hitting you full force. You visualize yourself just stepping neatly to the side while the emotion you want to avoid goes right past you. Whether you respond well to such exercises or not, the key is to do something to keep the patient's emotional reaction from hitting you. Then you will be able to understand it better, because you will not have the desire to protect yourself by becoming angry in return.

Be Encouraging

Patients need all the encouragement that you can offer. In an earlier chapter, I referred to a focus group participant who related the story of her experience in an orthopedics office. The staff members were so unsupportive that she was left feeling very discouraged. Fortunately, she is not the kind of person who gives up easily, or the comments she received would have caused her to quit trying, not something a patient in physical therapy should do.

There is a fine line between being unrealistically optimistic and openly pessimistic. Rather than focusing on how far she had to go, the staff members in the above-mentioned practice needed to focus on how far she had come. This patient had spent hours of pain at the hands of her physical "terrorist" ("Hate them now, love them later!"). She had graduated from a wheelchair, to crutches, to a cane, to no aid at all. Rather than commenting on her limp, which these folks did, they should have praised her for how well she had done. There can be no harm in doing that and it could have helped this woman a great deal.

Be Tuned in to Your Patients as Individuals

A nurse I interviewed told me about one patient, a farmer. On this occasion, after carefully explaining the side effects of a newly prescribed medication, the staff member had the clear impression that the patient had not understood. When he asked the patient if he had any questions, the response was, "Yes. I have to go home and feed the cows tonight. Will I be able to do that? I have to feed them cows you know." By being aware of the patient's life and what is important to him, this nurse could have addressed that concern first, thus opening up the chances that the patient would comprehend the rest of the message.

I realize that in busy practices, especially those in a city, firsthand knowledge of the patients may be difficult, if not impossible. In that case, it is important to avoid the opposite reaction—stereotyping. When you are unable to see patients as individuals, then you are quite likely to see them as a group. A lively discussion ensued between two residents at an inner city hospital who were attending one of my workshops. One of the residents said she was unconcerned as to why the patient in our case study had come to the hospital; this patient was, after all, just "one of those indigent city dwellers who don't know how to care for themselves anyway." All this doctor-in-training wanted to do was to treat the symptoms. Her point of view was challenged by a quiet young man in the corner who spoke softly but carried a big message: "I don't know, but it seems to me we have to care about why *this* patient is here. If her injuries are due to domestic violence, which they could have been, based on the diagnostic data, then it tells us a lot about the appropriate treatment." Being willing to know about the patients, to get to know as much as you can in the limited time you have, will help you to help them.

In an emergency, if you don't have the time to obtain personal information about a patient, learn all you can about that moment and that interaction. Watch their eyes, their facial expressions, their body language. A lot of important information will be carried in those nonverbal channels.

Don't Socialize or Argue in the Public Areas of the Office

When I asked a focus group to name one thing they would change about their doctor's office, I was amazed to hear their comments:

"I would stop the staff from socializing. They spend more time talking about what they are going to wear on Saturday night than they do talking to me."

"I am tired of hearing all that bickering. It makes me wonder about the kind of care I'm getting."

"I think in their attempt to create a relaxed environment, the staff thinks their social conversation will help. It doesn't. I feel ignored."

Save your social comments and your disagreements for the appropriate place and time: away from the patients.

Be Involved in Patient Education

Patients have many questions. They want to know about their condition, about their medication, even about their insurance coverage. The office staff personnel are often the ones to provide all of the above and more. Many times, the patients do not understand what the doctor tells them, and they are reluctant to ask him or her questions. So, after the physician has departed, it is not unusual for the patient to look at a staff member and ask, "What did he say?"

A part of educating patients is to give them honest answers to their questions. They want to know what is going to happen to them, if this procedure is going to hurt, if that medication is going to have side effects. They even want to know their prognosis. Honesty should start with the physicians. However, whether the doctors do it or not, the patients will look to you to tell them the truth, and, although some physicians might disagree with this advice, in most instances you should be willing to respond. Please read Chapter 14 for advice on how to do this, even when the news you have is not good. Perhaps the best rule of thumb is this: Do not volunteer information, but if a patient asks directly, give him or her a direct and honest answer. If you believe that even this advice might cause problems for you with the attending doctor, then at the very least convey to that physician the patient's expressed wishes for honesty.

One of the biggest sore spots with medical practice personnel is the load they seem to carry for the health plans. In my workshops, I hear this repeatedly. While many plans are doing a much better job of member education, there are some facts regarding insurance that are almost unavoidable. The truth is that most people, regardless of the type of insurance—automobile, home owners, or another type—don't really know how it works or the benefits they've purchased. Most of us don't pay much attention to our policies until we actually have to use them. Then we have lots of questions. Unfortunately for you, where do patients need their health insurance? When they are in the doctor's office. So, whom do they ask? The closest possible person. You.

In addition, you may be unaware of another fact: to many patients you are the health plan. In nonstaff models, most members do not actually see their health plan representatives, so they have no human face to connect with that organization. Thus, when they think of the health plan, it is understandable that they would think of the people they see, and those are the staff in the doctor's office.

I do have some encouraging words for you, though. If you are in an area that is just beginning to feel the impact of managed care, don't despair. Your colleagues in other parts of the country who have experienced managed care for some time report that patients do learn over time, and that terms such as *co-pay*, *PCP*, and *referral* have to be explained less often. Also, as I mentioned previously, many health plans are doing a much better job with member education. For example, Scott and White Health Plan in Temple, Texas, calls each new member to provide individual explanations, answer any questions, and provide a specific health plan contact person. Finally, most health plans want you to encourage patients to call the Membership Services Departments with their questions.

For the foreseeable future, however, at least some of the burden will continue to fall on the shoulders of the staff members in the medical practices. In Chapter 6, I offered some specific recommendations on how to work effectively with managed care. These suggestions will help you meet the needs of this new, secondary customer of your practice while also meeting the needs of your patients and providing ways to lighten your managed care load.

Listen to the Patients

As I indicated in Chapter 7, listening is the most ignored communication skill of all. It is even understandable why the staff members in a medical practice would fall into some bad listening habits. Probably the most prominent reason for tuning out a patient is that you have heard the story before. Sometimes the tale has been told by the same person over and over again, and sometimes many patients have very similar stories to tell. Often the result can be that you pretend to be listening when you really aren't, or you interrupt and finish the story for the patient, or you label the story as uninteresting and stop paying attention.

Yet, listening to the patient is key to building and maintaining a positive relationship. When the same patients tell the same stories over and over, stop and ask yourself "Why are they doing this?" Usually the answer is that they want someone to care about them and/or they want someone with whom to share their fears. By repeating the story over and over, they hope to find that reassurance they are seeking. When you have heard the same story but by different patients, try to remind yourself that it is the first time *this* patient has been able to tell his or her story *that* day. In short, when you understand *why* the patients are doing what they are doing and can empathize with their feelings, it becomes much easier to listen. Also, remember that a few well-placed questions can move the storyteller along and also show your interest.

Look the Part

Patients expect the staff in a medical practice to be clean, neat, and well groomed. They like to see uniforms, at least on the medical personnel. They do not want to see many pierced body parts nor do they expect to see jeans and T-shirts. They want to trust you. They need to trust you. Your credibility begins with how you look. (Review the section in Chapter 7 on Nonverbal Communication Tools).

BUILDING POSITIVE STAFF–PHYSICIAN RELATIONSHIPS

When interviewing practice personnel for this book, I asked one experienced practice employee what advice he had regarding a staff member's role in creating a positive relationship with the physicians. He responded, "Do it right, don't screw it up, and don't complain about it." In general, that response probably sums it up pretty well. However, I do have some additional and related suggestions that will help you do your part in creating a positive relationship with your physicians.

Know Your Physicians

Just as I advised the office managers in the previous chapter, resist the temptation to believe that all physicians are alike; they are not, and what will be right for one may not be right for another. As one nurse told me, "You have to learn each one and what they like and then try to offer it." Another put it this way: "It really is my responsibility to learn my doctors' preferences about things. I shouldn't expect them to adapt to me; I should adapt to them." Still another staff member told me, "I even have to learn how to talk to each one of my doctors. With some I can be direct and say exactly what I think and with others I have to be more subtle." By learning the preferences, communication styles, and personalities of each individual doctor, you can indicate your desire to meet their needs. In an interesting way, the doctor may be your most important customer.

Earn the Doctors' Respect

Respect is built on many factors, but one of the most important to most physicians is your professional expertise. The doctors expect you to be able to do the job for which you were hired. One physician told me, "I don't expect to have to teach the staff members what they should already know. I don't have the time for that. I expect them to know what they are doing." However, if you don't know something, don't be afraid to ask. Both physicians and staff members have underscored the importance of that step. One doctor said, "I'd rather have the staff member ask a question than to muddle through. But once I explain it, I expect them to remember."

Doctors tell me that one way you can demonstrate your skill is not just to meet their needs but to anticipate them. "I like it when I don't even have to tell my staff what I need; they *just know*." How do you just know? By knowing your doctor as an individual and by being proficient in your own job skills.

Another way to show your own expertise is to take good care of the patients. Although doctors don't get a lot of voluntary feedback from their patients, they do hear about problems with staff. One doctor told me, "I don't like to be bothered with complaints about my staff. I shouldn't have to be. If my staff members are doing their jobs, I won't be." While that may not always be the case, most of the time it is. If you are providing good clinical and nonclinical care to the patients, the chances are that the doctors won't hear negative comments. If they do, it will be the exception and will probably be seen as a patient-specific situation and not a chronic staff problem.

Don't Be Afraid of Your Doctors

In Chapter 8, I asked doctors not to be intimidating to the staff members. By the same token, you should not be afraid of them. This is probably more of a problem for new employees than for more experienced personnel. One staff member told me, "When I first started working here, I couldn't even talk. I had to get over that. Nine times out of ten doctors just want you to talk to them." Physicians want and deserve your respect; they don't want or need your fear.

Be Concise

Even though each doctor is a unique individual and should be seen that way, they do share one common fact: they are all busy. So, just as I advised the office managers in Chapter 9, you need to remember that when communicating with them. One nurse put it this way, "They've got 36 hours of work to do in 24. So, you've got to give them the facts, concisely and directly." Another staff member said, "They are pulled in all directions! The quicker you can give them the facts and tell them what you need, the better."

Be Positive

Doctors do not want to hear your complaints, nor do they want to hear employee bickering. In fact, the first important staff attribute mentioned by several physicians with whom I spoke was, "Pleasantness." One staff member explained: "If you never say anything bad about anybody else, then you never have to take it back." That's pretty good advice.

Be Interested in the Doctors as People

While that may sound like a blinding flash of the obvious, you may be surprised at how few doctors are viewed by their staff as just another human being. Sometimes due to the image associated with the professional status doctors have acquired, sometimes due to the doctor's demeanor itself, and sometimes simply due to the staff members' own insecurity, this fact becomes overlooked. While you will not and should not become buddies with your doctors, it does help your working relationship if you know some things about them as people. What is your doctor's hobby? Is the doctor married, and if so, does he or she have children? What unusually difficult stresses might the doctor be under at this point in time? Although no one in a medical practice has much time for social chitchat, it does help to be able to have some more casual conversations during the day. One receptionist told me of the interest one of her doctors had in sailing. So, she kept her eyes open for articles about this topic and brought them in for his perusal. She said, "He appreciated my effort to find out about him as a person and we have a wonderful working relationship."

Always Conduct Yourself as a Professional

What do I mean by that? The following list will touch on some of the so-called little things that go into creating that impression. Many of the ideas came from *The Ophthalmology Office Manual* and were preceded by this statement: "Little things can make the difference. Hundreds of details added together can produce a wonderful impression—or a disappointing one."

- Keep your uniform clean and well pressed.
- Abide by the smoking policies of your office.
- Practice excellent grammar.
- Give a friendly greeting to everyone.
- Call people by their names.
- No food or drinks should be visible to patients.
- Don't chew gum on the job.
- Close all doors and drawers completely.

- Wash your hands appropriately when with patients.
- Always have fresh breath and clean fingernails.
- Keep your working area clean and neat.
- Never complain in front of patients.
- Give each patient and staff member a sincere compliment every day.
- Make a written note of every problem situation—consult the Practice Administrator.
- Don't be satisfied with your present skills—insist on learning more from others in the office, from reading, and from lectures and courses.
- Never tell a patient "We are too busy to help"—find a way!
- Express gratitude to the patient for coming to the office.
- Don't engage in social conversation with other staff members in patient's presence.
- Do not talk about patients in any but a professional manner.
- Respect the importance of confidentiality and do not discuss patients in front of each other.
- Do not leave charts and files in plain view where they can be easily read by unauthorized individuals.[3]

While the doctors may not even seem to notice that you do these and other things, believe me they do. They are quick to point out the problems they have with staff, and almost always these complaints focus on areas such as these. Once in a while, doctors comment on a staff member's technical expertise or lack thereof, but most staff problems have to do with nontechnical kinds of behaviors, not the actual performance of the tasks involved with a given job.

BUILDING POSITIVE STAFF–ADMINISTRATOR RELATIONSHIPS

You can please your office manager by doing everything I've mentioned for so far in this chapter. You are the responsibility of the manager. How you relate to the patients and other customers, as well as how you interact with and support your physicians, will either make his or her life much easier or much more complicated. So, do your best to relate well to all those with whom you come into contact.

The *Ophthalmology Office Manual* outlined several guidelines for being an excellent employee, and I have added some of my own. If you follow them, you probably won't go wrong.

- Assist your office in providing excellent healthcare.
- Be supportive of the physicians' efforts.
- Keep lines of communication open.
- Utilize time to the fullest.
- Perform work accurately.
- Follow the rules of the office.
- Have a positive attitude.
- Do the best job possible in an enthusiastic, polite manner.
- Show interest in your job and take initiative to learn more.
- Assist your fellow employees whenever possible.
- Be gracious and helpful to all patients.
- Greet every person by name and in a friendly way. Adult patients should not be called by their first names unless the patient asks you to do so.
- Compliment others freely.
- Do not use harsh words—they accomplish nothing except to satisfy the ego of the angry person.
- Accept feedback in a positive manner.
- Inspire others to do the right thing.
- Let patients know they are appreciated.
- Promote the excellence of your practice's services to your patients and to others.
- Competence inspires confidence—do a great job!
- Do not talk about others behind their backs; do not tolerate that behavior in others.
- Providing excellent healthcare is the job of the practice. You are an essential member of the team.[4]

I hope you read this list carefully. I can guarantee you that if you incorporate these suggestions into your daily behaviors at the practice, you will have a positive relationship with your practice administrator as well as with everyone else!

One additional note: Learn how to receive feedback! In my workshops for office managers, one of the issues that comes to the surface quite often is how to give constructive criticism to employees. In Chapter 9, I offered some suggestions for doing that. A part of the success of this process, however, rests with you. Office managers have the responsibility of pointing out problems when they occur. You have the responsibility for receiving this feedback in the spirit in which it is offered: To help you become a better employee. By looking at such feedback as an opportunity to grow, you can help make this process go more smoothly for both you and the manager.

Some suggestions for positive reception of feedback are: (1) Listen rather than respond. (2) Avoid interrupting. (3) Acknowledge the sender's feelings. (4) Ask for specifics if they are not offered: examples, descriptions of the behavior, and so forth. (5) Avoid defending or justifying your behavior. (6) Ask for specific desired changes (staying focused on behaviors) if they are not offered. (7) Suggest an alternative behavior if appropriate. (8) Agree on future behaviors and the follow-up plan. (9) Apologize if appropriate. (10) Acknowledge the sender for giving you feedback.

Also, learn how to take a compliment! We are conditioned not to let such feedback into our psyches, or at the very least we are taught to discount it! I urge you to be open to the positive reinforcements offered by your managers and others. Take them in! And only respond with "Thank you. I appreciate hearing that!"

BUILDING POSITIVE COWORKER RELATIONSHIPS

I cannot leave this chapter on staff relationships without at least mentioning those you have with your colleagues. Although in Chapter 10 I will go into detail on how to work together as an effective practice team, let me list a few important items for your consideration at this time.

- Be willing to help each other in times of need.

- Don't gossip.
- Address differences directly and with a problem-solving orientation.
- Pull your fair share of the load. Do your job.
- Be friendly.

As coworkers, you need each other. I have seen too many small work units destroy themselves by violating the suggestions listed above. Yet, you can prevent a great deal of difficulty for everyone by following this advice.

The comments in this chapter may well sound like you should be all things to all people. To some extent, that's almost true. However, the most important person you should be all things to is yourself. Take good care of yourself. Believe in your own value and the value of what you do. Then, you will be able to be the kind of staff member that can impact, in a positive way, all of the lives around you.

END NOTES

1. "Don't Let Staff Push Patients into Malpractice Suits," *Medical Office Manager* 7, no. 1 (January 1993), p. 1.
2. John Edgarton, "Ten Rules We Don't Let Our Assistants Break," *Medical Economics* 71, no. 12 (June 27, 1994), pp. 66–68.
3. Frank Weinstock, *The Ophthalmology Office Manual*, (Columbus, Ohio: Anadem Publishing, 1993), p. I-8 (© Anadem Publishing, Inc. (800) 633-0055).
4. Ibid., p. I-9

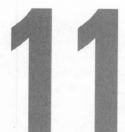

CHAPTER

Step Eleven—Create an Effective Practice Team

"**G**ive me a *T*! Give me an *E*! And an *A* and an *M*! What does that spell? Team! What? **Team!** Louder! **TEAM!!**"

Probably all of us have joined in with a cheer like this to cajole, elicit, or demand the kind of team play that would win a ball game. It also is my cheer to you as you bring about a medical practice that will be focused on service. It takes everyone, *each* one, working together in an extraordinary way to serve all practice customers.

CHARACTERISTICS OF AN EFFECTIVE MEDICAL PRACTICE TEAM

Actually, the use of the team approach is not completely new to doctor's offices. The medical personnel in many practices have formed "treatment teams," usually composed of a physician, a physician's assistant, nurse, and/or nurse practitioner, who work together to meet the patients' clinical needs. These teams are task teams and are similar to, although not exactly like, the type of team to which this chapter refers.

For my model, you will need to go back to your high school or college days when you were probably a member of, or cheered for, some kind of extracurricular team: athletic teams, debate teams, even chess teams. These teams were bound together by a common function, as are the task teams described above; however, they were also characterized by something more. These teams, if they were effective, had a sense of themselves as more than just a group of people gathered together to perform a task. They experienced an intangible sense of team spirit that transcended their common function. They also enjoyed a public perception of success.

If your practice is to experience that feeling of *team*, then you need to do more than share tasks. You need to feel pride in who you are as a practice, have a mutual commitment to your mission, and share a deep dedication to the reason you have chosen careers in healthcare. Several characteristics operationalize these attributes.

An Effective Practice Team Has a Clearly Defined Practice Culture

An *organizational culture* is defined as "the inner values, rites, rituals, and heroes that strongly influence the group's success, from top management to the secretarial pool."[1] Many of these aspects of your practice can be clarified in a well-organized, carefully crafted office manual, such as the one I've mentioned previously: *The Ophthalmology Office Manual.*[2]

Also, the culture is created by the unwritten but equally important norms that develop over time; they have not been written down, but are central to how things are done. In a team-building workshop I conducted for the American College of Medical Practice Executives, we talked about the importance of a *culture vulture* for new employees. This person usually emerges informally and becomes the source for the oral history of the team and the unwritten aspects of its culture. Whether assigned to an individual or allowed to unfold spontaneously, the sharing of common unwritten norms will provide clarification of behavior for existing members and accepted guidelines for new ones.

An Effective Practice Team Trusts

In Chapters 8, 9, and 10, I spoke to all members of the practice team, specifically talking about the responsibilities each person has for creating and maintaining effective office relationships. One of the most important components of these successful relationships is trust. Trust implies a suspension of reliance on what is known, and a willingness to leap into the unknown. In so doing, you relinquish control of a part of your life and give it over to someone else. Any time you release control, you are taking a risk—you risk that the trust will not be well-placed and that, as a result, you might be hurt. Once your trust has been broken, it is more difficult for you to trust again. The degree to which you feel safe and to which you believe the outcome will be positive determines your willingness to trust. At some point, though, trust involves a decision, a leap of faith. You ultimately have to *decide* to trust. Practice personnel need to trust each other. They need to believe in the competence, honesty, supportiveness, and understanding of each member of the team.

An Effective Practice Team Is Supportive of Each Other and Is Aware of Its Members' Interdependence

Team members need each other. A well-functioning team is aware of and appreciates this interdependence. In my workshops, I sometimes ask the participants to engage in a simple trust/team exercise: they form a circle or circles and then, when instructed to do so, each person sits on the knees of the person behind him or her. This exercise always stimulates a fascinating discussion.

One comment is made each and every time workshop participants engage in this exercise: "We are really aware of how much we relied on each other to accomplish this task." Another frequent observation is "I became aware of my responsibility to the person in front of me. I didn't want her to fall." This simple exercise demonstrates quite tangibly the sense of interdependence that must exist if a team is functioning properly.

Also, this exercise generates another observation when a member of the circle loses his or her balance and falls. Although no one has ever been injured when this happens, the group members respond in an interesting way. They quickly move to make certain that the fallen member is all right, offering help in regaining footing, and quickly incorporating the person back into the group. This demonstration illustrates how a team should function if one of its members is having trouble. Whether it is due to work load or personal life stresses, when a team sees one of its members falling they reach out to help.

One of my managed care clients demonstrated this notion quite vividly. The entire organization was undergoing a complete computer conversion which began just prior to the open enrollment period. Needless to say, the folks in the enrollment department were swamped with learning the new system, entering the new members' information, and transferring the old files. The marketing department heard of the problem enrollment was having and responded. The entire marketing staff, who were not as profoundly impacted by the conversion, donated three Saturdays to the enrollment department. They came in on their own time and helped input the information. That is what I mean by supporting one another.

An Effective Practice Team Has Clearly Defined Roles, Responsibilities, and Expectations

When all practice personnel know what they are supposed to do and what is expected of them, then no unnecessary duplication of effort exists, because people are not confused as to whose job it is to do what. Also, such clarity reduces the sense of turfism that prevents practice personnel from providing quality service, both internally and externally. Groups that have difficulty becoming a team probably have not clearly defined these aspects of the practice. A carefully written and constantly revised office manual is instrumental in providing this kind of clarity.

An Effective Practice Team Communicates Effectively with Each Other

Communication is the essential glue that holds any team together. With it, a strong foundation will be laid. Without it, the team will not be grounded. In fact, poor communication is at the heart of many practice management problems. Such problems can eat away at practice morale, negatively impact patient satisfaction, and even reduce practice profitability. Reread Chapter 7. The communication process described there as well as the tips for effective verbal and nonverbal messages and the suggestions for showing empathy, listening effectively, and managing conflict will help you with intraoffice communication.

An Effective Practice Team Has Clearly Defined Decision-Making Authority

In a practice that functions well as a team, doctors and administrators have clarified their respective decision-making roles, and staff members have been empowered to make appropriate decisions.

Practice personnel must be carefully informed about the areas in which they will be making decisions. Even trained people need to have very specific guidelines regarding advice given to patients. Vincent Fulginiti, M.D., who has studied major causes of malpractice suits, warns, "A number of cases have hinged on whether or not a staff member was empowered to perform a certain task, trained for that task, and monitored. You'd be surprised at the testimony I've seen about outlandish advice given to patients by office staff, presumably without the doctors' knowledge."[3] Actually, once the practice has clearly defined who decides what when, the likelihood of unauthorized personnel giving inappropriate advice will be greatly diminished. Everyone in the practice will know the boundaries of their decision-making authority and will know exactly who to go to for a decision that is not within their purview.

Whatever the boundaries, once the agreements are reached, management must support, not second-guess, every staff decision. Physicians and practice administrators should not reverse the decisions made by the appropriately designated personnel. On the rare occasion when that might occur, it should always be done after consultation with the original decision-maker, and should involve clarification of why the reversal appeared to be warranted.

An Effective Practice Team Has a Problem-Solving Orientation

A team that works well together will embrace problems and solve them, not hide or run from them. Although there are many elaborate methods for problem solving, I have found the simpler ones to be most effective in working with medical practice issues. Given the hectic nature of life in the medical practice, the easier the method, the more likely you are to use it. There are several useful models for creative problem solving, two of which are quite user-friendly.

The Affinity Process   This process takes its name from the notion that solving problems involves finding ideas that have an affinity for each other. By looking for the common thread that runs among many ideas, the group can find common ground. Rather than creating the division among team members that problem solving can sometimes cause, this process minimizes if not eliminates it. It also is an equalizing process, leveling all power and influence and making each team member's contributions of equal value. I have used the affinity process to identify perceived customer wants and needs, for finding creative solutions to practice problems such as an appropriate reward system, and for other important issues that require extensive brainstorming. (See the Appendix for Steps in the Affinity Process.)

The Six Steps To Creative Problem Solving This method leads the participants through a structured process for defining the problem, analyzing its scope, and brainstorming and evaluating solutions. (See the Appendix for Steps in the Creative Problem-Solving Process.)

Regardless of what approach is applied, the use of some structured format for solving problems will help bring order out of the chaos that often accompanies practice difficulties.

An Effective Practice Team Handles Conflicts Productively

Unexpressed conflict is a drain on the team's energy, while conflict, constructively handled, actually generates it. The truth is that unexpressed conflict undercuts the team's efforts. It saps the psychic and emotional and even intellectual energies of the people involved. Dealing with conflict removes the obstacle and allows the energy to flow again. Also, out of conflict comes creativity. When differences are expressed, it opens up the minds of those involved and unleashes their creative energies. If all team members thought alike, there would be no new ideas.

Finally, expressed conflict leads to new, stronger relationships. It is odd how this works. Even though we fear conflict, and even though we have suffered through some mismanaged situations, when we constructively and productively manage the conflicts that face any relationship, that relationship grows stronger. The realization that the relationship is strong enough to withstand disagreements, the gaining of the respect for the people with whom you conflict, and the realization that the team relationship is worth going through the conflict process—all of these make the expression of conflict a very desirable action. See Conflict in Chapter 7 for a review of the five conflict styles and see the Appendix for the process for effective conflict resolution.

An Effective Practice Team Has a Sense of Team Spirit

An elusive concept to define, team spirit is important nonetheless. You know when you've got it and you feel its absence when you don't. Team spirit has something to do with that sense of pride I mentioned earlier, and with excitement about being involved. On the old school teams, this spirit was demonstrated by enthusiasm, energy, and eagerness. Your practice team will display these same attributes if it is really functioning as a team.

Sometimes the manifestations of team spirit can be small but significant. A workshop I was conducting for practice managers and staff in Pensacola, Florida, was attended by six women who comprised the entire staff of one small practice. I observed how well this group worked together on the interactive exercises, and noted the fun they appeared to be having. I also noticed that they were attired in matching turquoise smocks. When I commented about their uniform appearance, they told me, with a great deal of pride, that "this was turquoise day." Each day of the week was allotted a different color. They were given free choice of which colors and even which style smocks would be worn, and the practice footed the bill. Based on the cooperative spirit and the obvious sense of *team*, I would say that the money was very well spent!

A Positive Attitude Pervades an Effective Practice Team

As a member of a medical practice team, you should have positive attitudes about the customers (internal as well as external), your medical practice, healthcare in general, and yourself. Your attitudes in any of these areas can and will impact how effectively the team communicates with each other and how well your practice functions as a team. Positive attitudes provide the basis for the team spirit mentioned above.

Maintaining a positive attitude can be one of the biggest challenges for practice personnel today. The major changes that are occurring in healthcare place physicians, managers, and staff under unusual pressures. These pressures make it difficult to keep your spirits up. It is beneficial to pause and focus on the positives. Remembering the best moment in your practice experience can bring a needed smile to your face and provide a reminder of what is really important. One office manager I interviewed paused a moment, frowned, and said, "I can't think of what makes me keep coming to work!" Then she smiled broadly and said, "I believe it's when we are able to help the children. I remember one little girl in long dark pony tails with red ribbons. When we were able to ease her pain, that made my day!" Conjure up your own examples. They will help you to remain positive.

Another method is to take a moment to see the world through your customers' eyes. By reminding yourself of their frustrations and often of their fears and pain, you can shift a negative attitude to a positive one. Review the section on empathy in Chapter 7. Remember, walking a mile in your customer's moccasins can be very enlightening.

An Effective Practice Team Is Seen by Important Others as a Team

Do others notice if your practice is a team or not? You bet they do. They notice if practice personnel know who has the authority to make certain decisions, they notice if there is a cooperative spirit; they notice if the practice personnel seem to work well together. I have heard this comment often from patients: "That practice has a real team effort." Conversely, when others perceive that your practice is loosely coordinated and awkwardly run, they conclude that a team does not exist. Comments such as, "No one knew what they were doing over there!" will indicate that your practice is probably not perceived as a team. This perception may well cause your patients to seek healthcare elsewhere.

An effective practice team will be noted for its team spirit, although probably not described as such. Comments such as, "They seemed to enjoy their work" or "Everyone was so positive" are usually referring to the perception of that intangible element known as *team spirit*.

An Effective Practice Team Experiences Increased Productivity

The notion behind this characteristic is captured by the following acronym:

T-ogether

E-veryone

A-ccomplishes

M-ore[4]

When an office functions well as a team, then each person will be more productive. All practice personnel will know their duties, their decision-making authorities, the norms, and the methods for effective problem solving and conflict resolution. They will not be bogged down in unnecessary work that only delays productivity, nor will they be harboring unexpressed conflict that steals from their time and energy. When the team's focus is on service, then customer complaints also will be reduced, thus freeing up the time formerly spent in handling them. As a team, the combined productivity makes the entire office more efficient and more productive.

Longevity Pervades an Effective Practice Team

A well-functioning team does not experience a high turnover rate. One office manager confirmed this when disclosing the secret of her effective office team: "The doctors started this practice 22 years ago, and we have doctors and staff members who have been here all 22 years." Now, clearly, just lasting a long time does not guarantee an effective team. However, it is important to note that on an effective team, key players have usually been together for years. In addition to the content of this chapter, see Chapters 8, 9, and 10 for discussions of how to create the effective intraoffice relationships that are important to keeping practice personnel on the job.

An Effective Practice Team
Successfully Incorporates New Members

Given the youth of most medical practice employees, the mobility of the American population, and the ceiling on advancement that is inherent in most practices, your practice will experience some turnover regardless of your team's effectiveness. So, it is important to know how to incorporate new members when this happens. An important step is the orientation training that was discussed in Chapter 9. At that time, the practice governing principles (vision, purpose, and core values), the polices and procedures, team commitment agreement, and the service promise (covered in Chapter 15) should be thoroughly discussed. These suggestions are designed to allow the new member as gradual an introduction as possible. During this process it is incumbent on all involved to remain patient and friendly and helpful. Sooner than you might think, the new team member will become an active, contributing member of your practice team.

An Effective Practice Team Has a
Clearly Articulated Sense of Itself

A practice that works as an effective team has clearly articulated the principles that it holds dear. One of the best such statements that I have seen is included in the *Ophthalmology Office Manual*:

> Our office is dedicated to providing our patients with the highest quality of opthalmological care. Every decision and every action by our employees should be aimed toward this goal. We believe that our patients are our most important asset. Without them we would have no purpose. We place great importance on remembering our patients' names and on treating them with courtesy, fairness, and respect. We believe that employees are the heart of the practice. The qualities which they convey to our patients have an impact much

greater than our office decor, our building, or our equipment. We believe that there is no place for rudeness by members of our staff. The ability to remain cheerful under pressure is equally important as attaining the maximum technical skills. We should strive at all times to be gracious and accommodating, both to our patients and to our fellow employees. It is our desire to have only staff members who will work together with a sincere spirit of cooperation and teamwork. We believe this is the ingredient not only in the success of our practice but in promoting a pleasant and rewarding work environment for our employees as well. We want our practice to be at the forefront of our profession.[5]

Another way of articulating practice principles is to create a three-part statement of governing principles, as described in Peter Senge's landmark work, *The Fifth Discipline*:

Vision: The What—the picture of the future you seek to create.

Purpose or "Mission": The Why—the practice's answer to the question of why it exists.

Core Values: The How Do We Want To Act—the description of how the practice wants life to be on a day-to-day basis.

Taken as a unit, all three governing ideas answer the question, "What do we believe in?"[6]

Unfortunately, it is possible that not everyone in your practice will embrace the statements that are articulated. Involving the entire staff or appropriate representatives in their creation will help establish a sense of ownership. However, practice leaders should be aware of the differing possible attitudes toward such statements:

Commitment: Wants it. Will make it happen.

Enrollment: Wants it. Will do whatever possible within the "spirit of the law."

Genuine Compliance: Sees the benefits. Meets and exceeds expectations.

Formal Compliance: On the whole sees the benefits. Does what is expected and no more.

Grudging Compliance: Does not see the benefits. But does not want to lose job. Does enough of what's expected, but also lets it be known that he or she is not really on board.

Noncompliance: Does not see the benefits and will not do what's expected. "I won't do it; you can't make me."

Apathy: Neither for nor against. No interest. No energy. "Is it 5:00 yet?"[7]

As should be clear by reading this range of responses, some are not acceptable behaviors if your office is to function as a team. Of course, it would be wonderful if every employee experienced *commitment*, and you can even function with a few in *enrollment* or *genuine* and *formal compliance*. However, any employees who refuse to budge out of *grudging compliance, noncompliance*, or *apathy* into the acceptable ranges should no longer be members of the team. They will only pull it down and destroy what others are trying so hard to build and maintain.

An Effective Practice Team Has a Clearly Articulated Way of Working Together

As a practice, you have control over how you want to treat each other. So, take time to sit down together and decide what will be important in your interpersonal interactions. By following a process called "Creating Your Dream Team," you can take control of this important aspect of your team experience. This agreement allows team members to design their own destiny and thus gives them ownership.

The staff of the American College of Medical Practice Executives created the following team agreement statement by using the process described in the Appendix, "Creating Your Dream Team."

> We the Staff of the American College of Medical Practice Executives are committed to:
>
> - Open, honest and respectful communication with one another.
> - Maintaining a positive and enthusiastic attitude.
> - Celebrating team and individual accomplishments.
> - Creating and implementing new ways to achieve our goals.
> - Sharing responsibility for implementing this Team Commitment.
> - Resolving conflicts in a timely and effective manner.
> - Trusting and listening to each other.

- Treating each other fairly.
- Providing adequate and timely information for the performance of our work.
- Having fun!

Such Team Commitment Statements provide powerful guidelines for desired team behavior.

HOW TO BUILD AN EFFECTIVE PRACTICE TEAM

Any medical practice can choose to become a team. Once that decision is made, however, it is helpful to have some specific steps to follow that will help you shape that desire into a reality.

Step 1: Place the notion of a team in context. I have seen organizations make a big mistake by the surface-embracing of the team concept. In such instances, people are called together and are told, "We are now going to be a team." No one bothers to explain why this is important or how it differs from what already exists. So, the people involved receive the message that what has been happening is bad and that somehow they are also bad. This mistake can be avoided by setting the team concept in the context of the Total Service Medical Practice. When all practice personnel understand the goal of, and the rationale for, such a practice and become committed to its creation, then they will also understand why the team concept is so important.

Step 2: Create your dream team. I am not talking about the Olympic basketball team or the defense attorneys for O. J. Simpson. Rather I am talking about giving your practice the opportunity to start from this day forward. By deciding together from the beginning of the dialogue about creating a team, this process allows all practice personnel to have a say in how you will interact with each other. The focus of the team commitment is on the future, and this process allows you to chart your own course. Creating the team commitment agreement early in the process of building your team is important because it will serve as a guide for all of the future interactions (See Appendix for "Creating Your Dream Team").

Step 3: Create a practice statement of "Who We Are." It is essential that everyone in your practice knows what *this* practice is committed to. When such a statement is clearly articulated, then it can be implemented. Earlier in this chapter, I included an excellent example of such a statement taken from the *Ophthalmology Office Manual*, and also suggested the three-part governing ideas state-ment. Such statements should be written by representatives of the physicians, the office manager, and representatives of the staff. All parts of the practice should have a sense of ownership of these statements. They can be written by following a process similar to that outlined in Chapter 15 and the Appedix for writing a "service promise."

Step 4: Build trust. As I mentioned earlier, the vital glue that holds a team together is trust. Thus, it is important to give this sometimes vague concept form and substance through open discussion. One way to facilitate this process is through the use of experiential trust games or exercises. The most successful that I have used is the one I mentioned previously: Have practice personnel form a circle(s) of no more than 20 people. After every one turns to their left, and on the count of "1–2–3", they are to sit on the knees of the person behind them. Following any such exercise the discussion should shift from the exercise itself, and the general discussion of trust and teamwork, to how it applies to your practice.

Step 5: Establish the importance of each team member to the success of the whole. If people are to see themselves as a team, then it is important for them to understand their interdependence. In addition to a discussion following trust exercises, Chapter 12 describes some excellent models for bringing the concept of interdependence to the performance of tasks. The "cycle of service" and the "internal processes model" show how each practice member, even those who may have limited customer interaction, impacts the customer's experience and impressions of the practice. When the team members see how they impact the total service experience for the customers, then they can feel more involved as members of the team. As a practice, then, chart the key cycles of service and internal processes as described in Chapter 12.

Step 6: Decide on tangible symbols of the team. Why do athletic teams wear uniforms? It's not merely so that one team can be distinguished from the other. It also gives members of the team a keen sense of belonging. Pride in the team's appearance and in membership on it is an important side effect of this tangible evidence of a team. I mentioned earlier that the patients expect the staff members in a medical practice to look the part. I also described the pride I saw on the faces and the cooperation I found in the behaviors of the practice team who attended my workshop on Turquoise Day. Perhaps a practice uniform would be worth your consideration.

If not that, and even in addition to it, be creative. Team members should decide on their own tangible indications of being a part of the practice team: a bumper sticker, a name tag, look-alike but named coffee mugs, even a practice song or cheer—all have come from the creative thoughts of practice teams. If the idea comes from the team, almost anything will have great meaning.

Step 7: Celebrate team successes. In Chapter 16, I discuss this notion in much greater detail. I mention it here because it is such an important part of cementing the sense of team spirit. Look for opportunities, large and small, to celebrate what the team has done together. For example, when the preschool physical examination crunch is over, celebrate! When the high flu and cold season has come and gone, celebrate! When the staff member who has been gone on pregnancy leave returns and the team has covered during her absence, celebrate! When you have completed any major part of this implementation process for becoming a Total Service Medical Practice, celebrate. And once a year, gather together as a practice team for a celebration of who you are and what you have done.

Step 8: Chart the practice's decision-making authority. Be certain that everyone in the practice knows what decisions they can make and under what circumstances. The following four steps will help facilitate this process: (1) Determine what decisions have to be made on a daily basis. You are looking for the most common ones that will fall under the headings of either clinical decisions or nonclinical decisions. (2) Assign to each person the decisions he or she is most often called on to make, clearly articulating the boundary of the authority: For example, receptionist can offer a no co-pay to a patient based on her discretion, but the amount cannot exceed the co-payment of $20. The office manager has the final say on any billing problems, but the insurance coordinator can decide on issues up to a specified dollar point. The scheduling clerk can squeeze in patients who have a timing problem, but the nurse will make such decisions if the rationale is medical. (3) Distribute a cohesive list of who decides what, when they decide, and under what conditions. (4) Decide who will be the final authority on which issues: usually the medical director on medical issues, and the practice administrator on business issues.

Step 9: Find appropriate ways to play together. A team that laughs together usually works well together. I say *usually* because sometimes the team becomes so focused on having a good time that they forget why they are there in the first place. One patient told me of a medical practice where the staff members seemed to enjoy each other so much that she felt like an intruder.

The kind of play I am talking about is easily defined. I mean the occasions that allow the team to step out of their professional roles for a moment and merely enjoy each other as people. Birthday parties, Christmas secret-Santa exchanges, even staff retreats—all provide the opportunities for play time that help the team enjoy one another.

The topics of *play* and *laughter* also raise an interesting issue: gallows humor. I am well aware of the need for levity in this serious business that you are in; however, I urge you to examine your behaviors. Any that exclude the customer or make the customer the butt of the joke should be avoided.

Step 10: Engage in annual staff retreats. I've mentioned the importance of orientation and ongoing training already, but that is not what I am talking about here. I am referring to an annual, one or two day off-site retreat for all staff members. Given the family demands that most team members have, it usually works better to hold the retreat at a local site. If possible, shut down the office on a Friday afternoon and start then with the retreat, continuing on Saturday.

When planning such an event, be certain that its content is worthwhile. A retreat for the sake of a retreat is not usually appreciated. But, such an occasion provides an excellent opportunity for revisiting team commitment and practice statements, for addressing problem areas that need to be resolved, for planning for the coming year, and for playing together as a team. If staff as well as physicians and the office manager are involved in the planning, the chances of having an effective retreat are greatly enhanced. Again, that sense of ownership is important to the success of this event.

It is essential that all practice personnel attend the retreat, including the administrator and all physicians who are not on duty. The message sent by the presence of the management team is a powerful one. It assures staff members that this meeting is important, as well as demonstrating management's commitment to the practice and the staff. Absence from such an event says just the opposite.

Step 11: Decide how conflict will be addressed in your practice. This may be done to some extent when you create the "team commitment statement." However, I urge you to think about and adopt a specific procedure for handling conflict. The steps I offered in the Appendix may work for you. I would suggest that this model, or something similar, be adopted and then practiced on hypothetical but potentially real issues. This calls for role-playing, and I am aware that this particular activity is not always viewed favorably by practice personnel. Their usual complaints are that the scenarios are not real nor is the role-playing itself realistic. The first can be countered by using actual potential conflict areas. The second can be dealt with by understanding that this is indeed a role-play and probably won't be completely realistic. However, with the commitment from each participant that he or she will do his or her best to make it as realistic as possible, the role-playing can provide important rehearsal prior to encountering real situations. Perhaps before beginning on personnel-related examples, you might start practicing with conflict scenarios that arise with your external customers.

Step 12: Create opportunities for team members to express their appreciation for each other. This can be done in a variety of ways. At the end of my team-building workshops, I order a couple of bottles of champagne, alcoholic and nonalcoholic, and I have the team members toast one another. We stand in a circle and toast the person on our right. In the toast, each person says what it is about the other that he or she appreciates. When each person has thus been acknowledged, it is time for open toasts. This means any team member can toast any other team member or the team as a whole. I have had such moments open up teams, bring them together, and even cause some tears. Find your own way to accomplish these ritualized expressions of appreciation, but find them. Team members need to know that they are valued and needed by their colleagues.

Step 13: Implement all the characteristics of an effective team that have not been covered in Steps 1 through 12. Go back to the first section of this chapter and make certain that your team has these characteristics. Then just *keep on keepin' on.* The efforts to be an effective team do not end with the completion of a series of steps. Rather, they must be exerted everyday you are in the practice.

Step 14: Eliminate and address any of the problems discussed in this chapter. Examine the next section of this chapter. Work to eliminate and avoid any of these problems.

ROAD BLOCKS TO TEAM EFFECTIVENESS

Any team can encounter difficulties. Sometimes they come in the form of individuals who are simply not committed to the team, and sometimes they are found in simple behaviors that undermine the team's effectiveness. Being alert to the following potential problems will help you correct them before they can have negative impacts on your office team.

Turf Protectors: Lack trust. May say *all for one* but aren't.

Weak Links: Some team members may lack the competencies necessary to be effective in their individual jobs.

Good Intentions: Mean well but don't know how to do it. Lack skill in planning, group problem solving, communication, decision making. Meetings are unproductive and direction is unclear.

Leadership Limits: Team is composed of capable people who do not have a leader who gives them direction/vision and freedom and support.

Misalignment: Roles of individual members overlap and responsibilities among team members are unclear. May also have differing interpretations of the vision. Results are duplication of efforts.[8]

Debrah Harrington-Mackin, president of New Directions Management Services, a consulting firm that specializes in team building in corporate America, described several behaviors that can be counterproductive for team members to exhibit. Among them are the following: attacking personalities rather than ideas, agreeing with everything to avoid conflict, inconsistency, chatting during meetings, chronic complaining, displaying hostility, displaying superiority, escaping (taking calls during meetings, etc.), frequent head shaking (as if to say "No way!" to any idea), glossing over problems, making decisions without team knowledge, missing meetings, not completing tasks on time, not participating in team decisions, not taking the process seriously, offering putdowns, raising false hopes, seeking sympathy as an excuse for not performing, speaking in *shoulds*, talking too much, withdrawing, and binding someone else's behavior ("You'll love this idea!" "You'll hate this idea!")[9]

In order to avoid problems such as those just described, every member of your practice team must be aware that they *can* exist. Then, keep your eyes open to spot and eliminate problems when and if they occur.

THE PHYSICIAN/PRACTICE ADMINISTRATOR TEAM

Within the larger framework of the practice team exists a smaller but essential one: the management team. Consisting of the administrator and the physicians (or a representative thereof in the form of a medical director) this team must establish the model for the rest of the practice to follow.

Before discussing how these individuals can work as a team, it might be helpful to understand why they might not. The biggest reason is that, often, administrators and physicians are very different. They frequently have different personalities and equally divergent training. Thus, they may develop suspicion of each other because they do not understand these differences. The physicians and the practice administrator can react like many other people do when faced with someone different: they can think that the other's way of doing things is not merely different, but wrong.

The contrasts between management and medicine often have been drawn. One of the best and still relevant discussions occurred in 1987:[10]

Management	Medicine
Designer	Doers
Group problem-solving	1–1 problem-solving
Proactive, with long timespans between results	Reactive
Long-term response	Immediate response
Delegators	Deciders
Collaborators	Autonomous
Participative	Independent
Organization advocates	Patient advocates
Interdependent professional	Independent professional

So, the first step to creating an effective physician/manager team is to realize that you may well have some very different perspectives and that those differences can be sources of strength at times, and, at others, sources of conflict that will need to be effectively managed.

In spite of all of these differences, the importance of shaping the physicians and the practice administrator into an effective team is becoming increasingly apparent. Diane Miner, the president of the Medical Group Management Association's Pediatric Administrators Assembly, urged, "Today in our busy and ever-changing medical practices, a strong leadership team consisting of physicians and practice administrator has become essential. Physician involvement in this leadership team is not meant as managing day-to-day activities—that is the job of the administrator. However, not even an aggressive and knowledge-able administrator can be an effective medical practice leader by himself or herself."[11]

Ms. Miner continued by outlining the following suggestions for effective physician/administrator teams:

- Set common goals through periodic strategic planning, not by day-to-day micromanagement.
- Regular communication between the leadership team is a must.
- Members of the management team must respect each other.
- Differing points of view should be encouraged. [12]

THE MEDICAL DIRECTOR/ADMINISTRATOR TEAM

Usually, regardless of the size of the practice, a medical director is elected or appointed to work closely with the administrator. Functioning almost as co-executives, these two individuals must also establish an effective teamwork relationship.

When working together, the medical director and the administrator each have roles to play and tendencies to be controlled. Sam Romeo, M.D., Dean of Clinical Affairs at the Medical College of Wisconsin, described some of them this way: "In my experience, the physician leader's tendency to resort to autocratic decisionmaking during times of crisis and stress, coupled with the administrator's fear of losing his or her job, is the single most critical issue in preventing proper development of the physician/administrator team. It also is the issue that is too often ignored." He continued by saying, "The physician/administrator relationship is built on trust. This relationship must develop through collaboration or else the personal success of team members and the group will be threatened."[13]

The practice administrator and the medical director should meet often, usually once a week. They should clearly define the scope of their individual roles and responsibilities, and should make these known to the other physicians and the staff. Above all, they should respect and support each other, projecting a partnership, not merely two people who work together. Dr. Romeo concluded, "As group practices grow in size and number, the critical need to have a physician/administrator relationship built on open communication, collaboration, and trust will continue to grow."[14]

Effective practice teamwork must pervade the Total Service Medical Practice. It is only through this kind of positive internal interaction that patients can receive the kind of quality in their clinical and nonclinical care that they deserve. Effective practice teamwork is also essential to the successful serving and interacting with the secondary customers that have become increasingly involved in providing healthcare to the patients.

END NOTES

1. Frederick Wenzel, "Conflict: An Imperative for Success," *Journal of Medical Practice Management* 1, no. 4 (April 1, 1986), p. 255.

2. Frank J. Weinstock, *The Ophthalmology Office Manual* (Columbus, Ohio: Anadem Publishing, 1993). © Anadem Publishing, Inc. Phone: (800) 633-0055.

3. Vincent A. Fulginiti, "The Big 8: Major Malpractice Traps in Pediatrics," *Pediatric Management* 4, no. 4 (April 1, 1993), p. 47.

4. Diane Hall Miner, "Physician/Administrator Teams: A New Necessity," *Primary Practice News* 1, no. 1 (Summer 1994), p. 10. Reprinted with permission of the Center for Research in Ambulatory Health Care Administration, 104 Inverness Terrace East, Englewood, CO. 80112-5306; (303) 799-1111. Copyright 1994.

5. Weinstock, p. 1–2.

6. Peter M. Senge, *The Fifth Discipline: The Art & Practice of the Learning Organization* (New York: Doubleday Currency, 1990), pp. 223–224.

7. Ibid. 219–220.

8. Carol Dubnicki, "Building High-Performance Management Teams," *Healthcare Forum Journal* 34, no. 3 (May/June 1991), p. 20.

9. Debrah Harrington-Mackin, *The Team Building Tool Kit* (New York: AMACOM, American Management Association, 1994), pp. 59–61.

10. "Can Doctors and Administrators Work Together?" *Physician EXECUTIVE* 13, no. 5 (September/October 1987), p. 14.

11. Miner, p. 10. See Note 4.

12. Ibid.

13. Sam Romeo, M.D., "Communication Collaboration, Trust," *MGM Journal* 38, no.4 (July/August 1991) p. 10.

14. Ibid.

FOUR

THE SYSTEMS, THE CYCLES, THE PROCESSES, AND THE MOMENTS OF TRUTH

Service in a medical practice is demonstrated through the nonclinical aspects of the customer's experience. As has been previously discussed, it is built on the positive relationships that are created and, as we will discover in this section, it is also demonstrated by the way things are done. By examining the systems, cycles, and processes, as well as the points of customer interaction, called moments of truth, you will be able to chart your course for improving service. In Chapter 12, you will discover some useful methods and models for examining how well service is done in your practice. Then, Chapter 13 will discuss how to manage a pivotal moment of truth for your primary customers: the doctor/patient interview. In Chapter 14, you will learn ways of handling the difficult customer situations that challenge even the most service-driven personnel.

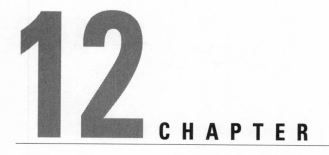

CHAPTER

Step Twelve—Analyze Your Systems, Cycles, and Processes

During one of my workshops for medical practice staff members, I encountered a young woman who expressed a frustration common among service providers everywhere: "I want to provide good service, but it seems like that the way we do things around here keeps me from it." What she and the others are referring to are the systems that are in place, the service cycles experienced by the customers, and the processes required for task completion. These ways of doing things are frequently at odds with the desires of practice personnel to provide quality service. They must be examined and often revised if your practice is to become one dedicated to Total Service.

ANALYZE YOUR SYSTEMS

Systemic problems are not a foreign concept for medical practices. You deal with such physical problems in your patients' bodies daily. Just as the human body can develop maladies within one or more of its essential systems, so can your practice develop problems within its organizational systems. If your practice is to be a healthy one, then careful diagnosis and treatment of any organizational systemic problems must be a priority.

Identify Your Systems

Your practice has four types of systems to be analyzed.

The Management System   This refers to the ways members of management interact with each other and with their employees. It also refers to the ways decisions are made and by whom.

The Rules and Regulations   Referring to the policies and procedures, this is probably the most troublesome of systems with which to deal. These codes become like unbreakable laws and, even though few if any practice personnel can recall why they are in place, they are often clung to with an almost religious fervor.

The Technical System   This system involves the hardware in your practice. All the way from the sophisticated equipment used in clinical diagnosis and treatment to the most basic office tool, the telephone, the technology in your practice impacts the service that is provided.

The Social System   This system involves the interactions among the practice personnel. Are the relationships positive? Who is influential? Does this influence come formally through job descriptions and stated responsibilities or does it emerge informally via personal qualities and characteristics?

Ask Two Key Questions

The service aspects of all these systems can be ascertained by asking and answering two simple but critical questions:

1. Does this system make it easy for your customers to do business with your practice?
2. Does this system make it easy for your employees to put the customers first?

In other words, are your systems customer friendly, and are your systems employee-friendly? If your answer to either question is "No," then changes need to be made. No system within your control that creates service obstacles for your customers or for your employees should be allowed to remain.

Your Technical Systems Revisited

Although analysis of all systems is critical to improving service to your customers, two technical systems warrant close and specific examination: the telephone system and the computer system.

The Telephone System

Literally the lifeline for some of your customers, your telephone system and its use must put the customer first. Check out that system. Be certain that it is user friendly. In addition to the quality of the system and its ability to handle the volume, several service concerns should be addressed.

■ Promptness of response. The old rule of answer the phone within three rings is a wise one. As we know from Chapter 6, immediate acknowledgement is one of the factors that is high on the customers' lists of important service items, and this extends to the telephone. The telephone company can do what is called a "busy audit" of your line for a week. It will tell you how long it takes to answer the phone, as well as how many callers become impatient and hang up, and after how many rings.

■ Friendliness of greeting. Customers report wanting to hear a pleasant, friendly voice on the other end of the telephone line. I wish you could call the office of my orthopedic surgeon just so you could be greeted by Josie. Her upbeat, warm, friendly voice makes me feel that she is really glad I have called, even before she knows who I am.

■ Permission to be put on hold. Customers have told me that the most annoying thing about calling a doctor's office is to be greeted with, "Dr. Smith's office. Will you hold?" followed by an immediate *click*. They unanimously agree that they would like the opportunity to say "Yes" or "No." Then they have a choice. More than that, because obviously the customers can hang up if they do not want to wait, they report that this pause for their responses makes them feel acknowledged as an individual and not just another telephone call. After observing many receptionists in action, I know that sometimes it seems all lines are blinking at once. However, taking that extra few seconds to afford the caller the opportunity to feel acknowledged is well worth the effort.

■ Length of time on hold. Many customers complain about the length of time they are kept on hold, listening to elevator music or some other type of music that they don't enjoy, or to silence. They report appreciating a check-back to see if they would like to continue holding. Again, although they have the option of merely hanging up and calling back later, customers feel more cared about when their response to the hold is solicited.

■ Skill and number of transfers. Once the call is being transferred from the switchboard to the appropriate party, customers often seem to encounter some service problems. They report that they are either being cut off during the transaction, or that they are transferred many times, each time requiring a retelling of their story. The solution to lost calls is to be certain that you have an employee-friendly telephone system and that all personnel are trained in how to use it. To solve the problem of numerous transfers, the person answering the telephone must secure enough information from the caller and must be familiar enough with who does what in the practice to make the correct connection.

■ Tactfulness of screening. Part of the job of any receptionist is to screen incoming calls. Physicians, for example, do not want to be interrupted with calls that can be handled by someone else or at another time. (Most physicians indicate that interruptions are not just permissible but desired if the caller is another doctor. They report that even patients understand the importance of such calls). The person answering the telephone must explain in a friendly, tactful manner why the party cannot take a call at this time and when the caller can expect to receive a call back. If this is a call that should be handled by someone else in the practice, this transfer must be made tactfully: "Actually, our office manager handles those questions. Her name is Alice Johnson. I'll put you through to her right now if you'd like." Note: In order for the caller to actually receive a return call at a specified time, the person on the switchboard must be informed about the hours for follow-up phone calls for each person, and these hours must be honored.

Keeping a list by the telephone, and updating the list daily, will provide ready reference.

■ Helpfulness of person answering the phone. The individual who answers the telephone in your office must have her finger on the pulse of the practice. She needs to know where the staff members are and when they'll be available for calls. She needs to know areas of responsibility so that she can transfer blind calls to the correct party. She needs to listen effectively and respond sympathetically.

The Computer System

Another part of your technical system is the computer: both the curse and blessing of modern life. Computers can be important timesaving devices that allow for easy storage and retrieval of information. However, they can also become obstacles to positive service if not handled correctly. Questions for your consideration are:

■ Do the computers physically obstruct interactions with the customers? Most frequently seen in the reception area, the computer itself can become an obstacle between the receptionist and the customer. Check out your front office. Where is the computer located? Does it obstruct the sight line to the door and sitting area? Can it be located elsewhere? Again, don't be afraid to ask the "Why" question: Why is it located where it is? One client of mine spent a lot of time telling me how difficult it was for the employees to input information with the computer located in a high traffic area. When I asked why it was located there, the answers were not very compelling, and the computer was moved. In Chapter 7, I discussed the importance of being aware of the messages conveyed by the semifixed space (those elements in your environment that can be moved). A computer monitor sticking up behind the check-in counter can communicate a message of distance and little concern for the customer's needs. One office manager told me of her decision to remove all computers from the front office area. All billing and ordering is conducted off-site, and scheduling is handled at a location near check-out, not check-in. She reported that this left the front office personnel free to greet the customers, escort them to the appropriate place, and take care of their needs. Incidentally, this office receives outstanding marks on patient satisfaction surveys for its friendly, personable approach.

■ Are practice personnel adequately trained on the current system? This should be an obvious requirement for the successful use of any piece of equipment. However, I have been surprised at how many office personnel confide that they do not feel comfortable with the computer system they are using, and would like to have more training. The reasons from a service standpoint are also clear. In order to respond to the customer's needs, the practice personnel must be able to access appropriate information. Also, having the information in the system is important to further serve the customer.

■ Does this system allow us to provide the information our customers need? Can it be supplied quickly and accurately? One specialist's office complained to me about the new computer system being used by a primary care physician's office. Although the system seemed to meet the PCP's needs, it did not allow the specialist's office to obtain the information they previously could access. When analyzing your computer system, ask yourself, "What impact will this system have on our customers?" Let the answer be your guide.

■ Has the computer become a substitute for human interaction? Be careful. In this day of computerized everything, you may well begin to see many uses of computers in new areas. Question each of these. The lure of saving time is the most seductive to any medical practice. However, what you may save in time may well be lost in dissatisfied customers.

Overcomputerization is not a problem unique to medical practices. It is a source of concern at a deep philosophical level to many people in our society: What impact is our increasing reliance on this technology going to have on human interactions? However, the concern becomes almost poignant in a medical practice, especially when dealing with patients. When patients come to, or even contact, your office, they are usually hurt or ill. At the very least, they are anxious. They need humanness, not coldness, at these times. Do not let an overreliance on computers come between you and your patient. Just because a task *can* be done on a computer does not mean that it always *should* be.

Another concern about overcomputerization is its impact on internal communication and service. The use of E-mail will save time and may even open up more frequent communication among practice personnel. However, it also can significantly reduce and even eliminate face-to-face, interpersonal interactions with your colleagues. Guard against this. You will need to make time for the face-to-face opportunities. Again, just because you have the capability to send all of your messages via the computer, it does not mean that you should.

■ Has the computer become a cover-up for poor service? "The computer is down" is one message most customers have begun to suspect. The medical practice personnel in my workshops around the country assure me that most of the time when this fateful message is delivered to their customers, it is the truth. And that raises another question about this part of the technical system. Customers have begun to wonder if it can possibly be down as often as it seems to be. If it the answer is "yes," then you need to do some serious thinking about the reliability of your current system. If it is not, then it has become an excuse for problems that need to be handled, not hidden. In either case, customers are reaching their limit on the computer excuse. Work to eliminate it from your vocabulary.

CHART THE CYCLES OF SERVICE

Identify Moments of Truth

Customers experience your medical practice through a series of interactions called "moments of truth." A term originated in Spanish bullfighting as *el momento de verdad,* or the final moment at which matador and bull face each other alone, these moments of truth for your customers are also pivotal events.[1] They occur whenever the customer contacts any part of your medical practice and begins to form an impression of your service.[2] For your organization, these moments of truth can make or break your practice in the customer's eyes. As one focus group participant put it: "If they [medical practices] could just understand the value of every single minute that they are in contact with the patient! If they could only realize that what may be a routine visit to them isn't routine to us at all. It involves our bodies!" Moments of truth in and of themselves are neither good nor bad.[3] Rather it is how they are managed and perceived by the customer that makes the difference.

Creating Positive Moments of Truth

Although many moments of truth in your practice involve a customer and a service provider, some may not. In Chapter 7, I discussed the importance of nonverbal messages, including those sent by fixed and semifixed space. Thus, customers can and do draw conclusions about the service aspects of your practice based on the nonverbal messages of such things as the appearance of your building, the parking lot, and the decor of the waiting room. Thus, you should examine the nonverbal messages sent during these moments of truth and make corresponding improvements where possible. If you are unable to alter the space, such as the imposing nature of the medical building in which your practice is housed, then you will need to do all that you can to manage the customers' perceptions in those moments of truth that are within your control.

As might be expected, the majority of your customers' moments of truth involve direct interactions, either face-to-face or via the telephone, with practice personnel. Since whether these moments of truth leave the customer with a positive or negative impression of your practice depends on what happens during these interactions, it is helpful to determine what can be done to increase the likelihood that the result will be positive.

Moments of truth that are viewed as positive experiences are characterized by several behaviors on the part of the practice personnel involved.

Create a Supportive Environment

To understand what constitutes a supportive environment, you must first examine its opposite: defensiveness. As human beings, all of us become defensive when we perceive that we are under attack. In fact, the tendency to defend ourselves in such situations can be traced all the way back to the days of the caveman. The instincts to fight or take flight when we are threatened run deep within us. Since you can't run out of the medical practice screaming, "I can't take it any more!" your only other instinctive choice when a customer seems to be on the attack is to want to fight back. By the same token, at the moment customers feel attacked, they too may well begin to defend themselves. So, defensiveness is a natural, instinctive response to a threatening situation. It also is one that can wreck any hope for a positive perception of service.

Also, defensiveness is reciprocal, resulting in a spiraling effect. Once either party in an interaction goes on the attack, the other will likely respond in kind. This response stimulates an even more hostile counterattack, and the situation quickly escalates out of control.

The good news is that defensiveness is caused by certain behaviors that can be identified and avoided. In fact, such identification can break the spiral just described, because for each aggressive behavior that is poisoning the environment with defensiveness, there is an antidote. Jack Gibbs originated the distinctions between defensive and supportive communication environments back in the 1960s.[4] The results of his landmark research have been borrowed by many communication scholars over the years. The distinctions will be helpful to you as you try to establish the supportive environment that will reduce defensiveness and create a warm, service-oriented interaction with your customer.

Defensive	Supportive
Evaluative	Descriptive
Controlling	Problem Solving
Game Playing	Spontaneity
Apathy	Empathy
Superiority	Equality

Let's examine each of these attributes more closely.

Evaluative versus Descriptive   People become defensive when they feel that they are being evaluated and found to be lacking. Implying an evaluation of the intelligence of the customer by saying, for example, "If you'd only read the information in your benefits package supplied by your employer, you'd know what your plan covers!" will have a very different impact on a patient than a more descriptive response: "Each benefits package is different, and so it is not clear what your plan covers without input from your insurance company."

Controlling versus Problem Solving   I asked a friend of mine who works in customer service for J. C. Penney's and handles upset customers all day what she does to defuse these situations. "The first thing I do is listen, and then I move as quickly as possible into a problem-solving mode: 'Let's see what we can do to solve this for you.'" Thus, for example, when the patient does not know his or her coverage, rather than immediately saying "No," which makes patients feel controlled, you can create a positive moment of truth by helping him or her find out. Many practices have accumulated thick books or extensive computer files on the various plans, and can answer the patients' questions. Others make the phone call to the health plan for the patient or at the very least provide the phone number and a telephone for the patient to use.

Game Playing versus Spontaneity Defensiveness arises when the customer believes that a game is being played, rather than that the staff is making a sincere attempt to help. Games become a part of the interaction when the service provider goes on "auto pilot" and fails to respond to the specific situation of the customer. It may be the 16th or even 60th time you've answered the question about the doctor's delay in returning from rounds, but for this patient it is the first time. "The doctor is still at the hospital" begins to sound like a game-playing excuse, even if it may be true, unless the patient feels some spontaneous concern for his or her circumstances.

Apathy versus Empathy Probably the most insulting defensive behavior is to convey a lack of caring. If, for example, patients pick up even a whiff of a "So you're sick" attitude, they become very angry. Return to the section in Chapter 7 on empathy. It is essential that your customers sense that you really do understand their feelings and what they are experiencing and that you are willing to express that understanding to them.

Superiority versus Equality No one appreciates being talked down to, and this approach will bring instant defensiveness. It is one criticism that patients level toward some physicians in particular. Perhaps brought about by the status differences perceived by the patients, and sometimes by the actual behavior of the doctors, the sense that the physician feels superior will make patients angry, defensive, and uncooperative. Although medical personnel do possess information and knowledge that the patients don't have, this must not be mistaken for superiority at a human level.

Problems can occur when the patient for one reason or another is judged as less than desirable by the healthcare worker, and is treated accordingly. Although it may be difficult at times to remember that such people are just people under whatever distasteful cloak they might be wearing, you must make every effort to do so. I remember walking down the street with a friend of mine who is a drug- and alcohol-abuse counselor. Each time we encounter one of his clients, whether they have been "using" or not, he always greets them with a warm, friendly, and most of all a respectful manner. The response he receives is a reward in and of itself as these people express, often very openly, their pleasure at being accorded a simple sense of human equality.

By exhibiting supportive behaviors, you can defuse and even avoid defensive situations. Even more important, your customers will have a positive service experience.

Listen Effectively

Identified in Chapter 7 as one of the most important communication skills anyone can develop, listening also is an important component for creating a positive moment of truth for your customer. Office manager Deborah Goodyear summarized it well: "I believe being listened to is more important than anything else. That starts at the front and goes all the way to the back. They [the customers] have to feel that their needs are being met and that we actually understand what they want." A physician in one of my workshops rather poignantly stated the importance of this skill when he said, "Personal contact, the need to say something to someone who is listening, is probably the top priority in medical care today." The suggestions for improving your listening skills covered in Chapter 7 will help you manage the moments of truth for your customers in a positive manner.

Ask Good Questions

The process of inquiry results in obtaining vital information. It also helps your customers feel valued and important. If ineffectively handled, however, asking questions can result in negative reactions. Patients report to me that their entire healthcare experience makes them feel like they are receiving the third degree: The doctors and their staffs ask questions, as well as the personnel at the hospital and at the insurance company. When these questions are asked in a rote, unfeeling manner, patients say they begin to resent the entire process. By merely focusing on your voice and manner, by trying to project sincere interest, even if the question is seeking the most basic demographic information, you can help create a positive moment of truth for the customer. Also, as I mentioned in Chapter 7, there are many different types of questions that you can ask. Review them as a reminder that you are not limited to yes-or-no inquiries. In addition, review the tips for effective listening.

One type of question that will help customers feel cared about and understood is the empathetic question. By placing this type of question in the midst of the more factual queries, you can make the entire questioning process more meaningful to the customer. When I was being interviewed by the nurse during a presurgical interview, not only did she ask the most routine questions with interest, but she paused as I was explaining how my arm had been injured to ask, "Were you alone when you fell?" When I confirmed that I was indeed alone, she responded with, "I think that would be so frightening. Was it?" Although she was a very busy lady with a full schedule, her expressed interest in what seemed to be the medically irrelevant circumstances, and the understanding she had of what I had experienced, made me feel cared for and created a positive moment for me in this very stressful experience.

Pay Attention to the Little Things

The old song, "Little things mean a lot" must have been referring to more than expressions of love. These so-called *little things* can make big differences in customer interactions. For example, pay close attention to how you word your sentences. Contractions such as *can't* sound softer than *cannot*. (*Unable* sounds even better and of course, "We'd be happy to do that for you!" is the best of all!)

Another important *little thing* has to do with appropriate forms of address. The formal use of "Ma'am" sounds rather distant and removed and can even sound insulting when said in a cool or, worse yet, condescending manner. In Chapter 13, I offer a rather lengthy discussion of the appropriate form of address for patients during a doctor/patient interview and will summarize it here by saying, customers like to be called by name and if you are uncertain as to whether that should be the first or last name, merely ask. Genevieve Finley, the manager of John H. Finley and Associates surgical practice in Southfield, Michigan, explained, "The first question I ask new patients is what name they would like us to use. I look at the patient form and say, 'So you are Elizabeth White. Would you like us to call you Elizabeth or Mrs. White?'"[5]

Several little tricks can come to your assistance should you be in a situation where you don't know or can't remember the patient's name. Meryl Luallin conducted personal observations of many medical practices while researching the quality of customer service. Acting as a mystery patient (pretending to be a patient when she was actually doing research) she reported being amazed when, while she was waiting in an OB-GYN practice in the Midwest, the nurse came directly to her in the crowded waiting room and softly called her name. When asked how she had known who Ms. Luallin was, the nurse explained that she and the receptionist had a little system. As patients arrived at the counter, the receptionist noted some distinctive item of apparel and jotted a description on a sticky note for the nurse to see. She then read the note, scanned the waiting room and found the appropriate patient, whom she now could address by name.[6]

Another way to personalize the interaction involves the use of staff members' names. Office manager Finley explains, "I always say . . . 'My name is Genevieve, and I can answer any questions you have' . . . I tell them 'Bridget will handle your insurance' and 'Julie will be right with you.'"[7] As I indicated in Chapter 10, staff members often don't realize their importance in the patient's experience, and thus don't believe that it matters if their names are known or not. I surprised the young staff member in a gynecologist's office by asking for her name. As we waited in silence for the doctor to arrive and conduct a pelvic exam, I asked, "And you are?" She actually jumped, and, looking startled, said, "Oh. I'm sorry. My name is Nancy." It only seemed right to me that if she and doctor were going to perform a very personal examination that I should at least know her name.

Another *little thing* has to do with your nonverbal communication while you are on the telephone. Since you are unable to be seen by the person on the other end of the line, at least until videophones become standard equipment, you may believe that it really doesn't matter if you are shuffling through papers, signing letters, checking charts or any number of other things that need your attention while you are talking on the telephone. Unfortunately, this work, although important, is a distraction and it prevents you from giving the person on the other end of the line your complete attention. Studies reveal that this distraction will show in your voice; the person listening can tell you are not focused completely on them. In addition, such distraction will also prevent you from listening with total attention and you may miss some very important information. One more point: remember that a smile on your face shows in the sound of your voice. Look pleasant when talking on the telephone to your customers. They will be able to tell.

Although most of the previous discussion has focused on patients, the same kinds of behaviors can create positive interactions with any customer. By creating a supportive communication environment, listening effectively, asking good questions, and paying attention to the so-called *little things*, you will be well on your way to providing a positive moment of truth, regardless of who the customer might be.

Analyze the Key Cycles of Service

Customers do not experience your practice in isolated moments of truth. Rather, they enter into a series of interconnected interactions that create a cycle of service for that particular encounter with your office. In Figure 12–1, you can see the visualization of this cycle as created by Karl Albrecht in his book, *At America's Service*.[8] As the model indicates, the customer enters the cycle, experiences his or her first interaction, and forms an initial opinion of the practice. When this interaction is completed, the customer moves on to the second point of contact, or moment of truth, and that initial opinion is either affirmed or not. Then the customer moves to the third point of interaction, and so on around the cycle, forming opinions of the service at each moment of truth. After the final interaction for this encounter, the customer then exits the cycle.

A specific situation will help you chart and analyze the cycles of service in your practice. Let's apply the following step-by-step

FIGURE 12–1

Cycles of Service

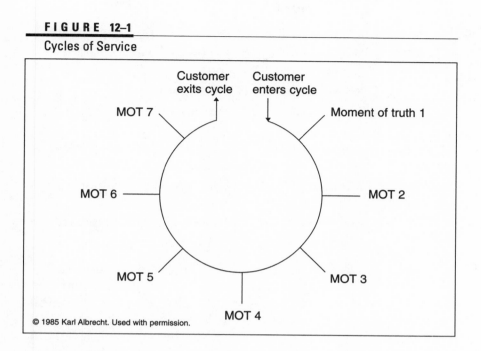

© 1985 Karl Albrecht. Used with permission.

analysis to probably the most important cycle in your practice: a patient visit. (The moments of truth reflected here are based on those offered by participants in my workshops. You will want to keep track of those pertinent to your practice.)

Step 1: Identify the cycle to be analyzed (A typical office visit).

Step 2: Identify the customer (A patient).

Step 3: Identify the moments of truth in the cycle. (Remember, not all moments of truth involve interaction with practice personnel; fixed and semi-fixed space also provide opportunities for customers to shape opinions.)

Moment of Truth 1: Parking the car.

Moment of Truth 2: Experiencing the building that houses uses your office.

Moment of Truth 3: Entering the reception area of your office.

Moment of Truth 4: Waiting in the reception area.

Moment of Truth 5: Going to the examination room.

Moment of Truth 6: Taking of vitals.

Moment of Truth 7: Waiting in the examination room.

Moment of Truth 8: Doctor/Patient interview and exam.

Moment of Truth 9: Checking out—making payment.

Moment of Truth 10:Rescheduling (if necessary).

Moment of Truth 11:Exiting the office.

Step 4: Evaluate each moment of truth from a service perspective. Revisit each moment of truth and ask yourself this question: "Are we able to manage this moment of truth in such a way so as to create a positive experience for the customer?" You can find the answers to this question in a number of ways, the most obvious of which is to ask, through patient-satisfaction surveys, patient-advisory boards, patient-feedback forms (brief forms completed before the patient leaves), and informal query, at each moment of truth. Another way is to experience the cycle yourself. Since most office personnel may well enter through a side or back door, you also may have no idea how the patient experiences your practice from the beginning to the end. Select someone from the staff and have this person go through the cycle as a patient would. A report on this first-hand experience will give you important information. A final source of data is to consider the complaints that are received. (See Chapter 14 for additional thoughts about complaints).

After this charting and analysis has been conducted, the steps to be taken will vary, depending on the autonomy of the practice. In smaller, freestanding practices, the next steps are fairly straightforward. Once any problematic moments of truth have been determined, you are ready to find ways to improve. In the office visit cycle for a small practice, then, the following three additional steps are necessary:

Step 5: Decide on a plan of action to resolve difficulties at any problematic moment of truth.

Step 6: Implement the plans.

Step 7: Check back to see if the difficulty has been resolved.

In larger group practices, where a different department may be responsible for each moment of truth, some slight differences in the analysis process will be found. First, the actual charting of the cycles will probably not involve every single member of the practice, but rather representatives of each department. Together these analysis teams will chart the major cycles of service. After determining problematic moments of truth in a given cycle, these teams will then decide on a plan of action to resolve the problem to be submitted to the management team or appropriate decision maker(s), and a decision will be reached. My advice to management: once you turn over this process to representatives of your staff, do everything in your power to approve the plans of action they recommend. Just as when dealing with advisory boards and suggestion boxes, nothing will deflate the spirits of these participants more than to have their ideas ignored or rejected. Also, it will be much more difficult to solicit their participation in the future.

As you are analyzing your cycles of service and moments of truth, be aware that repeated problems at the same moment of truth, regardless of the personnel involved, are usually indications of a systems problem. As a result, you can then examine the appropriate system to see how it can be corrected. Remember to ask the key questions: Is this system customer-friendly? Is this system employee-friendly? You want to be able to say "yes" to both questions.

On the other hand, an employee who has an inordinate number of troubling moments of truth or who experiences a major service explosion is probably sending out distress signals and will need counseling or coaching. Unfortunately, if this does not result in corrected behavior, this employee will quite probably have to be terminated.

Pay Careful Attention to Critical Moments of Truth

Customers are very much aware when they experience moments of truth cycles of service, although they lack the vocabulary to label them as such. During a patient focus group, one participant demonstrated his understanding of these concepts when he commented: "I think they should start looking at everything they do. From the time you park your car to the time you pay your bill, it matters what is happening to you and how you are treated." He continued, with great conviction, "Everybody in the whole darn place ought to be concerned with how they are serving you."

Although all are important, not all moments of truth in a cycle of service are equal. Some points of interaction for the customer are usually more critical than others. In a medical practice, probably the most important of all is the doctor/patient interview and exam, and this moment of truth is thoroughly discussed in Chapter 13. In addition, as in most cycles of service, three other critical moments of truth can be identified: the first and last points involving human interaction and any involving a waiting period. Let's look at each of these three in greater detail, and let's deal with the most problematic first.

Waiting Periods Probably the thorniest issue for most medical practices, this moment of truth is a critical one because patients intensely dislike waiting. They are not unusual; research in service indicates that waiting is a pet peeve of all customers regardless of the type of business with which they are interacting. In fact, research testing customer reactions to waiting indicated that customer satisfaction is inversely related to waiting time.[9] Left waiting for long periods of time, customers can become testy, angry, and generally difficult to work with once they can be seen. In medical practices, there is a direct connection between excessive waiting time and tendencies to file malpractice suits. Chicago pediatrician Jere E. Friedman, M.D., chairman of the Risk Management Committee of the Illinois State Medical Inter-Insurance Exchange, observed, "Chronic waiting room delay is a contributing factor behind patient antagonism toward the doctor, making [patients] more apt to seek legal action when an unexpected outcome occurs."[10] Patients have described feeling uncared about and unimportant as a result of long waits in the doctor's office, and others have a more colorful description: "I feel like I'm just in a herd of cattle!" was the way one patient reacted to waiting.

Since the office-visit cycle of service has at least two moments of truth requiring patients to wait, and often there are more, then it is important for medical practices to take action to reduce this problem. Begin by cutting down the number and length of the waits by taking the following four actions:

- Improve scheduling. Using the time-blocking method, you can reduce the waiting time for your patients. If, for example, the practice generally gets 25 percent to 35 percent of its appointments the same day, at least 35 percent of its slots should be left open to avoid overbooking. Also, measure the amount of time per typical problem and then schedule two long and two short appointments per hour.[11] Larry Gilber, M.D., a family physician in Santa Rosa, California, reduced the maximum wait in his office from 30 minutes to 15 while increasing the number of patients he saw each day from 28 to 32 by rearranging his schedule.[12]

- Increase the number of providers. The day of physician's assistants and nurse practitioners is on us, and their talents can contribute significantly to reducing patient delays. Some patients will need help in accepting treatment from anyone other than a doctor, but most find the PAs or NPs to be very satisfactory once they have a chance to experience them. In fact, one patient reported finding the nurse practitioners in her physician's office to be "more compassionate. They have more time and they do the basic procedures much more often than the doctors." One focus group participant described how his elderly mother's physician's office integrated PAs into her care. "They did an excellent job of educating her. First, she got a letter in the mail, telling her that they were starting a new approach that would help the practice respond more effectively to her needs. They were creating a patient case team, composed of her doctor, a physician's assistant, and a nurse—all of whom were to be up-to-speed on her case. Then when she went in for the next visit, a nurse sat down and explained it to her again . . . My mother is as happy as a bird!"

The office manager in a busy pediatrics practice, explained how both time-block scheduling and nurse practitioners have helped reduce the waiting time in her office. "We have one nurse practitioner who sees only sick patients during the day. She has no wellness appointments at all. As parents call in, appointments are scheduled with her for that day. She can see four in an hour. Other care providers have two hours a day that are set aside exclusively for sick patients as well."

■ Flexible scheduling. By having medical personnel available over a longer period of time, the patient load in any given time frame can be reduced. For example, opening the office at 7:00 A.M. instead of 8:00 A.M. and closing at 6:30 P.M. rather than 5:30 P.M. will provide a longer day in which to see patients. Flexible scheduling works for practice personnel too. Staggering the start and stop times not only accommodate patients' varied schedules, but also those of the staff.

■ Keep physicians on schedule. As I mentioned previously, many delays in the physician's office can be eliminated if the doctors will assume responsibility for managing their time more effectively. Industry estimates indicate that 80 percent of practitioners have problems managing their schedules. While some doctors create waits because they're chronically tardy or enjoy the pressure-cooker environment, most simply haven't learned to organize and maintain a schedule.[13] Office managers or scheduling clerks can help their doctors by faxing the next day's schedule to them each night, scheduling appointments in an appropriate manner, and nudging them along if they should fall behind during any given day. Doctors can take it on themselves to be more time conscious and to do their best to avoid unnecessary delays.

Regardless of all the best-laid plans, however, as long as there are doctors' offices, patients will experience some waiting periods. The emergency status of medical care, as well as the uncertain nature of other demands on the physician, are always going to play a part. Thus, it is important to know how to manage those moments of truth requiring waiting. Consider implementing the following suggestions regarding patients' waiting periods:

■ Label the area something else. Don't remind patients that they are experiencing a delay in their services by putting them in the *waiting room*. Consider doing as a participant in one of my workshops has done: label this area the *Reception Area* or *Patient Lounge*. Language does matter. If you call it a *waiting area*, patients will be more likely to focus on what they are doing. Also, they will receive the implicit message that patients must do a lot of waiting in your practice if you have an entire area designated for that purpose.

■ Show customers that you care that they are waiting. Apologies are important. Sincere ones, that is. When patients enter the reception area they should be greeted and told, with sincere apologies, when a wait is in the offing. Once they have begun to wait, whether still in the reception area or later in the cycle, someone should continue to check with them, again apologizing and seeing if they need anything. Patients report that this is especially important once they have been shown into the examination room and they are waiting for a doctor.

■ Explain the reason for the wait. An explanation often puts a patient's mind at ease. In fact, most patients are reasonable people, and once they understand that there is a good reason for their wait, they can live up to their title: they can be very patient. One woman in a focus group put it this way: "I know that something unexpected can come up, a surgery they think will take two hours ends up taking four. If that surgeon was operating on me, I'd want him to take all the time he needs!" Most patients understand that emergencies and complications can and do occur. Merely taking a moment to explain it to them will help ease the strain of waiting.

■ Allow customers a choice. Once it is clear that a wait, usually over 15 or 20 minutes, will occur, patients, like other customers in similar situations, want to be able to choose. The patient can be offered another appointment time, the option of seeing another doctor or a PA, or can choose to wait. Once they are given the alternatives, patients feel that they are back in control of their own lives again, and this reduces their stress over waiting. If the delay is known in advance, staffers should notify the patients by phone, giving them the option to decide prior to their arrival at the office.

■ Provide ways for the customers to occupy their time. Unoccupied time seems longer than occupied time. Thus, it is important to provide ways in which time spent waiting can be filled. The time-honored custom of magazines in the doctor's office is not an accidental one; however, take the trouble to keep them current, and keep the type that your patients will enjoy.

Noncoin telephones in the reception area are an excellent idea. They allow patients to conduct business, check on children and check in with other family members, and help rearrange schedules. Concerns about long-distance calls can be handled through the telephone company by either eliminating that function from the phone or installing a device that allows the long distance function to be turned off when no one is around. (Evidence from telephone companies indicates that these phones are hardly ever used inappropriately.) To get the best service advantage out of these phones, place them in a private area with a sign reading, "Available for our Patients. Free of Charge."[14] Of course, pediatrician's offices often have the child play area, but other practices could also have such a spot for the children of their patients. One OB-GYN office manager told me of the very popular recipe book that her patients have compiled. It contains favorite recipes and has a pocket in the front holding index cards and a pen for easy copying. This idea was originated by a patient advisory board and is in constant use. The mammography clinic I use has a professionally produced and very informative video on breast self-examination that is available for viewing while the patients wait.

■ Don't abandon a customer during a waiting period. Time alone seems longer than time in the presence of others. Thus, do all that you can to help the patients feel that they are not alone. Checking on them in the reception area or after they have gone to the examination room helps them feel less isolated.

Of all the potential moments of truth where waiting is problematic for patients, the wait in the examination room seems to be the worst. It is easy to understand why. The patients have disrobed, donned an odd little gown with a gaping hole in the back, and are usually surrounded by sterile equipment with only drawings of the human body for entertainment. They are more anxious at this moment, and anxiety increases the perceived time of waiting. They also report feeling completely alone at this moment, and they are. So, pay special attention to the patients you have waiting in those rooms for the doctor to arrive. As I've mentioned, check in with them to see if they need anything and to let them know when the doctor will be with them. As I discussed in Chapter 7, re-examine the nonverbal messages of the examination room itself and do what you can to make it warmer in tone and perhaps even in temperature. Probably the most innovative suggestion I've encountered for managing the perception of time in an exam room wait came from a participant in a workshop I was conducting. She explained, "We give each patient in an examination room a little clip board and a pen and ask them to complete the following question which is on a 3 x 5 card: 'What are the two most important questions you have for the doctor today?'" She reported that the patients found their waiting time in the examination room to go much more quickly, and the doctors reported that this process focused their interviews more readily, as well as reduced the "while I'm here" questions at the end.

First Moments
All customers report that their initial contact with a live person is a very important one. In the doctor's office, that moment usually is managed by the receptionist, easily the least-understood position in the practice. Begun in the days when all the receptionist was required to do was to meet and greet customers, this position in many organizations now involves much more. She often handles a complex switchboard, inputs information into computers, manages complicated scheduling, and is supposed to make the customers feel welcome. Since this initial contact is so important to the customer, the receptionist's position should be re-evaluated. Can the scheduling be handled by someone else in the practice? Can the computer be moved elsewhere so she can see and be seen? Patients report that even if the receptionist is on the telephone, they want some visible acknowledgement that they are present; a wave, a smile, a finger raised to indicate "I'll be with you in a minute"—all help the patients to feel recognized. Then, as soon as possible, the receptionist should speak to the patient, greeting him or her and, when appropriate, providing information regarding the waiting time to be expected. Merely allowing the patient to enter and sign in with no acknowledgement does not manage that important moment of truth very effectively.

Some practices have even begun the use of greeters. Although when I first heard of this in one of my workshops, my first reaction was "Sam Walton comes to healthcare!" I refrained from judging the idea until the participant had explained. She told of the use of senior patients who volunteered to spend a few hours a week serving as greeters in her office. She reported that they were very conscientious and were a great asset to the practice. They were able to meet the patients, bring them coffee or tea, sit and visit a while, provide reading material and keep it up to date, and assist the patient in other ways. Because these volunteers were also patients, she was able to screen them carefully and was also able to offer a small token of appreciation by absorbing the copayment for any of their visits to the doctor. In the same workshop, another manager told of similar use that she made of interns from the local high school and junior college. A nonpaid position, the young people were earning credit for their work in the practice, and part of their responsibilities included managing the reception area.

The Last Moment

Not often receiving much attention from medical practices, the last human contact the patient has is very important. Usually this moment is handled by either the person collecting payment or the scheduling clerk. Taking a few seconds to visit with the patient can go a long way to creating a positive moment. The scheduling clerk at Jackson Clinic in Jackson, Tennessee, said one day in a workshop, "I don't know, Vicky. Maybe I go too far with my job. The other day a little lady was leaving the clinic and she needed to schedule her next appointment. We talked about her current visit with the doctor and how things had gone and as she prepared to leave she burst out, 'I just love you.' Before I could stop myself, I answered, 'I love you too.' I don't know. Do you think I went too far?" Of course not. Such a spontaneous outpouring of affection was very natural for this particular woman and you can bet her patient left feeling warm and good. You do not have to tell every patient that you love them, however, to help them leave feeling cared for and served. A pleasant smile and a friendly voice helps the patient take away good feelings. (In Chapter 14, I discuss in detail how to create a graceful exit area, based on suggestions provided by Diane Palmer.)

A final thought: Remember that all moments of truth have the potential to be the most important moment of truth to any given customer. Thus, none can be considered unimportant.

Although, some moments of truth may be of greater importance to the customers than others, all are *equally* important to the practice personnel. What happens at any given moment of truth affects what happens in the next. Any negativity that may result from a moment of truth that has not been managed well will be carried over into the interaction that follows. Thus, it is incumbent on each person in the practice to do his or her best to provide a positive experience for the customer. Once understood, this kind of push from one moment to the next heightens the sense of interdependence experienced by practice personnel. Charting cycles of service helps people from different departments see how what they do impacts those from other departments. It helps bring a sense of unity to the entire process.

CHART THE INTERNAL PROCESSES

Although the most obvious opportunities for impacting service come through face-to-face interactions with customers, everything your practice does has service potential. Even the processes and procedures that are performed without direct contact with a customer can create positive or negative impressions of your practice. Laboratory tests conducted in-house, for example, involve processes that are conducted away from the presence of the patient, yet the results have a profound impact on their lives. Although the content of the results is beyond your control, the speed and accuracy with which the test processes are conducted frequently are not. It is important, then, to analyze the processes and procedures used to produce a product (a lab report, an X-ray, a bill for payment, etc.) to see if they are being conducted in a service-oriented manner.

Using the model in Figure 12–2, follow the steps listed below when charting the internal processes of your practice:

Step 1: What is the process being analyzed? (A lab test and report)

Step 2: What is the end product? (A lab report containing results of the test.)

Step 3: Who receives the end product? (The doctor and then the patient)

Step 4: From a service standpoint, what is important to the recipient about the product? (Usually, doctors and patients are concerned about the speed and accuracy of the test results and the accompanying report.)

FIGURE 12–2

Internal Processes Model

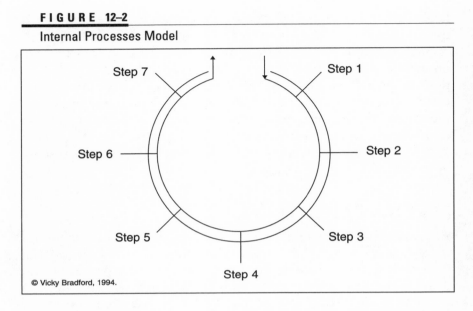

© Vicky Bradford, 1994.

Step 5: What are the steps in the process? (Identify each step that is necessary to conduct the test to find the results, and to prepare the report.)

Step 6: Do each of these steps enhance the desired service outcomes? (Examine each step to see if it meets the criteria specified in Step 4. In most cases, you will be looking for opportunities that will speed up the process without sacrificing accuracy.)

By analyzing the internal processes of your practice, you can also help employees who may not have a great deal of exposure to external customers to see their importance in the total customer experience. When working with one of my managed care clients, I asked a woman from the claims department what happened to a claim once she was finished with it. Looking puzzled, she said flatly, "It goes into a file cabinet." She had no concept of the idea that what she did in her little cubicle in the claims department had any impact on the member or on the physician's office. Look around at your practice. Is anyone working primarily on internal processes? Chances are that he or she may not realize how much what he or she does impacts customer service. Charting the Internal Processes will help this person understand the important contribution he or she makes to a quality service experience for your customers.

Also, the direct recipient of the product of internal processes often is an internal customer. Doctors are the first recipient of lab reports, for example, and so they become the customers of those who are performing that internal process. Charting internal processes, then, also helps improve the service provided to those customers within.

The quality of the service your practice provides is demonstrated through the systems, cycles, and processes that are in place. In order to make yours a Total Service Medical Practice, you should re-examine each of these and be willing to make changes. Without customer- and employee-friendly ways of doing things, even your most service-centered personnel will find it difficult to meet the needs of your customers.

END NOTES

1. Karl Albrecht, *Service Within* (Chicago: Dow-Jones Irwin, 1990), p. 12.

2. Karl Albrecht and Ron Zemhe, *Service America* (Chicago: Dow-Jones Irwin, 1985), p. 27.

3. Karl Albrecht, *At America's Service* (Chicago: Dow-Jones Irwin, 1988), p. 27.

4. Jack Gibbs, "Defensive Communication," *The Journal of Communication* 11, no. 3 (September 1961), pp. 141–148

5. "Spell Out Guidelines for Staff Interactions," *Physicians' Marketing and Management* 4, no. 11 (November 1991), p. 6.

6. Meryl Luallin, "Mystery Patient Shares Clues to Clinic Success," *Marketer's Guidepost* 2, no. 2 (Fall 1991), p. 9.

7. "Spell Out Guidelines for Staff Interactions."

8. Karl Albrecht, *At America's Service*, p. 16.

9. Mark Davis and Thomas Vollman, "A Framework for Relating Waiting Time and Customer Satisfaction in a Service Operation, *Journal of Services Marketing* 4, no. 1 (Winter 1990), pp. 61–69.

10. Paul Gerber and Marjolin Bijlefeld, "Ways Your Staff Can Lead You Down the Malpractice Path," *Physician's Management* 33, no. 1 (January 1993), pp. 98–99.

11. Harlene Ellin, "Practice Tune-Up," *American Medical News* 33, no. 49 (November 9, 1990), p. 9.

12. Ibid.

13. Ibid.

14. "Put a Courtesy Phone in Your Reception Area," *The Physician's Advisory* Leif C. Beck, Publisher 91, no. 12 (December 1991) p. 6.

CHAPTER

Step Thirteen—Manage the Key Doctor/Patient Moments of Truth

Troubling to some physicians and always challenging, the patient interview, sometimes called the patient encounter, is the time when doctors gather vital diagnostic information. It also provides the opportunity for building and maintaining positive doctor/patient relationships. In fact, the *Handbook of Clinical Psychiatry* calls patient interviewing the core skill in medicine, and stresses that good communication between the doctor and the patient is the basis of good medical practice. When discussing medical interviews in general, this textbook lists six purposes of doctor/patient encounters: (1) to obtain historical perspective of a patient's life, (2) to establish rapport and a therapeutic alliance, (3) to develop mutual trust and confidence, (4) to understand present functioning or condition, (5) to make a diagnosis or begin that process, (6) to establish a treatment plan.[1]

What do we know about doctor/patient interviews? Quite a lot, actually. Patients have been more than happy to discuss their likes and dislikes about these interactions. Doctors have been generous in sharing their opinions and experiences in published articles and in interviews. Researchers have focused their attention on these interactions in numerous studies. After synthesizing information from many of these sources, I have arrived at several suggestions for effective patient interviewing. By following these 12 steps, you can enhance the quality of the information you will receive as a physician, as well as create the kind of positive interaction that patients want to have with their doctors. Thus, this key moment of truth will be effectively managed.

THE TWELVE STEPS TO EFFECTIVE PATIENT INTERVIEWS

Step One: Prepare for *This* Patient.

Before you enter the examination room, stop and take a deep breath. Get focused on who is beyond that door. Look at the chart a moment to refresh your memory of past visits, of the clinical and nonclinical information you need to make this patient become a person to you. Also, discern the initial reason for the visit conveyed by the patient to your scheduling clerk. Prepare yourself, not for *a* patient but for *this* patient. Robert Tannenbaum, a partner in Tannenbaum and Berman Psychological Associates in Philadelphia, stated, "My bottom-line message is that you need to treat each one of your patients as an individual to the extent you can, given the time constraints that affect us all. If you succeed, your patient will come away feeling fulfilled, and feeling that you care, are competent, and are honest."[2]

During the last big push of writing this book, I realized that there was a gap in my methodology. I had not been a participant-observer yet, one of the most powerful tools in sociological research. So, I decided that I should become a patient with a mildly serious problem in order to see what would happen to me. Thus, I went for a walk one early spring day so that I could trip on a tiny bump in the sidewalk, fall on my hands and arms, and shatter the radial head of my elbow into four pieces. Well, all right, I didn't fall on purpose! Always an optimist, however, I realized that I could indeed use my experience for some firsthand research for my book. The following story tells of a skilled orthopedic surgeon who did not follow Dr. Tannenbaum's advice, and my impression of what it felt like not to be seen as a person, but as *the broken elbow in Examination Room 5:*

I have been blessed with good health all of my life, so this was my first major injury, and in spite of my familiarity with the healthcare scene, I was feeling very vulnerable and a little frightened. As I sat bracing my injured arm in the examination room that first day in the surgeon's office, I also felt anxious and nervous about what was ahead. Suddenly the door burst open and this bundle of energy bounded in, lab coat flying and X-rays in hand. Without ever looking at me (her eyes were already on the X-rays), she emitted her greeting: "Oh boy! OH BOY! OH BOY! You did it, didn't you." The irritation in her voice made me feel like a child being reprimanded for some irresponsible act. After a quick trip down the hall to look at a skeleton's elbow, we returned to the examination room whereupon, without pausing to allow me to sit down, she began to unwrap my aching arm. Standing there in the middle of the floor, I suddenly began to feel very weak in the knees. The doctor did not notice this at all as she mumbled something about, "Well, we'll definitely have to do surgery. I hate elbows." Not at all certain if I could remain on my feet, I finally asked weakly, "May I sit down?" For the first time in the 10 minutes or so that had elapsed since her entrance into the room, she really saw me, and said, "Oh . . . Well . . . Sure." Then with surprise she said, "You're really upset about this, aren't you?" When I confirmed that I was, she asked what about. I responded, "Everything. I've not been seriously ill or injured in my life. I've never even been a patient in the hospital, let alone had surgery. And my arm hurts! So, yes, I guess you could say I'm upset." To her credit, she had me lie down on the table and pulled up a chair by my side. Even though I'm certain she had patients waiting in the next room, she talked calmly to me about what was going to happen and how much she trusted the anesthesiologist and the entire surgical team at the hospital. By the time she left, I felt reassured, somewhat, and confident that I was in good hands. And surgically I was.

The service point of this story should be obvious. Although I am convinced that this doctor did not intend to be insensitive to me, she had shifted into autopilot, forgetting for the moment that she would be treating a whole human being and not merely a broken arm. If this physician had allowed herself to focus on me as a *person*, I think our entire interaction would have been much different. It would have certainly been shorter, because by the time she finally addressed my concerns, they had escalated to such a level that it took her a while to calm me down. Plus, she had to repeat much of what she had said earlier in the interview about checking in to the hospital, and so on, because I had been unable to attend to it at the time she first told me. From a patient's point of view, I really deserved to be treated differently. It was not necessary for me to go through this unpleasant and frightening experience, and it could have been avoided. So I urge you, take that moment outside the door to remind yourself that there is a *person* waiting for you on the other side. From a pragmatic as well as a humanistic point of view, patients should be accorded no less.

When preparing for a given patient, I also suggest that you check for any potential biases you might have and work to counteract them. What biases? Sometimes these are patient-specific and result from difficult interpersonal interactions in the past. If you find yourself thinking, "Oh no! It's Mrs. _____ again!" you are dealing with such a bias. Also, research has discovered that sometimes physicians hold more subtle attitudes about their patients, behaving more negatively (in effectiveness and/or in terms of services or information provided) toward minority, low-income, and female patients than toward white, higher income, and male patients, even within the same care settings.[3] An honest self-examination should reveal whether you hold such biases, and will be the first step to eliminating them.

This introspective process may not be entirely comfortable, yet it can be very helpful. I speak from personal experience. Years ago I was a college professor when research on gender bias in the classroom first became common knowledge among educators. I remember very clearly my certainty that this did not apply to me and also my discomfort when I began to identify some of my own previously unknown biases. Yet, that very self-analysis provided me with the opportunity to make needed changes in my interactions with my students. The same may be true for you in your relationships with your patients.

The focus on each individual patient that I am recommending may create a different rhythm in your day, at least for a while. Rather than the flow that can develop as you move from one diagnosis, illness, or condition to another, you will experience a sense of starting and stopping. Your professional life may feel like a series of jerks, and the pun is not intended! This is the result of shifting from autopilot to suddenly seeing each patient encounter as a complete communication situation with a beginning, middle, and end. Such starting and stopping takes energy. So, be prepared for a drain on your already well-tapped energy supply for awhile. In time, you will begin to find a new rhythm. You can even begin to like the variety and challenge of each patient encounter. Don't be impatient with yourself. This may be a new dance you are learning, and it takes time to become accustomed to the steps.

Step Two: Enter the Room

Yes, something as initially insignificant as how you open the door and walk into the examination room, and how you look while doing it, can communicate important messages to your patient. As was discussed in Chapter 7, if patients perceive you as frantic and harried, not only will they experience feelings of unrest and discomfort, but also their perception of time will be affected. The pause outside the door (recommended in Step 1) presents a perfect opportunity to slow down. Being aware of your kinetic behavior will help you control it as well. Paying attention to gestures, facial expressions, and the speed with which you walk will help you project the kind of initial impression you want the patient to have. The old saying, "First impressions are lasting impressions," certainly applies to patient interactions.

Immediate recognition is important to all kinds of customers, and patients enjoy this kind of greeting as well. A friendly demeanor, a smile even when the situation may be a difficult one, and a personal greeting using the patient's name will help create the kind of communication climate you want for the remainder of the interview.

The form of address you use is a small thing that means a lot to patients. The question is: When addressing a patient, should you use a first or last name? Opinions vary as to how this should be handled. Most older patients, certainly those older than the doctor, usually seem to prefer to be addressed by their last names, and may complain if it is otherwise. One woman said, "I'm old enough to be his grandmother! Where does he come off calling me Margaret!" A physician in one of my workshops related an incident that resulted in the patient's permanent departure from his practice, all because he called her by her first name. He said, "She was an older patient, but not that much older than I, and I decided that using her first name would be appropriate. I had no idea that this woman was a matriarch in the community and *no one* called her Alice. I would never have known why she left my practice if a colleague of mine hadn't told me. Apparently she told him I was disrespectful and rude. When he asked her why, she said, as if this would explain it all, 'Well, he called me by my first name.'"

The use of a first name for the senior patient population seems to be more acceptable by male patients when they are addressed by male doctors. Also, it seems to vary according to the length of the time the physician has known the patient. One man who has been treated by the same doctor for several years said, "It's OK with me if he calls me Dave. I mean, he's been looking down my throat for 15 years."

Probably the best advice is to ask the patients for their preferred form of address. It's easy to inquire during the first interview, "Are you more comfortable if I call you by your first name or your last?" This is also a question that can be asked by your appointments clerk or receptionist and noted on the chart: "We want you to be comfortable here with us, so it will help doctor to know how you would like to be addressed, Mrs. Jones or Betty. Which do you prefer?" Patients seem to appreciate attention to such seemingly small details and mention it as an example of superior service.

Remembering the patient's name is another trick at times. Eric Anderson, M.D., suggested that once you know the patient's name, repeat it immediately. The repetition will help you remember it and also will help you make sure that you can pronounce it correctly. Also, using it twice in the first two minutes of the interview will help cement it in your mind.[4] "So, Mrs. George, what seems to be the problem?" followed soon by "I see. About when did that pain start increasing, Mrs. George?" will not only help you remember your patient's name, but will also convey your personal interest in this patient to this patient.

Obviously not necessary when you already know your patient, introducing yourself is an important step to a new one. You need to decide how you want to be addressed, although you may or may not get your wish. Traditionally, patients have called their physicians *Doctor*, sometimes affectionately following the title with the first name. However, as with everything else in healthcare, the form of address from patient to doctor is changing, too. My advice and that of physicians who have been participants in my workshops is to be flexible. The workshop physicians report that while at first it was a shock to hear a patient use their first names, they soon became accustomed to it. Although I understand and perhaps even empathize with the rationale for the use of the title when patients address you, I agree with the Rhode Island physician who attended one of my seminars: "I'll admit I was startled the first time a patient called me by my first name, but I got over it. I mean, the issue is really about the patients' comfort, not mine. If calling me John makes them feel more connected to me and comfortable, then I really shouldn't object."

Step Three: Sit, as Close to Eye Level as Possible, With Your Patient

I have already mentioned the importance of this small but significant step in Chapter 7. Now let me explore it more fully. Sitting helps the patients feel that you care about them because it creates the perception that you have time for them, and this is an important perception! Vincent Fulginiti, M.D., chancellor of the University of Colorado Health Screening Center, stated in his article "The Big 8: Major Malpractice Traps in Pediatrics" "Complaints of physicians' rushed or hurried demeanor and their not listening, not making time for questions, and not taking time to explain a medical concept thoroughly dot many of the depositions I've examined."[5] Jack T. Patton, M.D., a family physician who has served on numerous committees to evaluate physician performance, found that even though the complaints received may not lead to malpractice suits, some doctors engendered patient dissatisfaction for no other reason than that they appeared to be rushed. Dr. Patton explained, "I'm not surprised patients complain. I've watched doctors and have seen them do it. They've never learned that no matter how hurried they feel, they mustn't convey that to the patient."[6] Perhaps one physician stated it most succinctly: "We have to learn. It doesn't matter if all hell is breaking loose outside that door, the patient must never know it." One of the easiest ways for a physician to convey an unhurried, caring demeanor is to sit during the patient interview.

As I pointed out in Chapter 7, sitting impacts the perceptions of time in another, related way: It also makes patients think you have spent more time with them than you actually have. In addition, patients report that when doctors sit, they experience a sense of equality and partnership in their healthcare and do not feel like passive observers of it. They also describe doctors who sit as more approachable, which results in greater openness in their disclosure of information.

Sitting helps the patient feel that you are listening, especially if you are sitting at the patient's eye level. As a result of his training in communication skills, my doctor makes a special effort to sit so that he can look me in the eye. If I am in a chair, he draws up one near me. If I am already on the examination table, I have seen him raise himself to sit on the counter. Even though I know what he is doing, it still makes me feel more comfortable and enhances my impression that he is really listening to me.

So, sit! It will help reap several important benefits.

Step Four: Make Some Personal Connection

Just how folksy this step becomes is a matter of personal style. Some physicians express their discomfort at what appears to be chitchat with their patients. They also complain that this kind of conversation takes time, time that they believe could be better spent. However, I am not talking about idle conversation. Rather I am referring to purposeful exchange. One patient told me, "I went to the same doctor for many years and I thought the world of him. When I first went in, he would sit there and make personal conversation. I'd been going to him for years, and then one day he told me about some training he had been conducting for younger physicians in the hospital. He said, 'I told them if you talk to your patients, touch them, get to know them, it will help you in their treatment and diagnosis.'" The patient laughingly reported, "I thought, 'That's what he's been doing all these years.' He got all of this information out of me and I didn't even know it."

Such conversations are important to creating a personal bond between the patient and the physician. Bernard Strauss, M.D., relied on his 25 years of experience when offering this advice,

"Don't hesitate to warm up to people. My patients do everything from collecting beer cans to piloting World War II vintage planes. In most cases, I wouldn't have found out these things if I hadn't asked. I note them on a separate sheet of paper in the chart and may bring them up at the next visit. When I do, the patient understands that I view him as a person and not simply as a disease process."[7] The importance of such doctor/patient bonding was discussed in detail in Chapter 2: It leads to higher levels of patient satisfaction, which in turn often result in increased compliance with treatment and the obtaining of more reliable data during the diagnostic phases of the interview.

Step Five: Identify the Chief Complaint

This step is accomplished through the use of several communication techniques, the most basic of which is the process of inquiry. The types of questions that are available to you were covered in the verbal communication section of Chapter 7. A review of those options will reveal that the open-ended question is usually the most appropriate type for use at this time. "What brought you here today?" will begin to focus the patient on the purpose of the visit, but leaves him or her plenty of room for responding.

I should also caution you to listen seriously to even the most ridiculous answer. A doctor in a workshop told me of a patient who answered the "What brought you here today?" question with the response, "The bus!" This doctor reported that his first reaction was to snicker and then he realized that the patient was not laughing. He probed a bit further and discovered that the patient was having difficulties with her husband, who refused to bring her to the appointment. This same spouse was also not encouraging the physical therapy the patient was supposed to be doing at home. What at first appeared to be a silly answer actually revealed a major concern that was on the patient's mind and a major obstacle to her compliance with the PT treatment plan.

Some physicians are concerned about the possible breadth of the response to open-ended questions. However, "Studies indicate that eliciting an opening patient narrative has little effect on the overall interview length and, in fact, improves the quality of the encounters by widening the scope of information received. Usually one to two minutes is sufficient for patients to feel that their story is being heard and understood. It also makes patients much more receptive to a detailed line of questions."[8]

Once you ask an open-ended question, you need to sit quietly and listen, something that is not the norm for most physicians. Remember the research that indicated, on average, after asking a question, physicians interrupt their patients after only eighteen seconds.[9] One physician reported a creative method for correcting this problem: he used a silent 90-second egg timer to force himself to listen. Much to his surprise, the technique has changed the tone of many of his encounters. "It has increased the sense of partnership, illuminated telling symptoms, and improved time management for new patient visits."[10] Risk managers also stress the importance of asking open-ended questions, allowing the patients to fully explain. They stress that doctors must avoid the temptation to interrupt.[11]

When patients pause, one of the most difficult listening behaviors to master is to merely sit and wait. This is particularly difficult for busy doctors who have a long list of patients needing their time. However, Eric Anderson, M.D., advised, that even when patients pause, physicians should wait quietly because patients often fill that time with some very important piece of information."[12] He further suggests another useful strategy: "The way to get better descriptions from the patient is not to rush in with yes/no questions once the patients run out of steam, but simply to repeat the patients' last words to jog their memory a bit and get them to continue with their train of thought."[13]

After asking an open-ended question and listening, without interruption, to the patient's story, the doctor should then ask a series of more guided questions, such as the following:

Direct Question: "How did that make you feel?" (Directing the patient to address his or her feelings.)

Indirect Question: "What do you think might have caused this pain?" (Guiding the patient to examine what has been occurring in her life that might have brought on the problem.)

Closed Question: "So, you started feeling bad last Friday?" (Verifying information, looking for a yes or no response.)

Building on each answer with another question can lead the patient through a description of physical symptoms, emotional impact, self-analysis, causes, and so on.

Another useful technique is the internal summary. At some points along the way, you can pause to paraphrase what you have heard thus far. These paraphrased summaries help you check your understanding of the story, move the patient more quickly through the story, provide the opportunity for you to clarify the complaint, and help crystallize what you will eventually write on the chart. Such a summary would sound something like this: "Let me be sure that I'm tracking with you, Mrs. Bennett. Last Saturday, you woke up with a pain in your right arm and a tingling in your right hand. As the day wore on, you begin to lose feeling in the fingers of that hand. That night, you took some Tylenol and went to bed and everything felt better until yesterday, when you experienced this same thing again. Is that the way it happened?"

The process of assessing the complaint is more than a linear collection of data. When done well, it can almost become a beautiful dance between the doctor and the patient as they move through its phases. It also is much like solving a mystery. The physician begins with only a limited piece of information— something brought this patient to your office on this day. Sometimes the answer is direct and simple—it's time for the annual check-up. Thus the mystery is short lived. However, often times, it is as complicated as any Sherlock Holmes story, and you, as the physician, must become the master sleuth, ever vigilant for the most subtle of clues. When it comes to the assessment of the complaint, nothing is "Elementary, my dear Watson."

Step Six: Comment on the Symptoms

Another tendency, usually caused by the pressures of time or merely just not realizing the importance of doing otherwise, is to move quickly after the patient has told his or her story to conducting the physical examination. Dr. Eric Anderson advised, "it is important to the patients' psyches that we reflect on the story we have just heard and make a comment. So often we record, without emotions, data that would knock even a priest off his feet.

Sure, we have to be professional and objective, but we often forget to show we recognize how disturbing those symptoms must have been for the patients. A statement to the effect, 'This must have been very distressing to you' goes a long way to legitimize the patient's concerns."[14]

What Dr. Anderson and I are really talking about is empathy. Empathy means that you understand the emotional message that the patient has conveyed to you. By expressing your understanding of not only the physical but the emotional impact of their health problem, you can show the patients that you are listening to their whole message and that you care. This creates a more trusting and less anxious situation for the patients, allowing them to provide better information and to comply more easily and readily with the treatment that is to come.

Some doctors find it difficult to express empathy, preferring to stay in the cerebral part of their minds. There are even understandable reasons for this choice. Consider what the following five physicians believe about the expression of empathy:

Doctor One believes that if he becomes emotionally involved with each patient, the resulting strain would be overwhelming. Although this concern is understandable, it is based on the misperception of empathy that I described in Chapter 7, that it has to be an almost magical experiencing of the emotions of the other. As I also indicated in Chapter 7, however, empathy does not have to be regarded in this way. It can be seen as a cognitive activity, requiring the understanding, but not necessarily the experiencing, of someone else's emotions. By accessing the recollections of how he felt when he was angry, hurt, frightened or sad, Doctor One could respond empathetically without experiencing the intense emotional roller coaster ride he fears.

Doctor Two believes that by being empathetic he will cause his patients to feel emotions they would not otherwise feel, and that this would not be good for them. My response to Doctor Two is twofold. First, Dr. Two, or anyone else for that matter, cannot prevent patients from feeling emotions. People will feel what they feel, and they will experience a keen sense of isolation while they do. Patients actually report welcoming the acknowledgement of their emotions by their doctors so that they will not go through it alone. One terminally ill patient poignantly described her gratitude to her physician, whom she called Edward, for his empathetic responses: "He is the only one who will allow me to feel what I feel and who will share it with me. My family members won't. I know they are trying to protect me, but Edward knows that isn't what I need. I always look forward to his visits so we can talk and plan what I have left of my life."

On the other hand, if Doctor Two is partially correct and the patients have not faced their emotions, *shouldn't* they? In addition to the cathartic release that comes with experiencing such feelings, these patients will be easier to treat and diagnose. Patients who do not acknowledge their feelings tend to be very passive or eternally sunny. They also may mask fear and sadness with anger. None of these emotional states allows the patients to provide useful information to a physician, nor do they allow patients to move through any painful emotions and into acceptance of their situations.

Doctor Three believes that an empathetic response is an unprofessional response. The problem here is with the definition of *professional*. To this doctor, technical expertise is the equivalent of professionalism. I urge this doctor to consider the following: the professional physician is the complete one: one who has the clinical expertise needed to treat the patients and the nonclinical skills to support them as human beings. According to this definition, then, empathy is one of the most important skills such a physician would possess.

Doctors Four and Five are uncomfortable with accessing their own emotions. Doctor Four has been trained in medical school to be objective, and has learned to control her feelings. When she felt something for her patients as a resident, she was ridiculed by her supervising physicians. Doctor Four has been heard to say, "My emotions have been programmed out of me."

Doctor Five is also uncomfortable with empathy. He became a physician because of his interest in the scientific process and is much more at home with the science of medicine. He finds, even in his personal life, that it is difficult for him to show his emotions. Because he is closed off from his own feelings, it is very difficult and uncomfortable for him to try to understand those of others.

To both doctors, I would say, "I know it is not your preferred mode of behavior. Yet, I urge you to stretch yourself to endure the discomfort. Your patients need it from you, and it, like any other communication skill, can be learned." Following the steps to achieving empathy, as discussed in Chapter 7, will help Doctors Four and Five learn how to make the empathetic response a part of their patient interactions.

All of the doctors described above can be found in medical practices across the country. However, they should not exist in a practice that has embraced the concept of total service. Empathy is a key to service, especially when serving those who are angry, frightened, or sad. The physician who does not choose to be empathetic will not be comfortable in a practice that is built on the extension of service to the customers.

Step Seven: Write it Down

Now is the time to record the comments made by the patient. Many doctors make the mistake of starting to write too soon. Not only does that disrupt the direct eye contact you have with the patient, and thus reduce the perception of effective listening, but it also will cause you to write insignificant details. By listening to the whole story first, you can reach the broader conclusions to be recorded and filter out the information that is irrelevant.

Another disadvantage of writing too soon is the impact that it will have on the length of the patient's story. Contrary to what you may believe, when the senders of communication messages perceive that the receivers are attentive and are listening effectively, they will take less time to complete their messages than if the receivers are not looking at them and appear not to be paying attention. Patients report that when the doctor is writing, they fear that he or she is not "getting" their story, and thus they repeat themselves. If you wait to write until after the patient has finished, you can actually shorten the interview.

During one of my workshops for physicians, a participant pointed out that in some cases he had to start writing soon. "These situations are complicated and there is a lot of information that I have to get correctly," he observed. This doctor raised a very valid point and one that can be easily handled. In those instances where you believe you must start writing fairly early in the interview, simply tell the patient what you are going to do and why, such as, "I'm going to be taking careful notes while you talk, Mrs. Jones, because I don't want to miss any of this important information."

This kind of statement will allay any concerns that the patient may have regarding your writing. In fact, patients report that they usually are not bothered by much of anything that happens to them in the practice as long as they are not surprised by it and if they understand why it is happening.

When you do write in the chart, please do so legibly, and concisely but completely. The old stereotype of the physician with unreadable penmanship is not too far off the mark for most doctors. When interviewing staff members in medical practices, and nurses who need to decipher your writing at the hospital, I discovered that one of their requests was that you write so that they can read it. Also, be sure to give enough detail that someone else can understand what the patient has told you and to refresh your memory when you read the chart at a later time. A doctor in one of my sessions offered an additional suggestion: Instead of completing paperwork regarding the patient in your office, do so while the patient is still present, telling him or her what you are doing. The physician reported that this simple act increased the patients' perception of time spent with them.

Step Eight: Conduct the Physical Examination

A most important moment in any patient interaction, how the doctor handles the physical examination makes a great deal of difference in the patient's reactions to it. While I would not presume to tell you what to do medically during this part of a patient encounter, I do have a few suggestions regarding its nonclinical aspects.

First, inform the patient that you are now ready to move into this phase of the encounter by telling him or her exactly what you are going to do. Although as a doctor you are given implicit permission to enter into their intimate space, patients report that it is still comforting to have a warning before you actually do so.

Next, explain what you are doing throughout the physical examination. Your explanation subtly demonstrates your competence to the patient; if you know what you are doing and can tell them about it, they are more likely to trust you. They also report a great deal of emotional reassurance when they know what is happening to them. Patients may not understand what is wrong with their bodies, but they can understand "Now I'm going to look into your ears."

Next, as may be fairly obvious, you should touch them. Of course, while you could hardly conduct a physical examination without doing so, there are some nonclinical reasons why touching is important as well. First, patients report their need for the kind and reassuring touch from their physicians in these moments of healthcare concern, even if it's merely a routine physical examination. For many patients your hands are equated with healing. Never underestimate the power of your touch as a doctor. While it may not actually bring about a cure to their healthcare problem, it does help assuage your patients' emotional anxiety.

Another and more pragmatic reason for physically touching your patients is its direct impact on patient satisfaction. Patients notice if you touch them or not. They come to see you to be examined. If you don't conduct some kind of a physical examination, even though it may not be medically necessary, they conclude that you have not given them good care. One patient in a focus group described just such a situation. When I asked the participants what made them the most upset about the nonclinical side of the care given by their physicians, this woman responded, "I couldn't believe it. He came into the room, looked down at me and asked, 'Are you still having pain in that knee?' I said 'Yes' and he told me to keep up my water exercise routine and then he left. He never even looked at my knee! What kind of a doctor is that?" Even if this woman's doctor may have discovered what he needed to know by the answer to her question, she didn't understand that; she wanted him to touch her.

Finally, demonstrate sensitivity and awareness during this most personal part of a patient encounter. Although most doctors know of the patient's vulnerability at this moment, many confess to having forgotten it. The physical examination becomes a routine part of a doctor's day. However, patient's report that this is the most difficult moment of their visit to the doctor. It is not an everyday occurrence for them to disrobe and don the odd little gown with the split in the back. Thus, they appreciate the doctor who remains aware of this vulnerability and acts accordingly.

The same sensitivity is equally important, perhaps more so, to patients who are chronically ill. Unlike those for whom the physical examination is unusual, these individuals are subjected to this undignified experience on a daily or weekly basis. I say *subjected* because no matter how often it occurs, this kind of repeated invasion into that highly protected intimate space is not pleasant. It may actually cause physical pain, and it most certainly attacks the patients' sense of personal dignity. Being aware of this fact and being sensitive to their needs for respectful treatment will help these chronically ill patients in this most difficult time.

I cannot leave this point without telling the story of Sister Grace. A large woman who looked to have the strength of two farm hands, she ruled the corridors of the small rural hospital where my father was a frequent patient. Based on her physical appearance alone, it would have been easy to judge Sister Grace as a poor choice for this field. Yet, when this nurse touched my father, her name's remarkable appropriateness became apparent. As I watched her gently search for a useable vein in his already pincushioned arm, or lift him from the bed to his favorite chair by the window, I saw firsthand her gentleness and genuine empathy for all he had been through. My wish for all healthcare professionals is that they too could have observed and perhaps learned from Sister Grace.

Most examples I have encountered of physician insensitivity during the physical exam result from doctors who have gone on autopilot and simply do not notice what they are doing. One doctor described his wake-up call regarding routine procedures. One day he was doing a simple examination of a patient—an agreeable woman he had known for years. After a while he began to take her blood pressure. She said in surprise, "Doctor, you've already done that!"

When doctors become caught up in the routine tasks, they run the risk of simply not being aware of what they are doing, as the above example illustrates. While this situation was merely embarrassing for the doctor, it might well have shaken the faith the patient had in him. I myself was treated by an insensitive physician during a routine physical examination. This doctor seemed completely unaware of my vulnerability and his behavior was inappropriate and embarrassing to me. Just as with my orthopedic surgeon, I don't think this physician had any purposeful intent, nor was he a particularly mean spirited-person.

Rather, I believed then and still do that he was merely unfocused on me as a person. This was not a major event in his life; it was just one more examination. However, to me, it mattered a great deal.

Another suggestion during the physical examination is to make encouraging comments as you go. The patient likes to hear "That looks good." "I like the sound of that." There is something about those words coming from the physician that makes the patient feel good. Even a nod of the head or a look of satisfaction means a great deal to the patient. If during this examination you discover that the patient has indeed followed your instructions from the last visit, now is the time to heap the praise on him. As Dr. Eric Anderson stated, "Give credit where credit is due. Compliment the patient. Tell him or her they've done a good job, but be sure you mean it."[15]

One additional little tip for keeping yourself on time: When you take a pulse during the physical examination, check the time as well.

Step Nine: Discussion of Diagnosis

Now it is time to offer information to the patients, which means it is time for you to offer some explanations, not something doctors tend to do very well. The American Medical Association, in a public opinion survey on healthcare issues, reported that only 42 percent of the survey respondents agreed with the statement: "Doctors usually explain things well to their patients."[16] Greg Carroll, the Director of the Miles Institute of Health Care Communication, described a study showing that doctors imparted information to patients for an average of little more than a minute during interviews that lasted an average of 20 minutes. When asked how much time they spent on patient education, the physicians overestimated by a factor of nine. The study also found that, in 65 percent of the cases, physicians thought patients wanted less information than they actually did.[17]

Failure to explain the material facts to patients is seldom the primary charge in malpractice cases, but it's a secondary element in many suits. A University of Rochester Highland Hospital study of 140 depositions in malpractice suits indicated that "failure to provide an explanation" was cited in 35 percent of them.[18]

Perhaps the biggest reason for the tendency to compress or even avoid explanations is that they are perceived to be time consuming. To a degree, that may be true, on initial explanations at least. However, as Eleanor Segal, a Stanford University professor affiliated with the geriatric division of the VA Medical Center in Palo Alto, California, stated, "It may take a little more time to explain matters in detail, but you save a lot more time down the road. If you inform patients at every step of the way, they won't return in a confused, miserable state because they don't understand what's happening to them."[19] Although there are places to reduce the time spent in a given patient interaction, explanations are not one of them.

So, it is at Step Nine that the process of detailed explanations begins. This also is the beginning of the process of informed consent. Lee Johnson, JD, counsel for healthcare law for New York City Medical Liability Insurance Company, said, "Doctors think informed consent is a form. They forget its just evidence of conversation. In most states, either by case law or statute, the patient is entitled to that conversation."[20] And that conversation begins with your explanation.

Even if you need the results of some laboratory tests before you can fully inform the patient of his or her condition, the patient wants to know what you have discovered so far. When discussing your diagnosis, be it final or tentative, the following six tips will be helpful:

1. Be clear. Don't speak in technical jargon, and if you must use a technical term, define it immediately. This is one of the biggest complaints of patients about their doctors' explanations.

2. Be honest. Don't hide the truth from the patients and don't speak in clever disguises. As gynecologist Debra Gussman told me, "If it's cancer I say 'cancer,' not 'a tumor.' They need to know from the beginning what we are dealing with." When interviewing nurses for this book, physician honesty was their first and most urgent request to the doctors: "Doctors should tell the patient the truth. If they don't, the patients will just ask us, and news about their healthcare should really come from the physicians."

When I was conducting a workshop for hospital interns, one young woman challenged this point, saying, "Patients may say they want honesty, but they really don't." My response to her was and still is: "There is a difference between brutal honesty and empathetic honesty." Delivering the bad news is never easy, and, in an effort to get past the difficulty of that moment quickly, some doctors deliver it in an emotionless, blunt fashion. Others understand the difficulty and, while still being honest, deliver the information supportively and empathetically. Most patients report that they want to know the truth, but they also report that they want to hear it gently.

In addition to the importance of honesty to the patients, it is also important for the doctor. As a part of the informed consent process, which is mandated in most states, the patients must be told the truth of their condition. They will be unable to knowledgeably give their consent for any treatment if they are not.

3. Be positive. Even if the news is bad, move quickly to treatment options. Dr. Gussman, the gynecologist referred to above, also said, "Once the news has been delivered, I move quickly into the steps we can take to deal with this situation."

4. Be thorough. One patient told me of her doctor, who sat down and went through every item on the checkup list. He then made a copy of the report for the patient to peruse at her own leisure. The patient described to me her great pleasure at having all of this information and noted that it did not require a great deal of time. Like this woman, patients like to know, want to know, and increasingly expect to know what you find out.

5. Verify understanding. Your job as a communicator is complicated, in the medical setting, by at least two types and perhaps all three types of noise, as discussed in Chapter 7. The patients' bodies are quite likely sending physical messages of pain and, at the very least, emotional messages of anxiety that vie with your messages for their attention. On occasion, the hustle and bustle of a busy practice may also provide environmental noise that can become distracting, increasing the likelihood that your message will be misunderstood. By merely asking the patients to express their understanding of important information, you may well prevent some serious problems later on.

6. Provide it in writing, too. To supplement the verbal explanations you offer, written materials can be quite helpful. They will provide excellent references when the patients are at home, attempting to remember what you said. In addition, patients report that having a doctor underline or highlight sections of a preprinted brochure helps to personalize the content. Doctors report that such preprinted material helps save time as well. I caution you, however, not to merely place the written material in the patients' hands; a thorough interpersonal explanation from you cannot and should not be replaced by the printed word.

Step Ten: Discuss Treatment Options and Instructions

Now the patient knows the results of your inquiry and physical exam. If treatment is necessary, you need to move into that phase and complete the process of informed consent. What I am talking about here is *shared decision making*. Even within the context of cost containment, most diagnoses carry a range of treatment options, and patients should have the opportunity to participate in the final decision. Benefits of this approach are reported by patients as well as physicians. Experts have stated that shared decision making enhances patient satisfaction, increases compliance, and reduces the chances of a malpractice suit if something goes wrong.[21] Physicians who connect with their patients through shared decision making enjoy practicing much more, because they no longer have to carry the entire burden of the decisions; also, the patients feel that they have some control over what should be done.

Of course, there are some patients who do not want to make this decision. Those people need to be encouraged to do so. Even if you merely offer the options, make your recommendation, and ask for their reaction to it, this will solicit their participation in their own healthcare and increase their ownership of it.

Once a treatment plan has been determined, then the physician must be certain to explain clearly what the patient's responsibilities are, how medication should be taken, how physical therapy should be done, and so forth. Also, instructions should be given on what to look for as side effects, desired results, or continuing or worsening symptoms.

Another reason for discussing treatment options and for providing complete instructions is the ever-present issue of malpractice suits. The Physicians Insurers Association of America, which has collected data on 96,000 malpractice claims, estimated that up to 30 percent charge a lack of informed consent or failure to instruct the patient properly.[22]

So, even though I am aware of some physician resistance toward using the shared decision-making approach, I am still recommending its use. Evidence shows that providing clear and thorough discussion of the treatment options and instructions for the chosen treatment is an important part of the patient interview, resulting in better medical care, higher patient satisfaction, better compliance, and a reduction in the filing of malpractice suits.

Step Eleven: Seek the "While I'm Here" Questions

These questions are the bane of most physicians' existence. Why, then, would I suggest that you invite them rather than run from them? First, because often these are the real reasons *why* many patients come to see you in the first place. These questions may contain embarrassing or difficult issues that patients just can't bring themselves to face directly. So, they will tell you they have come for some other reason and finally, just as you are about to conclude the interview and move on to the next patient, they say, "Oh, by the way!" Thus, these questions, while irritatingly impacting your already full schedule, are ones that in many if not most instances should be heard and responded to.

Secondly, by actively soliciting them, you can remain in control of the interview. Dr. Eric Anderson explained it this way: "Bring up the question of other problems before the patient does. If you initiate the discussion, then you can end it on your terms and, perhaps, quickly. Let the patient stumblingly initiate it and you've just lost the patient waiting next door."[23] You can stay in control of the interview by saying, "That question requires more time than we have today—let's schedule another appointment for next week to discuss it thoroughly." Most patients report that they do not mind when the doctor makes such a time assessment and indicates his desire to discuss the topic at a later opportunity. Most say, "I'd rather have the opportunity for him to go into detail than get a quick answer as he goes out the door." In Chapter 12, I offered a suggestion regarding how to focus the patient on those important questions and, as a result, increase the likelihood that they will mention them sooner.

Step Twelve: End the Interview

You are now ready to move on to the next patient. Do so quickly but not abruptly, and at least pleasantly and even warmly if that's your style. Make this patient feel glad that he or she came to you and, even more important, make this patient feel that you are glad too. Sometimes a reminder of what they are to do next is a nice way to end: "When you leave here get that prescription filled as soon as possible and get started on it tonight." "Let Janice show you how to use that breathalizer." "Stop to see Monica to schedule your next appointment." Making a comment that re-enters the patients into the cycle of service let's them know that this portion of their visit to the practice is over, and moves them on to the next moment of truth.

Also, urging the patient to call with questions is a nice way to end the interview. I know that this may sound as though I've taken leave of my senses. However, I promise you that not that many patients will take you up on it, and all to whom you make the offer will appreciate it. Most patients realize that you are busy and they will not bother you with questions that don't matter to them. Also, if they really do have a question, they should be encouraged to get it answered immediately. One doctor in a workshop I conducted expressed his frustration at a patient's noncompliance with his prescribed medication plan. He said, "She was told by the pharmacy that there were serious side effects to the medication and that scared her. She waited until her next appointment to tell me about it and so we were days and days behind schedule on her treatment." This doctor agreed that one way to help reduce such conflicting instructions would be to tell patients to call immediately with any questions. He could have allayed her fears if she had only been encouraged to contact him. You may think that patients will call you without being told to do so, but that is not always the case. In fact, frequently patients have told me, "My doctor is so busy. I didn't want to bother him."

Another excellent way to end the interview is to offer additional praise and encouraging words. When patients leave your office with positive thoughts in their minds, they are more likely to follow your instructions and to leave feeling satisfied with their visits.

SOME SPECIAL CASES

All right. There are some patients who will talk on and on! There are some with whom you simply disagree. Let me offer some suggestions for dealing with these individuals.

The Historian   These are the patients who talk and talk, giving all the details. Usually starting at the beginning and recounting every step that brought them to your office, these patients need some understanding and some guidance from you. Most of these people are looking for someone who will listen and empathize. They also can become stuck in their stories. The best strategy for dealing with them is: Listen attentively and then say, "I know you were unhappy and that must have been terrible for you. What can I do to help you today?" Repeat this often and you can guide the patient to the current problem.

The Disagreement   It is more than permissible to disagree with patients; often it is necessary. They may want something you can't give; they may be doing something that is harmful to their own health. As the healthcare professional, it is up to you to point these things out. The best strategy for doing this is directly: "You and I disagree about the appropriate course of action. I'm interested in your understanding of how these drugs affect you. Can you tell me more about your use of this medication over the past month?" You can make your disagreement known and then shift the patients into providing information that may well help you discover ways for pointing out their error. Many times you will be able to change the patients' minds or at least modify their opinions. The questions show your interest and your willingness to understand their point of view. It will also give you the information you need to correct any of their erroneous beliefs.

One final suggestion: make those follow-up phone calls. Considered by some physicians as the little extra "wouldn't it be nice if I had the time" gesture, others see these phone calls as a part of their usual routine. Dr. Eric Anderson stated, "The good will and public relations resulting from such endeavors is out of proportion to the time spent. The time is further minimized because patients are so pleased and surprised by the call that they let you hang up fairly quickly. More than anything, this will please your next new patient."[24]

If the physician is the heart of the practice, as I said in Chapter 8, then the patients are the blood that flows through it. You need them to have a function to perform. Your relationship with your patients is the most important relationship in your professional life. It may be the most important one for them *to* their lives. Conducting effective patient interviews is the key to building and maintaining positive doctor/patient relationships. It is also the key to creating a positive moment of truth for the patient, which will result in a positive impression of his or her experience in your office.

END NOTES

1. Harold I. Kaplan, M.D., and Benjamin J. Sadock, M.D., *Pocket Handbook of Clinical Psychiatry* (Baltimore: Williams and Wilkins, 1990), p. 7.
2. Robert Tannenbaum, "How to Effectively 'Grow' Your Practice," *Physician's Management* 34, no. 6 (June 1994), p. 54.
3. Judith Hall, Michael Milburn, and Arnold Epstein, "A Casual Model of Health Status and Satisfaction with Medical Care," *Medical Care* 31, no. 1 (January 1993), p. 93.
4. Eric Anderson, "20 Ways to Please Your Next New Patient," *Physician's Management* 34, no. 8 (August 1994), p. 26.
5. Vincent Fulginiti, M.D., "The Big 8: Major Malpractice Traps in Pediatrics," *Pediatric Management* 4, no. 4 (April 1, 1993), p. 48.
6. Eric Anderson, M.D., "The One-Minute Office Call," *Physician Management* 30, no. 9 (September 1990), p. 78.
7. Bernard Strauss, "Tips from My 25 Years of Successful Practice," *Medical Economics* 70, no. 3 (February 8, 1993), p. 68.
8. Gregory Carroll and Robert Engle, "Communication Techniques for Physicians," *HMO Practice* 7, no. 1 (March 1993), p. 41.
9. Ken Terry, "Telling Your Patients More Will Save Your Time," *Medical Economics*, 71 no. 14 (July 25, 1994), p. 52.
10. Carroll and Engle, p. 41.
11. Flora Johnson Skelly, "Communicate . . . or Litigate," *AMNews* 35, no. 25 (June 2p, 1992).

12. Anderson, "20 Ways to Please Your Next New Patient," p. 26.
13. Ibid.
14. Ibid.
15. Ibid., p. 29.
16. Christine Micklitsch, "Will Enhancement of Physician Communication Skills Improve Patient Satisfaction," ACMGA Unpublished paper, (August 10, 1993), pp. 3–4.
17. Terry, pp. 43, 46.
18. Ibid., p. 40.
19. Ibid., p. 46.
20. Skelly, p. 29.
21. Terry, p. 52.
22. Terry, p. 40.
23. Anderson, "20 Ways To Please Your Next New Patient," p. 30.
24. Ibid.

14

CHAPTER

Step Fourteen—Handle the Difficult Moments of Truth

Every service provider in any field is familiar with that knot in the stomach that comes when an interaction with a customer does not go well. That reaction can start as a small discomfort and swell until it seems to be all consuming. It can linger on and on, sometimes for hours or days, or even weeks, months, or years. In my workshops on managing difficult moments of truth, I sometimes ask the participants to describe their worst experience with a customer, and the length as well as the intensity of the aftermath never ceases to amaze me. One of the reasons that the impact is felt so keenly for so long is that these situations can escalate into intense confrontations, confrontations that could frequently have been avoided if the service provider had known what to do.

That difficult moments of truth exist should not be surprising. As I mentioned in Chapter 7, service is a most human activity, meaning that a complex human being is seeking service and an equally complex individual is providing it. Each person brings his or her own unique filters of attitudes, beliefs, values, experiences, emotional states, and so forth. Those filters will undoubtedly impact the entire service interaction. As a result, even though the goal of every employee in a Total Service Medical Practice should be to provide a positive service experience at *each* moment of truth for *each* customer, it is simply humanly impossible to make that happen. When we are dealing with human beings, we are not dealing with perfection.

In addition to the human foibles that may impact any given moment of truth, the systems (including policies and procedures) and processes within the practice can frustrate the delivery of quality service. Also, the rapidly changing healthcare environment itself poses challenges for even the most service-driven practice personnel.

How can you handle those difficult moments of truth so that the customer still feels cared for and listened to? The three-part process described in this chapter will assist you in doing just that. (Figure 14–1.) Although the focus here will be primarily on handling difficult situations with your primary customers, the patients, much of the advice is immediately transferable to handling difficult moments of truth with those in any customer population.

PREVENTION

Office Manager Arlene Stolte summarized the first step in the process for handling difficult moments of truth: "My mind-set is that you solve the problems before they start!" In your medical practice, this means being proactive in four different ways.

Educate Your New Customers

Many difficult customer situations occur in your practice because a new customer does not know how your office does things. This is especially visible when patients arrive for their first appointments. They often don't know what their insurance covers, where or how to check in, or even what their doctors look like. As a result, they may be feeling somewhat insecure, and, if they are injured or ill, they will also be feeling very vulnerable. All of this may make for short fuses. When patients are in that state, they are not able to listen and process information nor are they feeling particularly cooperative. So when you attempt to offer explana-

FIGURE 14–1

Three-Step Process for Managing Difficult Moments of Truth

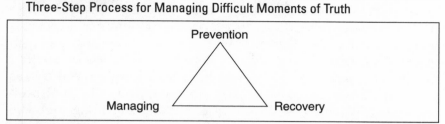

© Vicky Bradford, 1995.

tions or instructions, these customers may not be receptive to your message.

To avoid this *new patient* phenomenon, be proactive: send new patients a packet that will welcome them to the practice, introduce their doctors and other members of the team, and provide important information regarding a number of key areas. Well-known practice consultant Diane Palmer suggests a welcome packet that contains the following items:

- Personalized welcome letters from the practice.

- A physician biography containing the name of the patient's doctor, as well as pertinent medical education information (medical school, residency, etc.), years in practice, and any other items of interest.

- A new-patient form requesting basic demographic information plus a brief medical history.

- A self-addressed, stamped envelope if you are asking for the form to be mailed to you.

- An appointment card with time, date, and directions to the building in which your office is located and, if appropriate, the specific location of the office.

- Patient information sheet or booklet containing office hours, insurance information, as well as billing and scheduling procedures.[1]

With the electronic age on us, you will want to prepare a modified version of this packet to be sent via fax or E-mail.

In addition to this advance contact, you should continue the education process right through the first visit. Doctors should be scheduled to spend extra time on initial patient visits. Assuming the patient feels well enough, a staff member should be assigned to take the new patient through the office so that the environment becomes immediately familiar. If a tour of the office is not appropriate, each new patient should be met by an assigned staff member who will sit down in the reception area to provide a personal welcome as well as securing signatures on appropriate forms and, if it has not been completed in advance, assist the patient in filling out the information sheet. Procedures and policies can also be explained, always in a warm and friendly manner. After the doctor's interview and examination, the same staff member should have a few moments with the patient to determine if there are any questions.

A final point of contact with the new patient occurs after the visit. A follow-up phone call from the office manager, the staff member who spent time with the patient during the appointment, or even from the doctor, will allow the patient to ask questions and also to provide feedback.

Although these suggestions all require additional time, they will save time in the long run and help prevent many of those initial new-patient difficult moments of truth. The patients have the opportunity to become informed before they arrive at the practice, the chance to seek clarification while they are there, and to ask additional questions the next day. The old saying, "An ounce of prevention is worth a pound of cure" applies to avoiding difficult moments of truth through effective new-patient education.

Inform Existing Customers

Another potentially problematic situation occurs when existing patients encounter new policies, procedures, and personnel. Even positive changes in their doctors' offices are not welcome if the alterations are unannounced. Patients want to rely on what happens at the practice, and sudden surprises interrupt their ability to do so. Thus, it is important to keep your existing customers in appropriate information loops. You have four options for accomplishing this task.

■ Practice Newsletter. This type of publication has helped many practices stay in touch with their customers, particularly patients. The content usually includes updates on any changes as well as features on patients and staff, and informative articles about healthcare in the community or the nation. In addition to sharing information, the newsletter also serves as a reminder of the patient's medical care provider, leading to the scheduling of wellness appointments and periodic checkups. The newsletter should be published on a regular basis, usually monthly, and should be professional but approachable in appearance. The writing and production of the newsletter also takes time, but many practices report that it is well worth the investment.

■ Customer Notices. Another way to reach your current patient population is to send notices that are specifically designed to provide informational updates. A single page usually is all that is necessary. In order to make the information more palatable, as well as to catch the attention of the recipient, include a small gift. For example, one practice included a refrigerator magnet bearing the practice's name, address, phone and fax numbers, and office hours. This practice reports receiving calls of appreciation from their patients and that patient readily receive the information.

■ Telephone Communication. On occasion, you may have some time-sensitive information that needs to be communicated to your customers, and usually the best way to do that is via the telephone, especially when contacting a small pool of individuals. If you find it necessary to leave a message on an answering machine, please word your message in such a way so as not to worry your customer, especially if you are calling patients. An unsolicited call from their doctors' offices can produce anxiety, making the patients less receptive to your message. Although fax machines and E-mail may be faster, some changes should be communicated via a more personal manner; in these instances, opt for the telephone.

■ On-Site Update. When the existing customer is at your office, you can deliver your messages interpersonally. Plan ahead, however, so impending changes can be explained prior to their actual implementation, thus avoiding those upsetting surprises.

Develop Practice Responses

Many difficult moments of truth result from what customers perceive to be your lack of information or your inability to respond to their requests. They want answers and they want them now. When practice personnel stutter and stammer their way through explanations or are not able to make certain decisions and don't know who can, customers become irritable or worse. So, to avoid these situations, sit down as a staff and decide your practice responses to the following:

- What are the most frequently asked questions in each of our areas by each of our key customer populations? (Patients? Family members? Insurance companies? Hospitals? Other physicians and their staffs?)

- Do we have a "practice response?" (A response that any personnel has the authority to offer.) If so, what is it?

- If this question should be answered by a specific individual, who should that be? (For quick reference, list the name and perhaps the extension number by the question.)

- Do we know how to say "I don't know" without losing our credibility? If not, learn the following process:

  - Compliment the customer on the question and admit that you don't have the answer: "That's a very good question. You know, I'm afraid I don't have the answer to it."

  - Tell the customer that you will either find the answer, or you will have the person who knows call: "I will find out, though, and either I or the person who can help you more will call you back."

  - Secure the name and phone number and convenient hours for a return call: "Could I have your name and phone number and some times tomorrow that would be convenient for you to receive a call?"

  - Give the customer your name, number, and extension: "I'd like you to have my name and number. Please call me if you don't receive a response within 24 hours."

Once the practice responses are planned and shared with all personnel, then you can avoid many of the difficult moments of truth that arise from customers' frustrations at seeking information and/or decisions.

Do It Right in the First Place

The obvious way to avoid many difficult moments of truth is to provide good service in the first place. In the previous chapter, I discussed four important elements in creating a positive moment of truth: creating a supportive environment, listening effectively, asking good questions, and paying attention to the little things. In addition, by analyzing your systems, cycles, and processes and by making them as customer-friendly and employee-friendly as possible, you will eliminate many of the circumstances that cause a moment of truth to go sour. By creating your practice's customer report cards, described in Chapter 6, you will know what is important to your customers, and, thus, you can do everything possible to make them happy before problems can develop.

MANAGING THE DIFFICULT MOMENTS OF TRUTH
General Tips

Regardless of your good intentions and proactive efforts to avoid negative customer situations, they will inevitably arise. While problematic systems and processes usually can be corrected in the customer's absence, interpersonal encounters can not. On those occasions, then, you will need to be prepared to handle the situation in a customer-friendly way. After studying a wide variety of moments of truth in medical practices, I have identified several different difficult situations that occur frequently in this setting. Before discussing each of these in detail, I would first like to stress two general tips that will help defuse and even turn around many negative situations.

When I was first learning to ski, my instructor gave me advice that sounded absolutely crazy to me. If I wanted to make a turn, I was to lean downhill! Everything in my body and soul wanted to do the opposite. If I was afraid that I would *fall* down the mountain, why in the world would I want to *lean* down it? I have received the same reactions from workshop participants when I have told them that the key to defusing a negative situation is to lean into it, not away. Yet, office managers, service representatives, and customers themselves agree on two universal behaviors that will lay the groundwork for turning around a negative situation, and they are behaviors I have discussed before:

- Listening!
- Empathy!

Customers who are upset usually want someone to hear them out and to understand what they are experiencing. Although it is usually easier to listen and empathize when the situation is positive, these behaviors often require real effort when it is not. While at those difficult moments every instinct will tell you to lean uphill, away from the stressful situation that confronts you, it is at those very moments that you should lean down the mountain and into the storm.

Now, let's examine those specific difficult moments of truth.

Specific Difficult Moments

Handling the Customer Complaints

Before describing a process for handling complaints, I would like to dispel some old myths that exist about them.[2]

> Myth 1: No news is good news; we don't have that many dissatisfied customers.
> Reality: You should want to know when customers experience problems with your practice. If you don't know, how can you fix it? Remember, 96 percent of dissatisfied customers never say a word. They just don't come back. (Also remember if they believe they can't leave, as patients in narrow provider networks sometimes do, then they can make your life miserable.)

> Myth 2: One dissatisfied customer doesn't mean that much.
> Reality: A dissatisfied customer tells 9 to 10 people of the dissatisfaction; 13 percent tell more than 20 people. (This is especially true of healthcare.)

> Myth 3: Complainers represent the radical fringe.
> Reality: Complainers are usually "normal" people who have encountered a problem that they want fixed.

> Myth 4: We can afford to lose some customers—we'll replace them with new ones.
> Reality: Obtaining new customers costs five times as much as retaining existing ones.

Myth 5: Complainers are never satisfied.
Reality: Between 54 percent and 70 percent of the
discontented can be retained by resolving their complaints;
95 percent of this group will become loyal customers if their
complaints are handled well and quickly.

When the realities of customer complaints are considered, then, it can be convincingly argued that any organization, including yours, should not merely accept complaints, but welcome and encourage them.

Why, then, are complaints included in the chapter on difficult moments of truth? Because they are potentially explosive. I say *potentially* because not all complaints are leveled by irate customers who are out of control. In fact, most are not, and can be handled without a major explosion. However, every complaint carries the possibilities of high intensity, placing the complaint in the *difficult* category for most practice personnel.

In preparation for handling specific complaints, begin by studying the characteristics of those who register complaints in your practice. Twenty-four Health Stop Centers did just that and learned some interesting facts: Complainers differed significantly from noncomplainers in terms of three of the six independent variables tested. *Age*—Elderly (65 and over) were more likely to complain than younger patients, and they tended to write more often than to telephone. *Initial Visit*—Previous experience with the Center decreased complaints. *Cost*—The higher the bill, the more likely the patients were to complain. A summary of the results indicated "that complainers were significantly different from the typical patient in terms of age, previous experience with Health Stop, and size of bill. Complaints tended to come from older patients, who had not been at Health Stop before and who had a high bill."[3] These data can help Health Stop anticipate some of the common complaints and will allow Health Stop to prepare their best responses.

It is also helpful to identify common themes for complaints. In medical practices, common areas for complaints are:

- Perceived technical incompetence of the provider; usually these complaints are from patients who are experiencing pain.

- Ineffective interpersonal relationships with personnel, both nonmedical and medical—including physicians.

- Lack of access to appointments or other services.

- Perceived lack of coordination between different departments and providers.

- Poor handling of complaints.

- Financial difficulties.

- Customer-*unfriendly* systems (including practice-designed policies and procedures) and processes.

Again, knowing the common trends in your complaint data will help you to correct most problematic situations and to prepare responses should the complaints continue to be raised.

As I have mentioned, it is helpful for your practice to track complaints from its customers. However, care should be taken to avoid three mistakes often made when considering these data.

Mistake 1: Don't rely on complaints alone for feedback. If the only feedback that practice personnel receive comes in the form of complaints, they will become overwhelmed in negativity. Content of complaints should be used for finding trends in the data but not as the sole indication of how well the practice and its personnel are meeting the service needs of the customers. Rely on customer satisfaction and service-quality research, as described in Chapter 6, in order to determine that; both strengths and areas for improvement will be represented in those data.

Mistake 2: Don't count complaints as the measure of improvement. Remember, most people do not voluntarily complain, believing that it takes too much time and energy and that nothing ever changes anyway. Unless your practice actually solicits feedback, your customers will be reluctant to tell you when they have problems. In addition, as I indicated in Chapter 6, if and when your practice becomes known for its responsive handling of complaints the number received will increase almost automatically. Instead of counting complaints, measurements of improvement should be determined by comparing subsequent survey data with data discovered during benchmark customer-satisfaction and service-quality research, as described in Chapter 6.

Mistake 3: Don't restrict concern about complaints to only one or two people. Many practices have designated one or more staff members as patient advocates, service representatives, or some other title, and have assigned these folks the responsibility for handling complaints. Even with the resulting efficiency of this process, such designations must be made with the following qualifiers.

First, in a Total Service Medical Practice, all practice personnel must be empowered with the authority to handle specified situations on the spot. Next, all practice personnel should be involved in listing complaints as they are received, or your practice will lose an important method of tracking the milder, less explosive situations. Third, all practice personnel must be committed to the Total Service perspective, and sometimes the designated complaint staff can be seen as a way to pass on the accompanying responsibilities to someone else. Finally, the impact of handling complaints all day can begin to take its toll on the designated personnel themselves often causing burnout or a protective callousness, unless they have other duties to balance handling complaints and periodically are rotated out of this role.

Having said that, customer service representatives can and do provide a useful function in the practice. St. Joseph's Neuroscience Institute in Tampa, Florida, began using such personnel and have found them to be effective. Their jobs entail anticipation of patients' needs, making patients comfortable while they wait, putting patients in touch with whatever office services they need, handling complaints, conducting patient-satisfaction surveys and analyzing results, serving as a liaison between patients and physicians and between patients and staff, providing patient-relations education for other staff members, conducting employee recognition programs, and setting up programs to improve quality in patient and employee relations.[4] Again, if you decide to implement such a position or already have one in place, be certain that it does not become viewed by practice personnel as the only position where service matters.

When customers complain, they usually have an agenda. They want a problem to be solved, a difficulty to be corrected, and/or their voices to be heard. The following 10 suggestions will help you prevent the situation from escalating and can even turn this difficult moment into a positive one:

■ Listen. Already mentioned above, this is universally the first advice given across all fields by those who spend their days handling customer complaints. Often, all that the complaining customers want is someone to listen to what they are saying.

■ Acknowledge. Thank the customer for bringing this matter to your attention. This act alone will disarm many complainers. They will probably expect you to defend yourself or your organization. To have you express your appreciation for their feedback is a pleasant surprise.

■ Apologize. Don't be too proud to say, "I'm sorry." These two words will go a long way toward creating a positive out of a negative. If the customer is right, go farther than an apology; admit it: "I'm sorry, I found that you were charged incorrectly. I'll put through an adjustment immediately and I apologize for the confusion."

■ Probe. Ask brief questions to clarify the customer's position. This not only will assist you in understanding the complaints and buy a little time, but it also validates the customer's feelings and acknowledges his or her perceptions.

■ Restate. Restating what a customer seems to be saying can momentarily direct focus away from the issue and allow time to plan a response. In addition, this restatement assures that the problem has been understood. "If I understand you correctly, you're not questioning the amount of the charges, but the possibility that you had a test you didn't need."

■ Choose words carefully. Avoid using words that will push the customers' hot buttons or will imply incompetence on the part of others in your organization. Once, when registering a complaint to an airline ticketing-agent supervisor, I was told, "Dr. Bradford, I am so sorry that this has happened to you." This is masterful wording because it does not blame anyone in the organization, which you should avoid doing, and it still extends a sincere apology for the incident.

■ Ask the customer what he or she wants. Don't be afraid to ask, "What can I do to make this right for you?" or "What do you believe would be a fair resolution?" At first, fearing that if given the opportunity, customers will make unreasonable demands, many people think that it is foolhardy to give customers the chance. However, customers very, very seldom ask for more than you can deliver. They usually know exactly what they want, and often it is merely an apology. The perceived open-endedness of being allowed to specify their preferred resolution leaves customers feeling as though you are willing to accommodate their needs in whatever way you can, frequently resulting in not only satisfied customers but also very loyal ones.

■ Give the customer the benefit of the doubt. Don't debate with the customer who is complaining. Although his or her perceptions may vary widely from those of others, they are still valid because they are his or her perceptions. For now, accept the description of the problem as presented. If you feel more data are needed, by all means indicate that you will be happy to check into the situation and get back to the customer.

■ Document complaints. It is important for your practice to have a record of the complaints received. This record will help to determine common complaints that need organizational action to prevent their continued occurrence. Such information can also document for others exactly what was done to resolve the situation. These data can be useful in malpractice suits, as well as in less antagonistic circumstances. Documentation also tells supervisors what has already been done in order to attempt to solve the problem. At the minimum, record the name of the customer, the date and time of the interaction, a description of what happened as related by the customer, any additional information you gather on your own, what you did to resolve the problem, and the status of the situation as of the end of the interaction.

■ Follow up. For some simple, straightforward complaints this may not be absolutely necessary. However, for bigger problems that have taken time and energy to resolve, a follow-up phone call or letter is greatly appreciated. Even the little blips on the complaint radar screen warrant checking back.

Many customer service personnel report that they find handling complaints to be one of the most fulfilling parts of their jobs. They see these interactions as opportunities to make a difference for the customer, a challenge for stretching their own abilities, and a chance to be in charge. A receptionist in the pediatric unit at a staff-model HMO told me, "I like nothing better than turning a customer around. If patients come to me scowling and I send them away smiling, I know I've done my job." If practice personnel are going to view handling complaints in a positive light, however, they must be given the power to make on-the-spot problem-solving decisions.

Calming the Angry Customer

Anger is an interesting emotion. In the Anglo-American culture, many of us, particularly women, are taught that it is not acceptable to display our anger. Yet, other emotions that are more culturally acceptable are also more revealing. So, even though it may not be regarded as the thing to do, customers are more likely to show anger to strangers than to show other more personal emotions, such as fear or sadness. Every day in a medical practice, you encounter customers who appear to be angry. Remembering that this emotion is often a mask may help you defuse your own instinctive reaction to fight back.

Often the source of the anger may well be some entity, action, or policy that is beyond your control. Yet, because you are the closest available target, you frequently face the brunt of that anger. Knowing how to manage such situations will assist you in calming the angry customer:

■ Relocate. The angry customer should be removed from public view for several reasons. First, the action of walking from one spot to another will actually use up some of the customer's energy that was being poured into the display of anger. Second, by breaking the spiral of defensiveness triggered in you by such behavior, you too have an opportunity to calm down. Third, if you move the interaction into a private area, you move the customer onto your turf, so to speak, and this usually reduces his or her control of the situation. Fourth, by removing the customer from public view, you also take away the audience, and many of these people like to perform for a crowd. Next, by moving the customer to a spot where you or someone else can sit down and really listen, your practice implicitly demonstrates its desire to focus attention on this customer's wants and needs. Finally, it almost goes without saying that no practice wants other customers to witness such an angry display.

■ Listen. This is the most commonly recommended step to calming angry customers. Office Manager Marilyn Haley explained, "Nine times out of 10 when someone is angry, all you have to do is sit and listen. They run themselves down, and then they are ready to find a reasonable solution." Another seasoned office manager put it this way: "Just listen to them. Don't interrupt." Arlene Stolte said, "I just sit and listen. I let them vent their anger at me." Most angry customers merely want to be heard. Once they are given a chance to have their say, they often calm down.

■ Avoid giving orders, unless you are dealing with a customer who is completely out of control. The usual situation involving an angry customer will only be heightened in intensity if orders are given. (If a customer has spiraled out of control, however, then a firm voice giving a specific command can bring him or her back to reason.)

■ Allow yourself to feel empathy for the customer. Take a few deep breaths and step aside from the barrage of words that are coming toward you, and look behind them at the emotions. Place yourself in the customer's shoes and walk those proverbial miles. If you see the situation through the customer's eyes, you will be able to at least understand what is causing the anger and will probably be able to discern if it is really anger or a mask for some other more personal emotion.

■ Acknowledge the emotions. Once you have allowed yourself to understand the customer's feelings, verbally acknowledge them: "I can see why you would be angry about this, Mrs. Jones" or "All of this must be very frightening for you, Jamie." Be as specific as you can be in naming the emotion. If you are right, the customer will experience the sense of really being heard and will start calming down. The specificity of your attempt to identify the emotion will also show your sincere effort to understand; even if you are wrong, the customer will appreciate the effort. In addition, by hearing your label of the emotion, the customer will get a clearer image of what is really bothering him or her, allowing for such clarifications as, "Well, I wasn't so much angry as I was scared."

■ Don't debate who is to blame, and, if it's your practice, don't be afraid to admit it. As I mentioned in the section on handling complaints, be willing to give the customers the benefit of the doubt. If they are convinced of the reality of their complaints, you only make them angrier by denying the complaint. Don't hesitate to take responsibility for errors that are indeed the fault of the practice, but by the same token don't implicate other employees. The previously cited statement made by the airline supervisor is the best way to go: "I'm so sorry that this has happened to you." It implicates no one, accepts the customer's perception of the situation, and does not place the blame anywhere.

■ Avoid a defensive response. As I mentioned in Chapter 12, your natural instinct when under attack is to strike back. However, if you do not respond in kind, you can break the defensiveness spiral. Reexamine the ways to create a supportive situation, which was covered in Chapter 12.

■ Seek clarification. After the customer appears to start calming down, which most will when they feel they've been heard and understood, clarify the content of the message. The best method for achieving this clarity is to paraphrase your understanding of what you have heard: "Let me see if I understand your concern. You wanted to see your regular doctor, and, when you got here, you found that he wasn't available and that you would have to see someone else and that upset you. Is that it?" Or "Your concern is not so much that you will have to see someone other than your regular doctor as it is your fear that the new person won't understand your case. Is that it?" Such clarification allows both you and the customer the opportunity to make certain that you are talking about the same issue. It also enhances the customer's impression that he or she has indeed been heard, which also has a calming effect.

■ Be able to explain. If you are going to help resolve the problem, be able to offer explanations for what happened, if you can. Often customers are simply unaware of your procedures or policies. For example, one office manager told of her interaction with a very hostile customer who did not understand the timing of her refund policy. Expecting the refund to arrive on the first of the month, the customer became very angry when it did not. When the office manager explained that the refunds were posted on the first, mailed out on the second, and should arrive at his home no later than the seventh, he calmed down. The office manager went even farther: she told him to call her back on the seventh of the month if he did not receive the refund and she would check into the situation immediately. What began as a very hot situation was defused by explanations and offers to go the extra distance.

- Ask for what the customer wants. When the customer is sufficiently calmed, seek his or her input into what solution would be acceptable. A powerful device when used at the right time, interjected too soon it can result in an unreasonable demand: "I want that person fired, that's what I want!" However, after you have listened actively, experienced and acknowledged your empathy, and apologized for the customer's experience, you have probably defused the anger and the customer is able to engage in reasoned discourse.

- Form a team with the customer. As you brainstorm possible solutions, solicit the customer's participation: It's the two of you working to solve this problem you both face. Remember my friend who works in customer service for J. C. Penney! Her advice was "Listen and then say, 'Let's see what we can do to solve this problem.'" *Let's* is a key word here. It involves the customer in the resolution and creates the sense of partnership.

- Keep your sense of humor! Once in a while, an expression of your sense of humor can completely disarm the customer. One office manager told me of the man who was totally irate; he began a barrage of expletives that would make a sailor blush. Her response? "Excuse me sir, I couldn't hear all that. What did you say?" Her instincts were right! He saw the ridiculous nature of his tirade and laughed with her. My only warning here is to be certain that you read the customer correctly. Asked too soon, or of the wrong person, and her request might have gotten her even more of an earful.

Even the angriest of customers can be calmed by using the above strategies. Above all, listen and empathize.

When You Have To Say "No"

In a previous chapter, I made an important distinction that comes back into play when dealing with this thorniest of issues in a medical practice: The customer may not always be right, but the customer is always important. Thus, even in those situations when they must be told "No," customers should be treated with the utmost courtesy and understanding.

Under what conditions are you compelled to say "No"? Most fall into one of the following categories:

Confirmation of Denial: The customer has already been told "No" elsewhere, either by someone in the practice or someone outside such as an insurance company. The customer is merely checking with you to see if that is your understanding as well. Sometimes, you are in the uncomfortable position of delivering the news of a denial that has been made by someone else, but has not yet been communicated to the customer. For example, you may have to tell a patient that the insurance company has only approved a certain number of visits, and, after that, the patient will financially be on his or her own.

Correction of Information: The customer thinks he or she has an understanding of practice policies and procedures but does not. Also, frequently patients think they have information about what would be the best treatment for their conditions or what tests should be run. You may have to dispute their information and provide your own, which in effect is a denial.

Denial of Desired Action: The best example of this situation is also one of the most difficult: changing patients from one practice provider to another when the patient would prefer not to. When patients become accustomed to their doctors, in most cases they want to continue being seen by those providers. Thus, when they are denied that preference it can become a difficult moment of truth that must be carefully managed.

Life-Threatening Denial: Occasionally, you may find yourself in the position of having to say "No" when you realize that the results may threaten the life of your customer. Obviously applicable to patients, this situation can occur when you are dealing with catastrophic illness or an accident, the insurance maximum has been reached, and you are in a position of telling the patient that treatment will no longer be covered. Although most practices try to find a way to work with patients under these circumstances, the initial delivery of the denial can be painful and difficult for all concerned.

The stresses that accompany saying "No" escalate with the situation. Saying "No" for any reason creates a certain level of stress, because most us would like to make the customer happy. Understandably we also can harbor some fear around the uncertainty of the customer's potential response. Stress escalates again if you are in a position of having to say "No" repeatedly. Personnel who never have the opportunity of saying "Yes" face a high level of burnout and have to fight their own negative feelings about the organization for which they work. They also can project the negativity onto the customers, concluding that the customers are unreasonable and stubborn, a common symptom of burnout for any designated complaint personnel. The stress level jumps still higher if the denial is at odds with the employee's core values. It is often therefore very stressful for healthcare professionals to have to say "No" to patients, because everything in their training has told them to put the patient first. For example, during their training, nurses are specifically charged with being the patient's advocate. Thus, when the patient has to be told "No," it can go against all that they believe and have learned. Stress continues to climb when the denial elicits strong customer reactions. When the customer begins to shout or to cry or to make some other emotional display, your stress level increases. The most stressful moment of all is when the denial has a major impact on the customer's security, health, or life. No one likes to say "No" in these circumstances, and it becomes difficult not to take such situations home for some time to come.

The following tips for handling the situation of saying "No" to the customer will help you keep the stress level at a tolerable level:[5]

■ Be ready to explain the rationale behind any policies you have. These explanations should be carefully thought-out in advance so that they will make sense to the customer. Your practice should compile a list of the situations that commonly arise—such as requests for same-day appointments, requests to see a specialist, requests for antibiotics to be phoned in—and should determine a consistent rationale for denials on each.

■ Be willing to empathize with the customer. Empathy becomes difficult, especially if you are on the phones all day and have fallen into the pattern of, "just handle the situation and move on to the next." Although it may be the tenth time that week that you've had to explain why the doctor won't give any more refills without a visit, it's probably the first time this patient has heard it. Just as empathy helps calm angry patients, it also helps those who have made a request to feel heard.

■ Learn the sandwich technique. With this technique, the customer is given a positive message, followed by a negative message, followed by another positive one. In the case of patient interactions, the first part of the sandwich is a friendly greeting. The filling is the denial and its explanation. But the exchange shouldn't stop there. The last part of the sandwich is an attempt to reach a compromise, a suggestion of how your office will work with the customer.

■ Never be haughty with patients. Nothing brings customers to anger more quickly than snobby reactions to their requests. One doctor said, "I cringe when someone at my front desk tells a patient that my schedule is booked, and, she has a tone of pride in her voice when she says it. I know that being busy can be a sign of a successful practice but all patients care about is whether they can see the physician when they need to."

■ Be clear about what situations qualify as exceptions to established policy. It is very confusing for the customers to be told one thing by one person and something else by another. That usually occurs when policies are not clear or when the practice lacks clarity on the exceptions to them. If your practice is going to allow exceptions, and I urge you to consider doing so in appropriate circumstances, then everyone in the practice should know under what conditions these rules will be waived.

■ Determine where the buck stops and let everyone know. If a staff member is having trouble with a customer, it is important that he or she knows who is the final decision-maker on what issues.

Actually Saying "No"

The following 10-step format for the denial situation is helpful.

1. Acknowledge the request: "I understand that you want to see your doctor."

2. Acknowledge the emotions: "It must be very frustrating for you when he's not available."

3. Sincerely apologize: "I wish I could arrange for you to see him."

4. Say "No": "Unfortunately, I can't honor your request."

5. Brief explanation: "Dr. Smith is completely booked for today and simply has no more time in his schedule."

6. Offer alternative: "Here's what I can do. I can see if Dr. Jones can see you at 3:15 today, or I could schedule you with your regular doctor at his earliest open appointment which will be Thursday." Or, "In order to address your immediate need for medical attention, I would be happy to schedule you in with Dr. Jones at 3:15 today and then to call you if your regular doctor has a cancellation."

7. Seek acceptance of an option: "Would that work for you?"

8. Be ready for a customer comeback. In the case of the same-day booking, you should be ready to respond to a request for double booking: "You know, I'm concerned about you, and double booking won't really solve the problem. I can't guarantee you'd even be seen at all, and we want you to get the care you should have."

9. Thank the customer for his or her patience: "I appreciate your patience with us on this matter."

10. Exit the situation: "Good bye, Dr. Jones will look forward to seeing you at 3:15."

Being prepared for those times when you have to say "No" will help both you and your customer.

Handling the Customer's Financial Problems

As the content of many complaints and the stimuli for angry customer reactions, financial issues merit a discussion all their own. As patients attempt to unsnarl the complexities of managed care and wrestle with the costs of healthcare in general, the subject of finances creates many difficult moments of truth. Often the cause of patient dissatisfaction, economic problems have been known to push angry patients over the line and into the courtroom. Financial problems can impact patient care; those who are embarrassed by not being able to pay their bills may fail to return for follow-up treatments or may not buy prescribed medications.[6] In addition, collections and related financial issues can have a major impact on the financial stability of your practice. If these potentially difficult moments of truth can be handled effectively, it not only will help avoid customer dissatisfaction and benefit the health of your patients, but it also will help your practice stay financially solvent.

Consider the following suggestions for handling the situations when money issues must be discussed.

■ Project a respectful, accessible, friendly attitude. Money is one of the most difficult subjects for people to address under the best of circumstances. When patients must address issues of income and ability to pay, they can become defensive, angry, and embarrassed. What they need at this moment of truth is someone who cares, who treats the situation and them with respect, who appears to be approachable and friendly. These behaviors will help ease the almost instinctive tensions most people feel when money is being discussed.

■ Provide guidance in unraveling the mysteries. One of the most common reasons patients have financial problems with a practice stems from their lack of comprehension. Often an unhurried explanation of your practice's policy or processes can result in a new understanding, and the situation can be cleared up on the spot.

The policies and processes of insurance carriers are also the stimulus for frequent financial questions. Even though patients *should* know their own insurance coverage, practices that are focused on service will do all that they can to help educate the patients while helping them through the sometimes confusing ins and outs of insurance. One office manager put it this way: "Even if it might not be our job, when we help educate the patients about the way insurance works today, and teach them where and how they can find specific answers to their specific questions, we will save ourselves a lot of time in the long run. We also can show our willingness to go that extra mile to help them. Both are serious advantages as far as I'm concerned."

■ Allow customers to work with the same practice staff member throughout the resolution of the financial problem. Regardless of the type of business, customers complain, and rightfully so, about getting shifted around from person to person, each time having to retell their stories of financial problems. Errors are made, because each retelling may delete some important details, and, thus, each new staff member may not have the same understanding of the entire situation. By assigning a specific person to each case, a personal relationship can be built as well. Many practices have a financial counselor who works with patients on problem accounts. Customers report that they are much more comfortable when discussing financial problems with someone they "know."

■ Use lay person language. Customers usually do not understand accounting, bookkeeping, and even insurance terms and jargon. Examine what words you use in your explanations to your customers. Without talking down to them, speak in words that they can understand and be willing to explain any technical terms that you think are essential.

■ Make financial issues the responsibility of all practice personnel. Everyone in the practice should play a part in the collections process, thereby creating a coordinated effort. At the 1996 conference for the Professional Association of Healthcare Office Managers, Diane Palmer, who has graciously granted permission for the use of several forms found in the Appendix, conducted a workshop on collection procedures. She outlined the following responsibilities for each of the practice personnel:

■ Front Desk: Courteously inform new patients on the telephone at the time of scheduling if payment of any kind will be expected; complete registration forms, striving for zero error rate; greet patients with warmth and courtesy; if appropriate, ask for payment as patients check out.

■ Insurance Coordinators: Keep updated on all major insurance carriers and employer groups; educate the rest of the practice personnel, including the staff and physicians. File claims daily and verify coverage.

■ Business Staff: Collect co-pay at time of patient checkout, if not handled by the front desk staff; meet with patients to get all financial arrangements in writing; create and employ a consistent billing procedure; make calls on overdue accounts, unless handled by others.

■ Back Office (Clinical): Double check the physicians' encounter forms to be sure procedure codes are correct; escort the patient to examination room; deliver accurate encounter form to the front desk while escorting the patient to the front office area; don't give patients advice on finances and billing, but refer them instead to appropriate business personnel.

■ Physicians: Check off encounter form correctly for both procedures and diagnostics; don't advise about insurance companies or payments; direct patients to the appropriate practice personnel when there is a financial or insurance question.

■ Create a graceful-exit area.[7] Since patients prefer paying after they have been seen by a physician, their last stop should be at the collection counter. We already know that the final moment of truth in any cycle of service is an important one. Add to that the uncomfortable nature of finances for most people, and it becomes clear that this moment must be managed very carefully. Be certain the graceful-exit area is both customer and employee friendly. It should be neat and tidy as well as warm and inviting. It should be separate from the check-in area if possible, with a counter that is not crowded and is large enough to easily conduct business. No more than two patients should be left waiting in this area at a time; patients don't like to wait at any moment of truth, most especially at this one. Practice personnel should be able to see patients approaching the area so that they can be greeted with a smile.

■ Use a carefully planned time-frame for billing and collections. Guidelines should be established that will indicate very clearly when the initial bill should be sent, the timing of reminders by mail and telephone, and when the account should be turned over. (See Appendix for Diane Palmer's useful chart for this process.)

■ Be flexible; work with the customer. It's not just good service, it's good business to find a way to work with a customer who is having financial difficulty. Often, angry customers who do not believe that their specific situation has been taken into account refuse to pay anything at all, necessitating collection agencies and perhaps eventually write-offs. Being willing to work with the customer helps eliminate that cost in dollars and goodwill. Office Manager Stolte explained, "If patients don't have insurance or if they have reached the end of their coverage, then they come into my office and we work out some plan." In fact, of the 149 practices that responded to the MGMA Information Exchange question,

"Does your group offer time payment-plans to patients with outstanding balances?" all but one indicated that they did. The three optional payment-plans cited in the MGMA Exchange as being used most often were: budget billing—a monthly statement with a fixed payment; time payment—primarily for uninsured or delinquent accounts, involving a down payment with a fixed amount per month at no interest; credit cards—MasterCard, Visa, or Discover.[8]

■ Create a Customized Financial Agreement. When working out a time payment-plan with a patient, get in writing their commitment to pay. Although in some legal situations, such as bankruptcy cases, these documents will be inconsequential, the act of signing them ritualizes the patients' agreements to pay, increasing the likelihood that these commitments will be honored. Such documents also provide written records for your internal office use. (Sample forms created by Diane Palmer and Associates are included in the Appendix.)

■ Caring should apply to collection of overdue accounts as well. There are practical as well as humanistic reasons for this approach, and the AMA agrees that bill collecting should be handled carefully, recommending "that review of the patient's file by the physician [or final decision-maker] before it is forwarded to a collection agency will avoid inadvertent referral of those cases meriting consideration for special payment arrangements. In addition, the patient's refusal to pay is occasionally an indicator of valid dissatisfaction. Medical liability claims that might otherwise be avoided are sometimes filed solely in response to bill collection action."[9]

Your practice should make its own attempts to collect on bills before turning them over to an agency. Several office managers attending the 1996 PAHCOM conference described their practices' successful collection efforts. For example, one manager hired a special part-time staff who work five days a week from 5:00 P.M. until 8:30 P.M. This group is paid a high hourly wage with no benefits, and their work has resulted in a 98 percent collection-recovery rate. Other managers reported the similar success of their systems that rely on existing staff who are paid overtime and/or bonuses for their extra work in collections.

Collections calls should be well-planned and courteously executed. Ms. Palmer suggests the following eight-step process:

1. Make sure you are talking to the debtor. To protect patient confidentiality as well as to make certain you are speaking with someone who knows about this specific account, do not settle for speaking with anyone other than the responsible person, not even immediate family members. Of course, when the patient is incapacitated this guideline may have to be waived.

2. Identify yourself. Use your full name, if possible, and your title. "This is Jane Alexander. I'm the patient accounting coordinator for Dr. Crosby's office" sounds more official that "I am Jane from Dr. Crosby's office."

3. Be specific on why you are calling. In a few well-chosen words, ask for payment on the account.

4. Pause and listen. Allow the patient to respond. Take notes while he or she is talking.

5. Look for solutions you can offer to help the patient pay the account. Know what options you intend to offer before you call, if you can.

6. Work out a reasonable payment plan that you and the patient can live with. This will require the graceful art of negotiation. Keep in mind that your goal is to collect the money, and if it means allowing the patient to do so over time that should be acceptable.

7. Be specific on the parts of the payment plan. You should gain agreement on the exact amount of the expected payments, the exact time when the payments will be made, how the patient will make the payments (check, cash, credit card), and who exactly is going to make the payments.

8. Close the call with a positive statement. Ms. Palmer suggests the following wording: "Mr. Jones, I am so pleased that we were able to talk and work this out."[10]

When an account must be turned over, use a collection agency that is firm but fair. With appropriate work done by your practice, you should be able to keep down the number of accounts that are actually turned over to an agency. However, when this must be done, take care in its selection. Edward Grab, a consultant who advises practices on how to avoid malpractice suits, explained, "I see untrained people who think it is their job to beat up on patients. It's a big mistake to give your collection agency carte blanche . . . In fact, vigilantism in collections procedures could be enough to tip the scales against you."[11]

■ Avoid as many problems as possible by preventing them before they happen. Aside from inability to pay, the two most common financial problems in a practice center around payment policies at the time of service, and billing formats. Payment policies are sometimes difficult to convey in a tactful manner. Here are some suggestions that other practices have found effective:

   ■ Inform patients of your payment policies in advance. This can be done tactfully on the telephone at the time an appointment is made and reinforced, for new patients, in the new-patient welcome packet.

   ■ Secure patients' signatures on financial policy statements at the time of the appointment, especially for ongoing treatment.

   ■ Channel office-traffic flow through the check-out area. Including a stop at the payment counter in the usual cycle of service makes it a part of a routine visit. When a new patient is being toured through the office for the first time, the staff member can point out the payment counter and reiterate the practice policy.

Financial problems also occur when patients cannot decipher the bill. So, step back and take a good hard look at your statements. Better yet, ask a group of patients to take a look and to provide you with feedback. At the very least, patients should be able to clearly see the cost of the visit or service, what they have paid, and what is owed. As easy as that sounds, and as clear as your statements may appear to you, patients report that many times it is neither easy nor clear to them.

Many financial problems can be avoided. When they do occur, a carefully planned strategy for handling them can keep this difficult moment of truth from turning negative.

When the News Is Bad

A look of sadness and something deeper came to faces of the physicians I interviewed for this book when I asked, "What advice do you have for delivering the bad news?" I didn't have to define my terms; they knew what I was referring to. Said one physician, with a deep sigh, "It is the worst part of this job. I went into medicine to save lives, and it is so hard to admit that I can't always do that. And it's even harder to tell the patients."

Although the responsibility of breaking the news to the patient generally falls to the physician, the other members of the office personnel play an important part in providing support to the patient afterwards. Nurses, receptionists, scheduling clerks, even billing and accounting personnel—all interact with these patients and their families, and how you manage those moments of truth can make a big difference in how the patient handles the situation.

The following suggestions are useful for all practice personnel when dealing with patients who are receiving or have received bad news:

■ Be sensitive but not maudlin. Patients in these circumstances will appreciate your empathy. They will want your sensitivity to their feelings and your understanding of the situation they are in. However, they don't need nor want someone who is dripping with melancholy or who is overly saccharine in his or her approach. Patients report that they want someone with whom they can share this experience and who will understand without making them feel that they already have one foot in the grave.

■ Be supportive but not patronizing. Closely connected to the previous suggestion, this one refers to your ability to help without making the patient feel inadequate. Patients are able to do much for themselves and usually reach a point in their grief process where they want to. Medical practice personnel of all types can help them in that process by providing emotional and factual support, yet still asking the patient to contribute, too.

■ Be attentive but not smothering. Most patients who are dealing with bad news need more attention than others. They are working through their own inner struggle and that is a very lonely process. One nurse explained, "Sometimes I get told by the patient, 'They told me today that I have lymphoma.' You want to sit down and cry with them. I just stop what I'm doing and sit down and we talk. I try to be there for them at the moment and then get someone who can help on a longer-term basis (a counselor)."

Other times patients need some space to process what is happening to them. On those occasions, it is important to be available if you are needed, allowing the patient to determine if and when that is. One staff member told me, "I just let the patient know I'm there if he needs me."

■ Be honest but not brutal. Patients and medical personnel agree that honesty is important in these circumstances. However, take care in the way this message is delivered. You have to tell patients what is wrong, but you should say it with an explicit or implicit wish that it could be otherwise. A resident physician in one of my workshops made the comment, "Patients say they want the truth but they really don't." While that may be true for some, I suppose, the vast majority do want to know what they are up against. What they don't want is for that news to be told in such a way so as to leave them feeling uncared for. (See the next section, "Breaking the News," for suggestions on how to do this.)

■ Be optimistic but not unrealistic. It is important to keep the patient focused on what positives may exist. For example, "You are having open heart surgery but your heart muscle is in good shape and you should do just fine." Even when the diagnosis is terminal, there are usually treatment options available to reduce the pain or put a disease in remission. When you have done all that can be done medically, it is still important for the medical practice personnel to remain upbeat and supportive. One office manager told me of an elderly man who was diagnosed with terminal cancer and had reached the end of the treatment options. He looked at her with a twinkle in his eye and said, "Don't start treating me like I'm dead already. I'll still be giving you trouble until I take my last breath!"

■ Be problem-oriented but not cold. One way to keep the patient focused on the positives is to look at the situation as a problem to be solved. As I mentioned above, exploring the treatment options helps the patient begin to focus on what is still possible.

■ Be detached but not distant. For your own good, you have to develop a way to remove yourself from too much emotional involvement with these patients. In your field, these sad situations are encountered often. If you allow each of them to go to your own heart, you will not be able to survive. Yet, don't let your need to detach allow you to become distant. You have to become personally involved or you will come across as cold and aloof. One nurse put it this way: "I just try to think of how I would want to be treated and act accordingly."

■ Be patient-focused, not self-focused. An excellent guideline for the entire process of breaking the bad news, this advice was offered by gynecologist Debra Gussman. "The patient's comfort is what matters most here, not mine," she said. "I need to be tuned in to each patient and what she needs." This advice also includes asking the patients what they would like to know, rather than telling them what you think will be important to them. Remember the nurse who told the story of the patient who wasn't really interested in the technical explanation of what was wrong with his heart; his first concern was with who was going to feed his cows. Eventually, patients may want and need more technical information, but many cannot process that kind of data early in the process of receiving bad news. By asking, "What would you like to know?" you can address the patients' immediate concerns.

Breaking the News

"Each of us must find our own way to do this," one doctor told me. "It is never easy." I'm sure that this is true. However, I do have some thoughts that have been shared by patients who have actually been the recipients of bad news. The following format offers a suggested way to proceed, based on an assimilation of those thoughts.

For a face-to-face encounter:

1. Smile when you walk in! At least, look pleasant.

2. Sit down. Standing creates distance, and what patients need at this moment is closeness.

3. Make a brief connecting remark. A comment about the weather, the new dress, a new tie, something to break the ice. Patients report needing some warm connection to you before you move to the topic.

4. Move to the topic at hand. "I know that you have been waiting on the test results."

5. Describe the news. "I'm sorry, but the news isn't good."

6. Using the patient's name, specifically and clearly state the facts. "John, . . ."

7. Acknowledge the difficulty of the moment. "I know this is hard to hear."

8. Pause. This is hard to do because you will want to move on to the positives. However, the patient will need a moment to comprehend what you just said. Be silent.

9. Define what you mean. "The kind of cancer you have is called lymphoma. It is a disease of the lymphatic system." Keep the explanation brief and as simple as possible.

10. Plant the positive seeds. "We don't have to let this thing beat us though. There are several options we can explore." Don't attempt to give details at this point, although they can and should be offered later.

11. Again, acknowledge or solicit feelings. "I imagine this feels pretty frightening right now, doesn't it?" or "What are you feeling right now?"

12. Allow the patient to express his or her feelings.

13. Offer to answer the patient's questions: "Is there anything you'd like to ask me?" or "What questions do you have?"

14. Explain the positives in detail. "Let's look at the alternatives we have to attacking this problem. There are several things we can do."

15. Solicit the patient's participation in working with you. "We'll work together on this, John. You aren't alone. I'm going to need your help."

16. Be prepared to repeat yourself. Patients who have received bad news are upset and will probably need to hear parts of this message again.

Telephone Encounter:

Although most bad news should be broken interpersonally, there are occasions when you will need to deliver some bad news on the telephone. In those instances, the following steps may be helpful:

1. Identify yourself.

2. Express your pleasure at reaching the patient: "I'm glad I was able to catch you at home."

3. Acknowledge the patient's process. "You've been waiting on the results of your test."

4. Describe the news. "I'm sorry, but the news isn't good."

5. Give the patient a choice. "Would you like the details now or would you like to come in." One doctor told me she encouraged her patients to come talk to her in person but that most wanted to know something immediately. If that is the case, return to the face-to-face encounter and pick up the process at Step 6. Do everything you can to get the patient to come to see you if the news involves a terminal diagnosis. That kind of information should be delivered face-to-face.

6. Encourage the patient to seek immediate support from family or friends. Since you are not physically present to provide support at the moment, encourage the patient not to sit alone but to seek support.

Many physicians indicate that although it is difficult to actually tell the bad news to the patient, it is even harder to deal with the families. It is important to remember that many of the above suggestions will also help in talking with the family members of the patient involved. These folks also need sensitivity, supportiveness, attention, honesty, and optimism. Benjamin H. Natelson, M.D., chief of the neurobehavioral unit at the East Orange VA Medical Center in New Jersey, offered several helpful suggestions for breaking the bad news to a patient's family members:

- Use a social lead-in, such as, "I know that you have been worried about your son's condition."
- Acknowledge the problem: "I have completed my examination of him and there is a serious problem."
- Briefly describe the diagnosis: "Your son has _____."
- Acknowledge the family member's emotional reaction: "I know this is hard for you to hear. I wish it could be otherwise."
- Solicit any questions:" "Before I discuss the treatment options, do you have any questions?"
- Move to the treatment and its impact: "This is what we can do. It will have this impact." Start with the positive impact of the treatment and then move to any negative side effects, etc. Avoid being pinned down to a time-line in terminal cases. Any estimate should be labeled a guesstimate and that you hope to be proved wrong.
- Determine the family member's interest in assisting with the treatment: "Are you in a position to be involved with the treatment?"
- Specify what the family member can do to help, even if it's a simple make-work job: "I'm going to need your help with this. Your son can't do this alone." By getting the family

member involved, you return some power that he or she will feel has been taken away.

- Decide, with the family member, how to tell the patient: "When do you think would be a good time to explain this to your son?"[12]

Ronald Reisman, M.D., an Indianapolis internist who specializes in critical care medicine, has dealt with many families who are told the worst possible news. He explained, "Families in this situation are depressed and frightened. They're often angry at the healthcare system and disappointed by the failure to save someone they love dearly. Treating their pain is just as important as treating the patient's pain . . . Be patient . . . Let them work through their anger."[13]

When the news is bad, you do not have a pleasant job in front of you, no matter what you do. Your very human reaction may be to run away or to make the moment as brief as possible. Don't give in to those instinctive responses. Instead, as Dr. Gussman advised, put the patient's comfort first; it will actually make your task easier.

The Always Difficult Customers

Every practice has them! The customers who are never satisfied, no matter how hard you seem to try. When you see their names in the scheduling book or hear their voices on the telephone, you exchange looks with a colleague and say, "Oh no, it's Mr. Jones again!" You need say no more! In spite of this person's reputation, however, he is still a patient and you are charged with trying to, if not please him, at least help him. I have some suggestions that may assist you in this process. Although the following discussion applies to patients, many of these tips will help you to handle any chronically difficult customer.

- Get to know this patient. Abraham Lincoln is reported to have said: "When I see a man I don't like, I think, 'There's a man I don't know.'" These are wise words for any situation, and they provide a hint for dealing with even your most difficult customers. Take the case of the receptionist who could not seem to please one of the older male patients. She decided that there must be a way to reach him. So, she began by listing all that she knew about this customer. She consulted with other staff members and discovered that the man had a great interest in the local National Football League (NFL) franchise. The next time the troublesome patient stormed in the door demanding to see his doctor immediately, the receptionist tuned the conversation to the recent victory enjoyed by the local NFL team. This comment caught the patient completely off guard and he smiled! The two conversed a moment about the team's successful season, and then the receptionist said, "Why don't you have a seat over there by that nice sunny window, and I'll see how long it will be before Dr. Smith can see you." The report is that this patient was not a problem again. The old saying, "You catch more flies with honey than with vinegar" is true of patients too.

■ The handoff. Perhaps there is a clash between you and the patient that doesn't exist for others in the practice. Ask around and locate the staff member with whom this patient gets along. Allow that person to greet the patient, and, if possible, to move along through the cycle of service with him or her. This may sound like placating and it probably is. However, it is better for everyone to be able to move this patient in and out of the practice with as little upheaval as possible.

■ The hand-up. If a staff member encounters a person who knows it all, knows how the system works, and how he or she wants to be treated and by whom, and thinks that anyone who tries to explain the system is a jerk, the best strategy is to transfer this patient to the office manager or supervisor early in the conversation. People in positions of authority can set limits by telling the patient that this particular behavior is not acceptable. Also, when such people deal with someone they perceive to be in authority, they will often back down and begin to listen.[14]

■ The team approach. Another way to work with this patient is to try the team approach. All practice personnel who interact with this patient should sit down and brainstorm appropriate ways to respond. The team can be relied on during the patient's visit. By keeping him or her moving and handed firmly from one person to another, you can make the situation easier to handle.

■ Try tricks of scheduling. Most practice personnel tell me that always-difficult patients are handled better during the less hectic times of the day, usually toward closing. With fewer other patients around, they have a smaller audience for whom to perform, and the practice personnel can devote more attention to moving them through as quickly as possible.

■ The serenity prayer. Used to help alcoholics move toward acceptance, this simple prayer sheds light on how you might have to decide to deal with the always-difficult customer: "God grant me the serenity to accept the things I cannot change, the courage to change the things I can, and the wisdom to know the difference."

■ The termination option. You do not have to keep every patient who crosses your threshold. If this patient becomes impossible to handle, if you have tried all of the above suggestions and none of them work, then it is time to give serious consideration to termination. One office manager said, "Once in a great while, we encounter a patient who simply is impossible to satisfy. In those cases, I sit down with the patient and say, 'It is clear to me that we are not able to meet your needs in this practice. I will do all that I can to help you, but I believe it is time that you seek your healthcare elsewhere.'" Of course, you want to keep every patient you can, but there is no shame in admitting that once in a while the match between this patient and your practice is a poor one. Everyone concerned will be happier if this patient goes someplace else. Be sure to follow a well-documented procedure for termination of care. Failure to do so can result in claims of malpractice due to "abandonment."

The Abusive Patient
Bearing in mind that these patients represent a very small percentage of your total patient population, these few people can present a great drain on the psychic energy of the practice personnel. Thus, they must be handled.

"The abusive patient is one who threatens and demeans the staff, usually verbally . . . They scream at the staff, swear and call them names, and intimidate those whom they believe to be inferior to them."[15] Such behavior is beyond what any practice personnel should be expected to tolerate, and even a practice dedicated to serving its customers has a right to draw the line. The following tips should help you deal with these situations:

■ Be firm. Sometimes these people only need to have someone call their bluff. One nurse told me about a patient who was a chronic problem. He had been dismissed from practice after practice for his behavior. One day he was especially abusive. This nurse told me, "I really lost it, I'm afraid, but he settled down. I looked him in the eye and said, 'Mr. Jones you have a choice. You can either sit here and be quiet and let us take care of your problem, or you can go home. It's as simple as that.' It was amazing. After that, he did everything I said."

■ Relocate. Just as with the angry customer, the very act of moving this patient into another area in the practice usually has a calming effect. Plus, abusive patients are frequently performing for whatever audience they can find. By removing them from that spotlight, you can also change their behaviors.

■ Shift the situation to a higher authority. Often these individuals need to be told by someone whom they perceive to have power in the office that their behavior is unacceptable, that it will not be tolerated, and that it could lead to potential termination. The only two people who can deliver this message are the office manager or a physician. Whomever is called on to perform this task must do it. Staff members will suffer heightened abuse the next time the patient comes in, if the person in power has not stood behind them initially. Physicians, in particular, need to be aware that abusive patients are like leopards who can change their spots at will. They can be meek, mild, and even friendly with an authority figure, especially physicians, and can treat the rest of the staff in a hostile, demeaning fashion. The word of your staff should be trusted in these cases, not your perceptions of the patients. If you have a very good reason to believe that the staff member's perceptions may be in error, delay your response to the customer by saying, "I will look into this situation and get back to you by (specify a time within the next 24 hours)."

■ Set limits. The abusive patient needs to know exactly what his or her limits are. One strategy for preventing another occurrence is to conduct a joint conference with the patient, the doctor, the manager, and the staff member who was confronted by the unacceptable behavior. The purpose of the meeting is to establish for the patient what he or she must do in order to remain a patient of this practice. Regardless of whether behaviors are determined by a team or by the person in charge, specific behaviors must be described, those that you expect the patient to demonstrate and those that are unacceptable.[16]

■ Discharge, if necessary. As in the situation of the always-difficult customer, the abusive customer can also be subject to being discharged. I should mention here that you will need to handle this situation carefully, making every attempt to provide a suitable recommendation, to thoroughly document the entire situation, and to follow all legal requirements. However, no one in your practice has to be subjected to abusive treatment, and if it does not stop, then discharge is your only alternative.

The Violent Customer

Clearly the extreme case for most practices, the patient who becomes violent presents a clear and present danger to himself or herself, the practice personnel, and other patients. Even though such behavior is usually rare, the best way to deal with it is through advance planning. Your practice should have specific policies and procedures for dealing with it. Also, local law enforcement officials should be invited to meet with the staff to discuss concerns and potential alternatives and to provide some basic self-defense training to the staff. Specific guidelines for implementing 911 should be established. A crisis team can be formed with a team leader who is the contact person for assessing the situation and for developing the team strategy for handling it.[17]

After the incident, arrangements need to be made that will vary. They can include "(1) requiring the patient to change physicians and/or facilities; (2) a warning that such incidents can result in termination; (3) a behavioral contract with the patient for future interactions with the [practice's] staff"[18] and (4) actual termination of care with specific documentation within three days of the incident.

Even though they are uncommon incidents, such emergencies must be anticipated and planned for. Otherwise, your practice will be caught off guard, and the result could be tragic.

Three More Thorny Moments

Sexual Harassment   A somewhat loaded topic in today's corporate environment, the potential for this behavior by customers themselves or for claims made against organizational personnel by customers is even greater in a medical practice. Medical and on occasion nonmedical personnel must enter a patient's intimate space in order to do their jobs and to meet the customer's needs. Such situations invite inappropriate behaviors from patients and provide the opportunity for claims of harassment from them as well. Thus, care must be taken in all circumstances.

If the patient behaves inappropriately, making sexual comments or gestures to staff or other patients, action should be taken. It should be reported immediately to a supervisor, manager, or physician. The authority figure in the practice should then talk to the patient, making clear that such behaviors will not be tolerated and could lead to termination.[19]

The best protection against claims of sexual misconduct against practice personnel is to prevent potential situations from developing in the first place. The most vulnerable individuals for such claims are the medical personnel who are conducting physical examinations. Thus, precautions should be taken, such as asking for an assistant to come into the room during certain examinations, maintaining a professional demeanor (not to be confused with cold and distant), and keeping casual conversation appropriate in nature. If a claim comes, then you will have an unquestionable record, and this will help when it becomes a case of your word against the patient's.

Noncompliance   Probably one of the most frustrating situations for a physician is to try to solicit compliance from a patient who seems bent on ignoring the physician's best advice. As I mentioned in Chapter 2, an amazing number of patients don't comply, but there are ways to increase the likelihood of compliance, as specified by Eric Anderson, M.D. He offers eight methods that have worked for him.

1. Get a feel for the patients. Be observant, listen to what they say. Do they reveal that they are in denial about their illnesses, have a money issue, or have a chip on the shoulder?

2. Don't overreact. Don't rise to the possible baiting or probing of your defenses. Try to see the difficulties from the patient's point of view. What does he or she believe is wrong? Does he or she have a secret concern or fear? Listen!

3. Win the patient's trust. Gradually over time, show that you can be trusted. Didn't you set the broken arm so that

it healed nicely? Didn't you live up to your promise to have him or her in and out of your office on time?

4. Keep slogging away. Keep repeating, patiently. You never know when a chance comment might suddenly work.

5. Anticipate the problem. Why are these people noncompliant? Because patients don't see the benefit of compliance, they enjoy their bad habits and accept the consequences. Or they have a long-term disease and are tired of being medicated. They don't feel a lot better.

6. Use other resources. Solicit the help of the patient's family, and don't forget that others in the practice may be able to gain the patient's compliance. One nurse who was especially successful at this explained, "I behave as if I'm their granddaughter. And I show I care."

7. Don't overanalyze the failure. Try to identify why noncompliance occurred, but sometimes you can become too introspective. Sometimes there is no real answer.

8. Discharge without anger. When you reach the end of the road with this patient, sometimes the sensible thing to do is to document the situation in the medical record, then confront and discharge the patient. One doctor said that he explains where the patient is headed if he or she doesn't change. Then he says good-bye, hoping all of this will help the next doctor.[20] Again, be sure to follow specific procedures, so as to avoid claims of abandonment.

When dealing with a noncompliant patient, be sure to document everything. When dealing with no-show appointments, for example, staff members should make every effort to reschedule them. The receptionist should keep clear, specific records of both the missed appointments and the efforts to follow up. If, after repeated attempts, the patient cannot be reached by phone, a letter should be sent to the patient requesting that the patient reschedule, and copies should be kept in the patient's file.[21]

Referrals When the patient arrives at your office without the proper referral papers in place, it is always an awkward moment of truth, at best. Although office managers seem to agree that there is no magic formula for making it otherwise, the following suggestions have worked for many of them:

1. Develop a clear procedure for seeking approval and transferring the appropriate forms.

2. Develop a friendly, professional relationship with the practices with whom you do a lot of referral business; have interoffice brown-bag lunches, referral appreciation coffees, and other such functions.

3. Develop a friendly, professional relationship with the appropriate personnel in the major insurance companies on whom your practice and its patients rely.

4. Work at educating your patients about their responsibilities in this process.

Regardless of the type of difficult moments of truth you are facing, there are specific steps you can take and suggestions you can use to manage the situation successfully. Remember, the effective handling of these situations often results in not only the retention of the customer but also in the development of strong customer-loyalty.

RECOVERY

Staff, managers, and/or physicians who have to face difficult moments of truth should find ways to recover. In fact, they must do so or the stress produced by these situations will stay with them, draining them of productive, positive energy. You are in a high-stress profession anyway, and workers who deal with distressed people as a basic part of their jobs tend to take on the bad feelings of their clients to some extent and often empathize with the clients to the detriment of their own positive feelings.[22] Add to that the intensity of feelings that result from negative customer interactions, and you have a situation that has to be handled. People in high-stress jobs, such as those in healthcare, must learn ways of managing and reducing their stress. So, I challenge you to use the suggestions made in this last section of this very important chapter.

Recovery from difficult moments of truth for you, the service provider, must be done on a short-term basis as well as the long term.

Short-Term Recovery

To recover in the short term, you need to be able to move past any given difficult moment of truth. The following seven-step process will allow you to reflect on what happened, learn what you can from it, and then let it go.

1. As objectively and unemotionally as possible, replay the situation either verbally or in writing (recounting exactly what happened as best you remember it).

2. As honestly as possible, answer the following question: "What, if anything, did I contribute to making this moment difficult?" Be honest with yourself. You can't learn what not to do next time if you don't acknowledge what you did in this situation.

3. As perceptively as possible, answer the following question: "What, if anything, did the customer contribute to making this moment difficult?" Stay out of the attack or counterattack modes when recounting the customer's behaviors. Try to stay objective.

4. As accurately as possible, answer the following question: "What, if anything, did the system (often policies and procedures) in which we were interacting contribute to making this moment difficult?" If you find systemic problems, make a note of these to be referred to later in this process.

5. As accurately as possible, answer the following question: "What, if any, contribution did the content of the situation have to do with making it a difficult moment?" If the content itself was the cause, such as when delivering bad news to a patient, awareness of that will help you understand why it was hard, and this understanding will assist you in reducing your stress about it.

6. Answer these three final solution questions:

- "If I encountered a similar situation again, what, if anything, would I try to do differently?"
- "What, if any, additional skills and knowledge do I need to gain?"
- "What, if any, changes need to be made in the systems, policies, and procedures that I am empowered to change or that I can bring to the attention of those who are?"

7. Move on! You have taken the most proactive action possible: you have learned from even a difficult situation. There is nothing more you can do about it. Let the energy go.

Long-Term Recovery

Over time, what can you do to help manage the tension that builds up from handling difficult moments of truth and other job-related stresses? I asked other healthcare professionals what advice they could share with you. The following is a summary of what they told me:

- Know what causes you stress. Is it the phones that are constantly ringing? Is it your fear that in all of the rush around the practice you might make a mistake? Or is it the result of the mistakes you have already made? Is it the long hours? Or is it that patient you couldn't seem to please? Maybe it's all of the above and more. Somehow being able to identify what causes you stress can help you recover from it. Giving it a name removes it f r o m the vague category of *pressure,* and that seems to help.

- Remember why you are in the healthcare field. Remind yourself that one motivation for your choice of a career in healthcare was to help people. Refocusing on that can help you get your priorities in place and help you handle the stress that comes with the territory.

- Focus on the positives. One office manager told me with a wry smile, "Some days you don't think you're helping anybody. Then, I have to remind myself, 'Well, Monday was a good day!'" Be even more specific than that. Remember the woman whom you helped obtain Medicaid and the little girl who smiled happily after her obstructed ears had been opened. Reflect on the good judgment call you made when you told the anxious parent to bring in her child and he had needed immediate attention. Recall the spontaneous little gifts and cards from patients who want to say "thanks." Even remember how you were able to hold the hand of and provide comfort to a patient's family member after the news of a terminal illness had been shared.

- Realize that you can't please everyone. No matter how hard you try, some customers will insist on being unhappy.
- Realize that nobody is perfect. No matter how hard you try you won't always make the right choices.
- Keep your sense of humor. Remember that it takes many more muscles to frown than it does to smile. One nurse told me, "You have to develop a sense of humor, just laugh some of it off. If you get mad, you can't be effective. And you know anger is like an acid. It destroys the container it's in. It'll eat you up!"
- Learn how to detach. There is a delicate balance between caring enough to be there when the patients need you and not so much that it eats you alive. As one woman told me, "You have to learn to detach yourself. You have to have empathy for the patients and care about them as people, but you can get so tied up that it makes the whole rest of your life miserable. You can go home at night with nothing left to give to your own family."
- Learn to leave it behind. A nurse I interviewed in Kansas City put it this way: "On the way home from work, you have to find a spot on the road and leave all of your problems there until the next day. There's this billboard on I-470, and when I reach it I say,' OK, that's my dumping spot. I'm not going to think about any of this until I come back tomorrow.'"

In addition to these very insightful suggestions, I urge you to look into other ways of managing your stress. Locate and attend workshops on stress management and performance tuning. Check your local bookstore for helpful books on managing stress. Find something that works for you and then do it, regularly and faithfully. Just knowing about how to manage stress won't help at all, unless you put that knowledge into practice.

Why is this the longest chapter in this book? The answer is twofold. First, moments of truth are those interactions that will make or break your practice, and the difficult ones are potentially explosive. Handled with skill, often the negativity can either be avoided altogether or turned into positive experiences for all concerned. Second, difficult customer interactions are a constant drain on the energy of the practice personnel. They usually cause stress and create tensions, and often will burn out even the most dedicated employees. Thus, the three-part model presented in this chapter—prevention, managing, and recovery—is one of the most important contributions I can make to you, your practice, and your customers. It makes sense, then, that it would take considerable time and space to cover this important information.

END NOTES

1. Diane Palmer, "Collections in a Managed Care Era," Workshop, 1996 National Conference, Professional Association of Health Care Office Managers (May 9, 1996), Austin, Texas. Contact at: Palmer Associates, Inc., P.O. Box 717, Lake Tahoe, Homewood, CA 95718. Phone: 916-581-0187.

2. Randall Luecke, Virginia Rosselli, and Jody Moss, "The Economic Ramifications of 'Client' Dissatisfaction," *Group Practice Journal* 40 no. 3 (May/June 1991), p. 10.

3. David Hemingway and Alice Killen, "Complainers and Noncomplainers," *Journal of Ambulatory Care Management* 12, no. 3 (August 1989), pp. 19–27.

4. "Customer Service Rep Enhances Office Quality, Florida Administrator Says," *Medical Office Manager* 2, no. 7 (February 1993), pp. 7–8.

5. Suggestions adapted from C. Carolyn Thiedke, M.D., "Teaching Staff to Say 'No' Graciously," *Family Practice Management* 1, no. 8 (September 1994), pp. 84–86.

6. Paul Gerber and Marjolin Bijlefeld, "Ways Your Staff Can Lead You down the Malpractice Path," *Physician's Management* 33, no. 1 (January 1993), p. 105.

7. Diane Palmer, Workshop, May 9, 1996, Austin, Texas.

8. "Patient Credit and Collection," MGMA Information Exchange (IE), #4567, (June 1994).

9. Gerber and Bijlefeld, p. 100.

10. Diane Palmer, Workshop, (May 9, 1996), Austin, Texas.

11. Gerber and Bijlefeld, p. 100.

12. Benjamin H. Natelson, *Tomorrow's Doctors: The Path to Successful Practice in the 1990's* (Plenum Press: New York and London, 1990) pp. 246–251.

13. Ronald Reisman, M.D., "Help Your Patients' Families Accept the Inevitable," *Medical Economics* 66, no. 8 (April 17, 1989) p. 178.

14. Liz Osbourne, *Resolving Patient Complaints: A Step-By-Step Guide to Effective Service Recovery,* (Gaithersburg, Maryland: Aspen Publishers, Inc., 1995) p. 97.

15. Ibid., p. 96.

16. Ibid., p. 97.

17. Ibid., p. 107.

18. Ibid., pp. 108–109.

19. Ibid., p. 98.

20. Eric Anderson, "Ways to Get Cooperation from Noncompliant Patients," *Physicians Management* 31, no. 8 (August 1991), pp. 130–132, 137.

21. Gerber and Bijlefeld, p. 105.

22. Karl Albrecht, *Stress and the Manager: Making It Work for You* (Englewood Cliffs, New Jersey: Prentice-Hall Inc., 1979), pp. 93–98.

FIVE

CONTINUATION

The first 14 chapters of this book have led you through the steps to establishing a Total Service Medical Practice. The last three will tell you how to keep the process going. In Chapter 15, the methods of cementing commitments to service though practice service promises and personal service statements are described. In Chapter 16, the techniques for the reinforcement and, thus, continuation of quality-service behaviors are discussed. In Chapter 17, I offer advice for maintaining Total Service as a way of life for your practice.

Good luck!

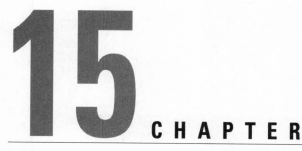

CHAPTER

Step Fifteen—Put Your Commitment to Service in Writing

It is difficult to capture in words the impact of the creative process described in this chapter. When members of any organization, including yours, sit down together to articulate their commitments to service, magic can happen. Suddenly the sometimes vague service concepts will be removed from the stratosphere of your imagination and will be brought into the world of your reality. I have seen faces illuminated with a new understanding. I have witnessed eyes filled with tears of emotion and smiles of confidence tinged with pride as these written commitments to service are read aloud. Whether creating the practice service promises[1] that put service into operation for the entire practice, or personal service statements that express deep individual commitments, the process of putting all of this in writing is one that will leave you and your practice changed.

In order to reach this point of near nirvana, however, you need to know the basics of what and how. Because, you see, this is the chapter where the rubber meets the road. You are ready to say to the world that your practice is dedicated to putting its customers first. As an individual and as a member of your practice team, it is now time to put your commitment to service into words,

words that will be shared with your colleagues and with your customers. To help you accomplish this task, I'd like to answer a few fundamental questions.

WHAT IS THE DIFFERENCE BETWEEN PRACTICE SERVICE PROMISES AND PERSONAL SERVICE STATEMENTS?

Practice service promises are of two types: The unified statement that expresses your practice's commitment to providing quality service experiences for all of its customers, and the separate service promises made to each of your key primary and secondary customer populations (usually four or five) on which the unified promise is based. Regardless of the type, service promises are created through the collective efforts of practice personnel and are made public to the customers so that they know the practice's intentions to serve. They also provide goals for all practice personnel to meet.

Personal service statements are more private. Created individually and then shared within the practice, these statements describe specific actions that each person plans to take, actions that will help provide for the nonclinical aspects of the customers' experiences with the practice. Personal service statements assist each individual in seeing how he or she plays a part in the Total Service experiences of all practice customers.

PRACTICE SERVICE PROMISES

Why Should Your Practice Create Service Promises?

There are several reasons any organization, including yours, should take the time to articulate its commitments to service through service promises. Let's look at the benefits for the practice personnel first. To begin with, the actual process of searching for the specific words needed to write these promises helps clarify the service intentions of the practice. Also, the discussion that accompanies the creation of service promises make more, meaningful the sometimes vague service words, such as *courtesy, respect,* and even *friendliness.* This process also lets all practice personnel participate, either personally or through an appropriate representative, in the creation of the promises, thus enhancing each person's buy-in to them. By putting the ideas and concepts of service in writing, the commitments made in service promises take on a reality that they might otherwise lack. It is easy to talk about service as something that should be done, but when the commitment appears in black and white it becomes an expected standard.

Written practice service promises also provide a major benefit to the customers. Because these statements will be made public, they allow customers to know early in their contact with the practice whether this is an organization with which they want to do business. For patients, it is an even more critical decision— they will have an early indication of whether this is a group of people in whose hands they are willing to place their lives. Service promises, then, permit the customers to obtain an early understanding of what they can expect in their interactions with the practice, allowing them to make well-informed and educated decisions.

What Are the Characteristics of Practice Service Promises?

Four characteristics describe well-written practice service promises.

■ Well-written practice service promises present achievable yet challenging service goals for all practice personnel. Service promises should not commit your practice to more than it can deliver. Repeated failures to meet unrealistic service goals will ruin your credibility with your customers. By the same token, service promises should not aim for mediocrity, because you undoubtedly will hit your target. Service promises, then, should present achievable but challenging goals for all practice personnel.

■ Well-written practice service promises should be reasonably brief. Unlike mission statements, which tend to be lengthy and cover many aspects of organizational visions and philosophies, practice service promises are brief and to the point. They need to grab the attention of the customers, be customer-friendly and, thus, memorable, and have a direct focus on the service to be provided. The overall implicit message should be that the practice aims for quality service.

■ Well-written practice service promises should focus on the nonclinical aspects of your practice that are important to your customers. Remembering that *service* in a medical practice involves the interpersonal relationships and the way things are done (your systems cycles and processes), your practice should create service promises that articulate its intentions to provide positive experiences for its customers in those areas that matter to them. By returning to the items listed on your customers' report cards, described in Chapter 6, you will be able to incorporate those items of importance into your service promises.

■ Well-written practice service promises should focus on specific customer populations. Each practice service promise should clearly identify the customer it is addressing. Thus, your practice should create the following separate service promises:

■ Promises targeted for each of the practice's key external customer populations.

■ A single, unified promise created after the more specific promises have been written, incorporating the common themes that run through them.

■ Practice service promises should be made public to the customer populations they address. Whether framed and displayed on counters where patients and often family members check in, or conveyed in a letter to contacts at hospitals, insurance companies, or other physician's offices, practice service promises must be shared with your customers. When your practice goes public with its service promises, the commitment made by practice personnel intensifies. As mentioned previously, this publicizing also helps customers know what to expect from your practice, providing them with important information for necessary decisions.

What Do Practice Service Promises Look Like?

Regardless of the population addressed, practice service promises usually have three parts to them:

1. The recipient of the service is stated or very clearly implied.

2. The service value or contribution that will be provided to the customer is stated.

3. The means and the circumstances for providing the service will be included.[2]

As you peruse the following sample promises, please keep in mind that they are offered only to show you the range of possibilities, and are not necessarily models for replication. The explanations following each promise provide insight into their intent.

Sample 1: A multispecialty clinic with 25 physicians.

(A unified promise to all customers)
"We promise to create and maintain a customer-friendly climate in which we respond with sensitivity and in a friendly, respectful manner to our customers' wants and needs."

The key words and phrases are:

create and maintain: This phrase is important because it indicates that the creation and the maintenance of service are two separate processes.

customer-friendly: This phrase serves as a reminder to the practice personnel as well as an announcement to their customers that this practice intends to make it as easy as possible for its customers to do business with it.

climate: This word is defined as *the customers' interpersonal interactions with practice personnel* as well as *their experiences with the practice's systems, cycles, and processes.*

sensitivity: This word conveys to all customers that they will find empathy and understanding in their dealings with this practice.

friendly: This well-known word is operationalized by behaviors, such as smiles, direct eye contact, unobstructed views of customers and vice versa, pleasant vocal quality, helpful attitude, and so on.

respectful: This word also is operationalized with a variety of behaviors, such as forms of address, confidentiality, language, and so forth.

customers: This familiar word stands for all customer populations and implies an understanding of their common characteristics as well as some of the unique features among the different populations.

wants and needs: The use of these words indicates an understanding of the difference between them. Also, their inclusion opens the discussion of when those wants and / or needs could not or, on occasion, should not be met.

Sample 2: A specialist's office with five physicians.

(A promise to patients)
"Caring for you physically is our profession; caring for you personally is our pleasure."

A little more poetic and a little less descriptive, this practice promise is certainly memorable. The key words and phrases are:

caring: Although used twice in this promise, this word is defined differently in each instance. The first usage refers to the clinical aspects of the practice, more specifically to diagnosis, treatment, and health maintenance.

physically: Again, this is a direct reference to the clinical aspects of the patients' experiences. Although it is somewhat unusual to include this in the service promise, it works in this instance because it provides a nice contrast later with nonclinical aspects of the patients' experiences with the practice.

profession: This word was included to refer to the expertise of the practice personnel.

caring: In this instance, this word refers to all *service* aspects of the practice.

personally: This word indicates the practice's commitment to seeing each patient as an individual—that each patient's personal needs will be attended to.

pleasure: This word presents the desire of the personnel to serve the patients. It also conveys friendliness, warmth, and enthusiasm.

How Do You Write Practice Service Promises?

The steps for writing practice service promises are included in the Appendix. In preparation for writing these promises, blocks of no less than two hours per promise should be set aside. To write the separate promises, all practice personnel or representatives of appropriate practice departments should meet with a single objective in mind: to write a practice service promise. Once the promises targeted for the specific external populations have been completed, they should be contrasted to locate any conflicting goals which will need to be resolved as well as for any unique aspects that will need to be departmentally implemented. When this process is completed, these separate promises should be compared in order to find the common themes that can be used to write the unified practice service promise applying the same steps provided in the Appendix.

How Should the Practice Service Promises Be Made Public?

A number of methods are available for publicizing both your unified practice service promise and the separate promises aimed at each key customer population. The most obvious way to let your patients know of your official commitments is to place copies of these promises in a high-traffic area, such as at the reception desk or on the wall nearby. Another place for them is in the new-patient welcome packet described in Chapter 14. A third is on the letterhead or billing statement form that your patients receive.

To reach the secondary customers with your promises for them, you will need to examine the means of communication you have with those populations. The promises should be conveyed in writing in a letter, on the letterhead itself, and/or on other correspondence you have with these customers.

Practice service promises should be available in written form to all employees, whether they are directly involved with implementing each of them or not. Some practices place their service promises on small, laminated cards that the employees can carry in their purses or wallets. Others frame them, placing them in high-traffic employee areas.

Departments that primarily serve internal customers can create "department service promises" of their own. For example, an information systems department might have a promise similar to the following:

> We will assist all clinic personnel in serving their customers and completing their tasks by providing highly reliable, up-to-date,

responsive data processing service and technical support. We will treat all of our customers with courtesy and respect.[3]

Departmental service promises such as this one will remind employees of their responsibility to provide quality service. Taking this idea one step farther, your practice could consider writing "internal service promise," similar to the unified promise for all external customers, that would describe the kind of internal service that the practice personnel will provide to one another.

The benefits of written practice service promises go farther than might first be thought. The actual process of creating them, and their function as reminders to the employees themselves, will keep the service commitment of your practice front and center in the minds of all.

PERSONAL SERVICE STATEMENTS

Why Should Practice Personnel Write a Personal Service Statements?

Remember, these are statements written by each member of the practice: physicians, the front- and back-office staff, the office managers, and the supervisors. These statements offer each person a chance to reflect on and commit to what he or she is willing to do to make service happen in your practice. As with the practice service promises, the act of putting these intentions in writing increases the individual's commitment to them. Personal service statements are shared internally by a public reading. As each statement is heard, the idea that service is indeed a way of life for the practice becomes cemented. The overall benefit of writing and sharing these personal service statements, then, is that they demonstrate each person's involvement in the ultimate goal of quality service for the customers.

What Are the Characteristics of Personal Service Statements?

Personal Service Statements should *do* or *have* the following:

- Well-conceived personal service statements will reflect their authors' authority and expertise. When writing your own personal statement, think carefully of what your duties are. Your statement should reflect those responsibilities.

■ Well-conceived personal service statements will be based on specific moments of truth or steps in a process. In addition to thinking about your authority and expertise, also reflect on where you fit in the cycles of service or internal processes. (Return to Chapter 12 for a refresher of these models.) The part that you play in these cycles and/or processes will be represented in your statement.

■ Well-conceived personal service statements will indicate specific action. Sometimes called *personal action plans*, these statements should indicate specific behaviors you will demonstrate and actions you will take. They will state what you are going to do to provide service.

■ Well-conceived personal service statements will indicate the recipient customer population. Since cycles of service and internal processes involve specific customer groups, you should state the customer population to whom you are making your promise.

What Should a Personal Service Statement Look Like?

Even more personal and individualized than practice service promises, the content of personal service statements will be unique to each member of the practice team. However, each statement will contain the following parts:

1. Who the customer is.

2. Identification of the cycle of service or internal process.

3. The action you are committing to take.

4. A cosignature of a colleague who will serve as your partner.

The sample promises are offered for your consideration only. As I said above, yours will be uniquely yours.

Sample 1: An insurance coordinator

In my precertification interactions with insurance companies, I will be organized, patient, friendly, and timely.

This statement shows an awareness of the insurance coordinator's part in making precertification efficient and effective. It indicates her responsibility to have her facts of the case specifically organized, to work without impatience, in a warm and cooperative manner. It also demonstrates an awareness of the need to be timely with requests to insurance companies.

Sample 2: A receptionist

In my interactions with patients at check-in (during an office visit), I will be prompt in recognizing them, friendly in my demeanor, and helpful in my attitude.

This statement reflects the importance patients place on immediate recognition. It also shows an appreciation of the patients' desire for warm greetings, especially those who are feeling particularly anxious. In addition, it shows a willingness to be available to answer questions, to help the patients complete forms, and so on, thus preventing service problems from arising later in the cycle.

Sample 3: A physician

In my patient interviews, I will listen empathetically, ask good questions, explain clearly, and demonstrate a friendly, approachable demeanor.

This statement concentrates on some of the key elements of an effective patient interview. It serves as a reminder to listen without interrupting, to show understanding of the patient's situation, to ask a variety of questions, and to offer thorough explanations. It also offers a description of the demeanor the doctor intends to show, thus serving as an additional important reminder to her to do so.

Sample 4: A lab technician

I will complete the processing of the patients' blood tests for the physicians in an accurate and timely manner.

This statement also serves as a reminder. It reminds the technician that there are indeed people who are dependent on him to perform his job. The inclusion of *accuracy* and *timeliness* reflects an awareness of the service impact of this internal process.

How Do You Write a Personal Service Statement?

Each member of the practice team—that's everyone who works there—should write his or her own personal service statements.

Following the creation of these statements, they should be shared with the entire practice or department.

How Should Personal Service Statements Be Made Public?

There is two-step process for making these statements public.

Your Service Partner: After you write your personal service statement, select someone else in the practice with whom to share it. After you read and explain your statement to your partner, it should be sealed with a ritual signing process: you sign the statement and your partner cosigns as a witness. Then this sharing process is reversed, so that you become the witness for the other. You and your partner should then support and encourage each other in the implementation of the behaviors described in the statements. When you begin to feel comfortable with your performance of this statement, then you can write another one.

Your Practice Team: When each person has written his or her personal service statement and has shared it with a partner, then the entire practice, or in a larger clinic-setting of one or more departments, should meet together. Each person should read aloud his or her personal service statement followed by a brief explanation, if necessary. Imagine the impact of publicly sharing your own personal service statement with others in the practice. Your commitment to it will be intensified. Also, imagine the impact of hearing each person in your practice making his or her own personal commitment to service. When the series of personal service statements are heard together, the impact is quite moving or even dramatic. When you actually hear person after person make this kind of public statement of their intentions to serve in very specific ways, everyone develops a real *can-do* feeling. The public sharing intensifies feelings of teamwork and interdependence: *one for all, all for one!*

The cycle-of-service and the internal processes models provide interesting tools for unifying these individual service statements. As you remember from Chapter 12, each cycle is composed of moments of truth for the customer, and each internal process involves steps leading toward the production of an end product. When a cycle of service is charted and the individuals who are responsible for managing each of the moments of truth are asked to share their personal service statements, several outcomes will occur. The practice personnel will gain a new appreciation for the teamwork that is necessary to provide quality service throughout the cycle. Also, the act of hearing all of these interconnected personal commitments to service is inspiring in and of itself. Finally, it will help you to determine and then to correct problem points in the cycle, where service has been allowed to suffer. By charting the internal processes and identifying the steps that are necessary for their completion, you also set up the opportunity to share the personal service statements of those involved. As occurred with the cycle of service, this sharing also cements the notion that all are needed to help this process meet important service goals. It also reminds practice personnel of the service nature of even these internal processes.

As you can see, the written, public commitments to service made by your practice as a group and by each individual draw on all of the concepts discussed in the previous chapters. It is here, in these promises and statements, that service in your practice is operationalized.

END NOTES

1. The idea for the service promise was stimulated by Karl Albrecht's discussions of service strategies. These can be found in the following three publications: Karl Albrecht, *At America's Service* (Homewood, IL: Dow Jones–Irwin, 1988), Karl Albrecht and Ron Zemke, *Service America* (Homewood, IL: Dow Jones–Irwin, 1985), Karl Albrecht, *Service Within* (Homewood, IL: Dow Jones–Irwin, 1990).

2. Albrecht, *Service Within*, p. 145.

3. Adapted from a statement offered by Albrecht, *Service Within*, p. 145.

16

Step Sixteen—Reward and Recognize Service

I vividly remember the tired and beaten expression on the face of a practice staff-member in one of my workshops. I was completing a discussion of the importance of rewarding positive service behaviors when she raised her hand and said, "I'm a good worker. I know what I am doing and really want to do a good job. But, no one ever appreciates it. No one ever cares." This frustration is not reserved to people in staff positions alone. Those in leadership roles also often suffer from a deficit of positive feedback. At first, this absence of appreciation may seem strange, because the rewarding and recognizing of service performance is vital to its continuation. As noted behavioralist B. F. Skinner recognized, positive reinforcement helps develop desired responses rather than merely reduce the chances of undesired ones.[1] All members of the practice personnel want and need to know that their efforts are valued and appreciated. If quality service is to be continued in your practice, then rewards and recognitions must become an important part of the way you do business.

CATEGORIES AND TYPES OF REWARDS

Rewards fall into one of two categories: *informal* or *formal*. Informal rewards are those spontaneous, low- or no-cost rewards that can be given on a moment's notice. They are based on the perceptions of one individual, usually, and appear in the form of a "thank you" or an "atta boy" by managers or colleagues. *Formal* rewards are company or practice initiated. "Although studies have shown that they are not as motivating to individual employees as more . . . personal forms of recognition, that does not mean they are not important. Such programs are useful for formally acknowledging significant accomplishments, especially as they cover a long period. Formal rewards can also lend credibility to more spontaneous, informal rewards used daily."[2]

Within these two categories, you will find two types of rewards. *Tangible* rewards are more traditional, usually items such as money, plaques, or jewelry, and usually, although not always, are presented in some organization-wide forum. *Social* rewards, sometimes called *butterflies*, consist of informal personal messages of appreciation, formal events or celebrations, or other more unusual rewards, such as some suggested later in this chapter.

CRITICISMS OF REWARD SYSTEMS

There are several reasons rewards are frequently overlooked or consciously eliminated, none of which I believe are strong enough to justify the absence of recognition. The most common is the scarcity of that precious resource: time. Many practices are so busy that no one takes or makes the time to acknowledge positive behaviors. People are often hard-pressed to offer the suggestions or directions needed to correct or prevent deficient or erroneous behaviors, and so the positive behaviors slip by without apparent notice. Yet, to keep the process of service going, you must make time for this important step. Remember that many of the rewards people want don't require a great deal of time to supply.

Some people believe that employees should not receive additional rewards for doing what is expected of them. An office manager in one of my workshops said, "Why should I reward the staff for providing good service? That is what I expect them to do." On the surface, that argument even makes some sense. However, when we balance that reasoning with what we know about motivating people, we can quickly see that even expected behavior needs to be reinforced. Most people, probably even the office manager who spoke those words, need to know that their efforts are appreciated. A recent survey by the Minnesota Department of Natural Resources found that recognition activities contributed significantly to employees' job satisfaction. Most respondents said they highly valued day-to-day recognition from their supervisors, peers, and team members. Sixty-eight percent of the respondents said it was important to believe that their work was appreciated by others; 63 percent agreed that most people would like recognition for their work; and 67 percent agreed that most people need appreciation for their work. Only 8 percent thought that people should not look for praise for their work efforts.[3] If the office manager cited above wants the positive service behaviors of her staff to continue, she needs to reward them. If she does not do so, I predict that it will be just a matter of time before the staff in her office, and perhaps she herself, will suffer from a lack of motivation and burnout.

Another reason for the scarcity of positive reinforcements is the belief that money is the only acceptable reward. Some people still subscribe to the Theory X explanation of motivating workers, which postulates that employees will only respond to a carrot-and-stick methodology, operationalized by money.[4] While most employees need to make a living wage, beyond that they have other needs that dollars and cents can't meet. I don't mean to say that lots of *thank-you's* gives your practice permission to pay ridiculously low salaries. As one staff member grumbled, "*Thank you* doesn't pay the rent." However, it would be a mistake to assume that money alone buys motivation. It does not. In his very helpful book, *1001 Ways To Reward Employees*, Bob Nelson indicated, "What tends to motivate [employees] to perform—and to perform at high levels—is the thoughtful, personal kind of recognition that signifies true appreciation for a job well-done. Numerous studies have confirmed this."[5]

Still another reason for the lack of rewards is an uncertainty of what kinds of rewards to offer, other than money. Earlier in this chapter, I delineated between the two major reward-categories, formal and informal, and the two types of rewards found within these categories, social and tangible. Within both categories and types, many nonmonetary rewards exist, some of which will be specifically discussed later in this chapter. The point is: Rewards don't have to carry a high price-tag, and there are many such options from which to choose.

Sometimes individuals are not singled out for their superior service behaviors, because management fears it will serve as a de-motivator for other employees. While the total quality management (TQM) gurus often argue this position, most people in the service field believe otherwise. Perhaps the difference lies in the Japanese influence that the TQM perspective brings to bear. Although conceived by American Edwards Deming, the application of TQM began in Japan, a society in which individuals abhor being singled out and in which they thrive on being part of a group. Japanese workers tend to be embarrassed by individual recognition and usually are not motivated by it. What pleases them instead is to have their work teams rewarded, and that is what TQM advocates. American employees are different. Although team membership is important to us, ours is a society based on individualism, and we aspire to receiving acknowledgment for our individual efforts. A recent survey by the Council of Communication Management confirms what almost every employee already knows: "that [individual] recognition for a job well done is the top motivator of employee performance."[6] Since both team and individual recognition have unique motivational advantages, an effective reward system will include both kinds.

Some people believe that reward systems are too cumbersome to be utilized effectively. That is not necessarily the case. Later in this chapter, the STEP Program of the Bristol Hospital in Bristol, Connecticut, will be discussed in greater detail. It serves as an excellent example of a simple but effective formal reward system. Also, remember that many of the rewards that employees want come from the informal reward system and are not complicated at all. For example, a simple "thank you" means a lot.

Finally, some people complain that the standards for rewardable behavior are difficult to determine. This criticism can be aimed at the formal reward systems where the quantitative standard of measurement needed to warrant the reward can be too arbitrary. It also can be leveled at the more informal systems where individual perceptions of behaviors are subject to incomplete or inaccurate information as well as the perceptual filters that can cause distortion. Even though these reward systems may be vulnerable to the above criticism at times, appropriate standards are not impossible to set, and they will be discussed in greater detail in this chapter.

So, although there are arguments against rewarding positive behaviors, they are not compelling. More than that, the benefits of rewards outweigh the potential disadvantages.

BENEFITS OF REWARDING SERVICE BEHAVIORS

There are several reasons why your practice should reward positive service behaviors. First, as has been mentioned already, rewards are high motivators. Employees not only want but need this kind of figurative pat on the back. Without it, they can easily begin to feel like the staff member I cited at the beginning of this chapter: "Why bother? No one cares." This is especially true in medical practices where all personnel tend to be working at maximum capacity or beyond. If tired people believe that their efforts are not recognized and appreciated, many will stop trying, reducing, if not eliminating, the positive service behaviors. If, however, they realize that their efforts are valued, they will find ways to carry on.

A closely connected second benefit has to do with the impact the above motivation has on the Total Service process itself. When you, as well as your team as a unit, are reinforced for providing quality service experiences to the customers, you will be motivated to repeat these behaviors, establishing the kind of ongoing process that your practice's commitment to Total Service requires. If Total Service does not become thus ingrained into behaviors, then it will be nothing more than the trendy saying of the year.

The result of this ongoing process of repeated positive service behaviors is the creation of an organizational climate and culture that is characterized by quality service. In such a climate, positive service experiences do not merely occur in isolated instances; they become a part of the fabric of the practice itself. When this transition has occurred, when quality service has become the expectation not the exception, then your practice has truly reached the zenith of its journey to Total Service.

In addition to this rather complex but essential process of behavioral integration, rewards also offer other benefits to the practice. For example, they can provide opportunities for practice celebrations and can increase the sense of team work. Many times rewards are fun. I am reminded of the good time had by all when one of my HMO clients discovered this fact. When employees were asked what they would like for a reward after a certain organizational goal had been reached, they said they wanted to be entertained by their executive team. So, at the annual Christmas party, all six of the top executives in the company—from the CEO on down, granted that wish. The marketing department wrote parodies of several well-known songs, and each executive, dressed in appropriate costume, sang to the assembled employees. The hit of the evening was the CFO, who had been criticized for being coldhearted when he had to say no to requests for funds, attired in a long auburn wig and a formfitting dress, he offered what must have been a most memorable rendition of "Feelings!" According to the reports, when he sang, "Feelings. Sometimes I have feelings," the crowd burst into applause. Many said that this was the best reward they could have ever imagined.

THE CONTROVERSY OVER INDIVIDUAL REWARDS REVISITED

Most experts agree that rewards should be given. Major disagreements center around whether or not individuals should be singled out for recognition, due to the aforementioned concern about potential demotivation of other employees, and whether if individuals are rewarded, it should be done in private or in public. I have already made my case for the motivational impact of individual recognition. Moreover, I believe that most employees want to see their deserving colleagues appropriately acknowledged, and find anything less to be unacceptable. A friend of mine told of the low-key, 22-minute acknowledgement reception that was held for three of her colleagues at the university where she is chairing the communication department. After the brief and halting presentation of the awards, a faculty member was heard to comment: "Well that was very dispiriting, wasn't it."

The criticism of individual rewards seems to revolve around the word *deserving*—some people receive rewards that others don't think they deserve. When that happens, the value of the reward can be diminished and the feared de-motivation usually occurs. So, is there a foolproof system that will never allow anyone to receive a reward that he or she does not deserve? No. Does that mean, then, that no rewards should be given? I would argue that would be like throwing the baby out with the bathwater. Even employees are quick to say an occasional glitch in the reward system is preferable to eliminating it altogether. Also, if your system is carefully conceived and constructed, if it clearly places value on tangible and social rewards from both the informal and formal categories, the chances of the undeserving being inappropriately acknowledged will be greatly diminished.

The bottom line is that people need to be rewarded for their hard work. Without these reinforcers, people will give up. With them, they can climb mountains.

CHARACTERISTICS OF AN EFFECTIVE REWARD SYSTEM

As you consider establishing or revising a reward system to make certain that it provides acknowledgment for positive service behaviors, the following characteristics will guide you in the process:

■ An effective reward system will include rewards from both the formal and informal categories. Even though the traditional formal rewards may be more familiar and do still have a purpose, it is important to remember that the informal rewards are found to be more motivating by most of today's employees. It would be a mistake, however, to shape your reward system exclusively from the informal category. Just as employees need those spontaneous, usually individual, responses to their efforts, they need to see the formal organizational commitment to service at work as well. Bob Nelson recommends the following rule of thumb: "For every four soft (informal) rewards (e.g., a thank-you) there should be a more formal reward (e.g., a day off from work), and for every four of those there should be a still more formal reward (e.g., a plaque or formal praise at a company meeting), leading ultimately to such rewards as raises, promotions, and special assignments."[7] Although I am not suggesting an arbitrary tabulation of formal and informal rewards, the above ratio should be helpful in determining how to balance the mix.

■ An effective reward system will include both tangible and social rewards. Employees need to be able to touch, see, hear, and experience their rewards. By mixing the types, you will satisfy these various needs and introduce an interesting variety into the reward system. Remember that social rewards are powerful and can be given often, usually with relatively little cost of time or money. Tangible rewards are important, too, and some should definitely be a part of the reward system in your practice.

■ An effective reward system will match the rewards to the recipients.[8] Although when rewarding a team for a joint effort, group rewards are recommended, when it comes to acknowledging individuals for individual performance, the jelly-bean approach to motivation—giving the same reward to every member of the organization—does not work. Not only does it not inspire employees to excel, but it may actually damage performance, as top achievers see no acknowledgment of the exceptional job they have done.[9] Janis Allen, performance management consultant and author of *I Saw What You Did and I Know Who You Are*, advocates having all employees—staff, managers, executives—complete a reinforcer survey of things they like.[10] For a gesture of appreciation to be seen as a reward, it should meet the employee's definition. What is rewarding to some may not be rewarding to others.

■ An effective reward system will match the rewards to the achievements. Effective reinforcements should be customized to take into account the significance of the achievement. An employee who completes a two-year project should be rewarded in a more substantial way than one who simply does someone a favor. The reward should be a function of the amount of time available to plan and execute it and of the money available to be spent on it.[11]

■ An effective reward system will be timely and specific. To be effective, rewards need to given as soon as possible after the desired behavior or achievement. Rewards that are delayed for weeks or months do little to motivate employees to repeat the desired action. The reason for the reward should always be stated. People need to know what they are being rewarded for, if they are to be able to repeat that behavior.[12]

■ An effective reward system will reflect the values and culture of your practice.[13] When your practice places value on service, then the reward system should recognize service behaviors. This may mean that an existing reward system will need to be modified so that recognition for positive service behaviors becomes integrated into it. In other practices, a reward system will need to be created from scratch. In either case, the rewards given should reflect the value on both internal and external service.

■ An effective reward system will be be both public and private. The formal rewards, those planned in advance by the organization, will usually be public. The informal rewards, offered spontaneously from employee to employee or manager to staff, are often private, although on occasion a spontaneous public acknowledgement in a meeting can be gratifying to the recipient and motivating to the others.[14]

■ An effective reward system will include both team and individual rewards. As mentioned previously in this chapter, both individual and team rewards are necessary to meet the motivational needs of practice personnel.

GUIDELINES FOR STRUCTURING A REWARD SYSTEM

Since each reward system should be unique to the practice it represents, I won't go into details on the structuring of specific methods of recognition. However, there are some guidelines that will help you no matter what forms of rewards are chosen.

■ Clarify the types of data that will be relied on for particular rewards. As I discussed in Chapter 6, there are two types of data: quantitative and qualitative. When using the former, you are quantifying with numbers, and when using the latter, you are relying primarily on quotations, descriptions, and other language and perceptual-based data. Both kinds of data can be relied on to justify service rewards.

Although quantitative data can be powerful, don't let a compulsion to quantify blind you to the importance of the qualitative data. Keep your eyes open to catch others in your practice providing good service (or listen for reports thereof), and take the time to acknowledge them for what they did. Whether you are in a supervisory role or in a peer relationship, your colleagues will appreciate your acknowledgement.

■ Articulate the standards that will constitute rewardable behaviors. For some rewards, reaching a certain quantitative goal constitutes the standard by which positive service behaviors are measured. Sometimes the desired number will be low and sometimes it will be high, depending on what is being measured. For example, the desirable number of rings before a phone is answered is low, usually no more than three, and when that standard is reached and after it has been maintained by the receptionist, he or she should be acknowledged for it. On the other hand, the desired number of positive responses to items on a questionnaire is usually high. When that standard is reached or exceeded, and/or improvement is shown, rewards usually should be given. For example, if a physician's scores are high on the patient communication items on a survey, some appropriate acknowledgement is warranted. If that score is lower than the predetermined acceptable standard, however, there is work to do. When that score improves or the predetermined standard is reached or exceeded, then appropriate acknowledgement should be accorded that physician.

Since unsolicited perceptions, such as letters from customers, are usually offered unexpectedly, there is no clear standard that indicates how many warrant reward. Although these data are not used for formal rewards, they provide superior data for informal ones, and I would argue that one positive unsolicited perception warrants recognition. For example, when a supervisor receives a compliment from a managed care company regarding the pleasant, efficient approach of the practice's insurance coordinator, that coordinator should receive praise and acknowledgement from the supervisor.

One final thought on this topic: Don't fall into the "quantity equals quality" trap referred to previously. Although some quantifiable standards can be helpful or even essential when determining salary, bonuses, or formal organizational acknowledgement, it should be remembered that more does not necessarily mean better.

■ Allow employees to participate in the reward process. Practice personnel should participate in the design of the formal reward system and be involved in its implementation. The ownership that results is amazing. This involvement reduces the potential for the criticism of undeserving recipients as well. I asked several staff members how they felt about rewards to individuals. They agreed that when the staff themselves had a part in it, it made a significant difference. One staff member told me, "I liked it the way we used to do it. We were involved in the nomination and selection processes for outstanding employee awards. When they took it away from us and put it in the hands of the management team, it became political."

The staff members also indicated that nothing can replace the soft, informal rewards that practice personnel provide for each other as well. Peer appreciation is highly valued, as one staff member indicated: "It means a lot to me to receive compliments from my colleagues when I do a good job." Such rewards offered by managers, physicians, and supervisors are important too. One staff member told me, "I was on cloud nine the other day! One of the doctors stopped me and told me I was doing such a good job with the senior patients and that he really appreciated it. I felt like I was flying all day long!" Another said, "Our office manager puts little notes on my desk whenever she catches me doing something good. It makes me feel great and I try harder!"

- Give rewards to the practice team as a unit as well as to individuals. Although you may have thought I was arguing against team recognition earlier in this chapter, I was not. There I was making the point that team recognition should not replace individual rewards. However, it is still important to reward and recognize the entire practice and/or departmental team when it is warranted. Sometimes the decision to reward can be based on the quantification of some functional task. For example, one practice was aiming at a wait time of no longer than 15 minutes. When they were able to achieve that goal for a week, they celebrated. (To their credit, they also examined the patient response cards during that time to see if the push to move patients through had a negative impact on the quality of the experience. In this instance, it had not.)

Meeting a quantitative standard is not needed for a team celebration, however. As I mentioned previously, when a practice has made it through a rough flu season and can see a letup ahead, that is a perfect time to celebrate! At the university where I taught, our dean instituted what he called the February Doldrums party.

Its purpose was to help the faculty through the often difficult stretch after the newness of the semester had worn off and before the Easter holiday rolled around. It was to reward us for doing a good job and to encourage us to keep it up. That event was often the best attended and most enjoyable function of the year.

■ Service rewards usually should involve the customer. The most obvious way to involve customers in the reward process is to include their feedback in the selection process. Customer surveys, focus groups, letters, and comment cards—all contain customers' perceptions of service. Some practices actively solicit nominations from their customers for the service champion awards. Even the quantified number of telephone rings are based on the customers' indications that they like to have quick responses.

Sometimes other practice personnel may observe a colleague handling a customer situation in a positive way. Those observations can also provide grist for the reward-system mill, either through formal or informal recognition. At other times, a staff member may make a suggested change in an internal process that will impact the service goals—making it quicker without reducing accuracy, for example. Such people should also be acknowledged for their positive service ideas and for changing processes and systems to be more customer-friendly.

SUGGESTIONS FOR SERVICE REWARDS

Bob Nelson's book offers many interesting examples from a wide variety of industries. I recommend that anyone involved with the formation or restructuring of your reward system read this small but excellent volume. Also, practice personnel might be encouraged to read it when formulating their reinforcement lists. Keeping in mind that the best suggestions for rewards will come from the practice personnel themselves, please consider the following suggestions as examples only. I include them more to whet your appetite than to provide a comprehensive list.

Individual Rewards

■ Service Reward Cards: Given a wide variety of names such as bravo cards, caught-in-the-act-of-service cards, and others, these cards are awarded by supervisors and/or peers, depending on the specifics of your reward system, to employees who are observed or heard offering positive service to either internal or external customers. Usually, when an employee receives a certain number of these cards, they can be cashed in for some larger reward. The Everett Clinic in Everett, Washington, cements its very successful service initiative with HeroGrams. This program allows staff members to recognize one another and other departments by awarding a HeroGram after observing outstanding service. All recipients are listed in a weekly bulletin, and multiple recipients receive further recognition, including service excellence name badge emblems, gift certificates, and time off.[15]

■ The Accolades Bulletin Board: Located in a high-traffic employee area, this bulletin board serves as a location for placing letters, pictures, or memos, in which individuals are recognized for providing excellent service. Some bulletin boards are divided into internal and external service champions, and all are devoted to recognizing individuals for providing quality service. One word of advice: If your practice uses this approach, someone should be assigned, as a part of his or her workload, the maintenance and updating of this bulletin board. Torn, discolored, ragged items will soon be ignored. An easy way to keep the board current is for the person who is in charge to place the date that the item should be removed in the upper right-hand corner. Then, without having to reread each item, old ones can be removed, making room for new ones. One practice places the removed items in a scrapbook, forming a record of the positive service behaviors demonstrated by practice personnel.

■ A Behind-the-Scenes Award: Taking any of a number of appropriate forms, this reward is given to those who offer primarily internal service and those who work most often in internal processes. It recognizes the importance of the sometimes overlooked internal service behaviors and should be just as substantial as those given for similar external service behaviors.

■ Let's-Do-Lunch Reward: There are a wide variety of ways this reward can be played out in your practice. The following are just a few:

  ■ Staff Lunch with a Doctor: On a regular basis, each doctor takes a staff member to lunch.

  ■ The Office Manager Treats: On a regular basis, the office manager rewards deserving staff members with a coupon for a free lunch at a nearby restaurant.

■ Bag It: The service champion receives a free gourmet sack lunch for a week or longer.

■ Post-It/Note-It Reward: This reward system can be adopted by any member of the practice—physicians, managers, staff. All it requires is a supply of Post-it® notes and the desire to acknowledge people for providing quality service. When you become aware of someone in the practice who provides good service to you, some other internal customer or an external customer, take a few moments and write a note of appreciation. Just leave the note affixed to a computer screen, telephone receiver, appointment book—some place where the recipient will find it easily. These little surprise tokens of acknowledgment often mean more than the larger, more elaborate methods of appreciation.

■ Put-This-in-Your-File Reward: A close cousin to the above method, this reward technique is more formal. Instead of a quick note on a Post-it, write a letter of appreciation, detailing specifically what behavior is being acknowledged and why. A copy of this letter should be placed in the recipient's personnel file and/or mailed home so that spouses, parents, children, and additional significant others will know also.

■ A-Rose-By-Any-Other-Name Reward: A nurse told me of this meaningful and yet simple reward: On Nurses' Day, she and her colleagues were greeted at the office door by the doctors who enthusiastically wished them a "Happy Nurses' Day!" Each nurse was given a corsage of roses to wear for the entire day. (See the Team Rewards section of this chapter for a variation on this idea.)

■ The Bradford Award for Innovative Individual Reward System: This unofficial award goes to the STEP Program at the Bristol Hospital, Bristol, Connecticut. This nonprofit, acute care community hospital wanted to improve patient satisfaction by communicating to the 950 employees that service was important and of value to the organization. By taking four key words from the hospital mission statement—service, teamwork, excellence, and professionalism—the hospital management team with advice from the employees created the STEP Program. Three types of rewards were given, each leading to the annual outstanding Service Star Award:

■ STEP Cards: Employees receive STEP cards (small laminated cards) when middle managers catch them in the act of providing good internal or external service. The recipients of a specified number of STEP cards are rewarded with a STEP coffee mug or some other appropriate item.

- Quarterly Awards: Offering peer-based recognition, this system features Outstanding Service Awards. Employees are nominated by their peers, and nominees are honored at a breakfast and are featured in the hospital internal newsletter.

- Outstanding Service Award: Given to one employee annually, this award receives a lot of attention and press coverage. This person also receives a diamond pin, an engraved watch, and his or her name engraved on a trophy in the lobby. The recipient is chosen from all individuals nominated throughout the year.

How effective is the STEP Program in improving patient satisfaction? I'll let the numbers speak for themselves. In one year, the Press Ganey Associates, Inc., firm that specializes in patient-satisfaction research showed the hospital jumping from the 26th percentile to the 88th percentile in patient satisfaction. Patients who said they would avoid the hospital in the future dropped from 26 percent to 12 percent. Market share was up from 55 percent to 59 percent.[16]

Team Rewards

As has been mentioned previously, teams need appreciation too. When your practice team has completed a big project or has successfully survived a crunch period, celebrate! Once in a while, when the task at hand is difficult and draining, stopping at midpoint to acknowledge the progress so far can encourage the team to keep going until the process has been completed. The following are some ideas for team rewards:

- Take-Me-Out-to-the-Ball-Game Reward: If your practice is near a city with a professional athletic team, tickets can be purchased for the entire staff. The location of the seats often is not as important as the fun the group has together at such an event. Physicians and office managers should attend. The spouses, or significant others, of practice personnel can be invited.

- There's-No-Business-Like-Show-Business Reward: An outing similar to the one above but with a different destination, this event also enables the team to play together, an important part of team building, as well as serving as a reward for work well done. The destination can be live theater, a movie, or even a well-chosen comedy club. Enjoy!

■ Amuse-Yourselves Reward: Staying in the same vein but acknowledging that the personnel in your practice may well have small children at home, a trip to the local amusement park for all personnel and families would be a nice reward for a big project completed. Usually such projects require extensive time away from home for the employees, and by including the families they are also being acknowledged for their support.

■ Employee-Appreciation-Week Reward: Rather than honoring each segment of the practice team during special weeks, you could copy the idea of the University Health Associates, the medical practice plan for the West Virginia University School of Medicine. Held in addition to its formal winter holiday party and a summer family picnic, this week takes the place of all other special recognition days for various professions. The week's festivities are planned and coordinated by central administration, which consists of an administrator, director of nursing, and the medical director. Each day of the week is marked by a different event: Day 1—Each employee is awarded a special gift to kick off the celebration, such as flowers, a mug filled with candy and emblazoned with the name of the corporation, or a credit-card-sized pocket calculator inscribed with the corporate name and logo. Day 2—Breakfast is served from 7:30-9:30 A.M. Day 3—Central administration serves lunch to all employees. Day 4—Cake is served during the lunch hour and early afternoon. Day 5—The grand finale is an ice cream/frozen yogurt bar all afternoon, served by the central administration and corporate chief executive officer. While serving, these folks express their personal appreciation to the staff.

A week-long scavenger hunt has been added to the daily events in more recent years. Employees from each specialty suite serve as a team. Teams pick up a list of questions in the morning. The following day, the completed answer sheet, along with the representative items, are returned to the central administration for cumulative scoring. At week's end, the team earning the most points wins a free lunch for all employees, served to them in their suite.

Medical Director Norman D. Ferrari, III, M.D.; Vice President for Operations and Ambulatory Services James Craig, and

Administrative Assistant Barbara Bartlett, observed that "employees look forward to the week with excitement and anticipation." Regarding the scavenger hunt specifically, they also indicated that "the employees commented on the team building that resulted . . . and said they learned about the corporation and medicine while solving the questions."[17]

■ Annual Banquets: Sometimes considered a yawn by some people, if time and care is put into the planning, these events can be quite special. I was the guest speaker at one of these events, and the attendees appeared to be having a great time. They were dressed to the nines, and the event was held at the local country club. The team was acknowledged by the event itself and by several tributes offered by appropriate individuals during the evening. No individual rewards were offered that night. It was the team's night to celebrate what they had accomplished together.

■ A Symbol of Team Excellence: Creating a symbol that captures something special about this team—T-shirts, coffee mugs, pens—can provide tangible reminders of the team efforts required to serve customers.

■ A-Picture-Is-Worth-a-Thousand-Words Reward: A photo collage depicting scenes from a successful project is another good idea. Providing a visual reminder of the team effort required, this collection of photographs could include pictures of the people who worked on the project, its stages of development, and its completion.

■ The Bradford Award for the Most-Innovative-Team Reward: This honor has to go to the executive team of my client HMO. From taking the risk to ask the employees what they wanted all the way to their good-spirited honoring of that request, these executives proved their desire to recognize their employees in a meaningful way. By being willing to relax and have some fun, perhaps at their own expense, these executives deserve acknowledgement and recognition themselves.

Practice personnel should be rewarded for their positive service behaviors. You should be reinforced when you do the expected and lauded when performing the exceptional. The efforts of your practice as a team should also be acknowledged and recognized, too. Rewarding the behaviors that should be repeated is essential to the continuation of quality service in your practice.

END NOTES

1. Gerald Goldhaber, *Organizational Communication* (Dubuque, Iowa: Wm. C. Brown Publishers, 1979), p. 67.

2. Ibid., p. 159.

3. Bob Nelson, *1001 Ways to Reward Employees* (New York: Workman Publishing, 1994), p. 19. © Copyright 1994 by Bob Nelson. Reprinted by permission of Workman Publishing.

4. Goldhaber, p. 77.

5. Ibid., p. xv.

6. Ibid.

7. Ibid., p. xvi.

8. Ibid., p. xv.

9. Ibid., p. xvii.

10. Ibid., p. xvi.

11. Ibid.

12. Ibid.

13. Catherine Meek, a Los Angeles compensation consultant, quoted by Nelson, p. xvi.

14. Nelson, p. xvi.

15. Brenda Hull, "Service Standards Hallmark for Practice Marketing," *MGM Update* 34, no. 11 (November 1995), p. 7.

16. "Stepping toward Quality Service," *Profiles*, no. 52 (March/April 1993), pp. 28–32.

17. Norman D. Ferrari, III, M.D., James Craig, and Barbara Bartlett, "Recognize Employee Team Efforts with Special Week," *MGM Update* 35, no. 1 (January 1996), p. 4.

17

CHAPTER

Step Seventeen—Make Service a Way of Life

Reaching this chapter is a milestone. If you have been working your way through the process described in the previous 16 chapters, you are probably ready to celebrate . . . and I hope you do. You also may be feeling quietly reflective as you look back on what has transpired. The kind of commitment that the steps toward Total Service require has caused you to look within as well as to expose yourself to the scrutiny of others. This kind of introspection and exposure contributes to your sense of quiet reflection now.

Also, you may be realizing that the journey you have taken is not over. In truth, it never will be. In Chapter 3, I referred to the "Are we there yet?" question asked by many organizations who embark on this kind of journey. The answer to that query is both *yes* and *no*. *Yes* because you have completed the steps and have arrived at what appears to be a destination. *No* because that destination is a mirage. There is no such place as the Kingdom of Total Service. It is, instead, a state of mind. Total Service is more than a way of *doing*. It is a way of *being*. That kind of commitment to service comes from deep inside. You know it when you've got it, and your customers know it when you don't.

So, yes, you've reached a milestone. Just as milestones function as but markers on a path, so is this one a marker on your journey. The best is yet to come.

PARTING THOUGHTS

If I left you with only the heartfelt words above, you would probably feel cheated, and rightfully so. I can't just lead you through the steps to Total Service and then say, "good-bye." I have an obligation to guide you as you prepare to go on down the path alone. In parting, then, I have three final pieces of advice that will help you to make service become a way of life.

Be Willing to Go over the Edge

Yet another skiing analogy provides helpful advice. When I was first learning how to ski, I felt awkward. I had to keep focused on every detail: Were my knees bent? Was my back straight? Did my ski suit match my goggles? In all seriousness, anyone who has learned a new sport, regardless of what it is, can understand what I mean. You become so aware of all the *parts* that you somehow can't see the *whole*. My ski instructor kept telling me that one day it would all come together. Some day, he promised, I would *go over the edge* and everything would just flow. It would become instinctive. I doubted him very seriously as I snowplowed my way across the mountain. Then, one day, it happened. I didn't have to think any longer about arms and legs and poles. I was skiing effortlessly down the slope. Of course, it still helped to stop on occasion to analyze form and style, but I had reached the point where the entire process of skiing had become a part of me. I'd made it mine.

The same applies to you and this process toward Total Service. At first, even now, you may feel the awkwardness of just learning it. However, as my ski instructor kept urging me, don't give up. Learning any new skill takes time and practice. I promise you that one day you will look up and find that you have gone over the edge. Without even realizing when it happened, you will be skiing.

Keep the Process Alive

Now that you have completed Step 16, you need to start all over again. On this trip, you will not have the same *creating-the-wheel* mentality that was needed the first time through. Instead you'll now need a willingness to course-correct. The steps to Total Service should not be revisited only when problems appear, however. Just as your patients come to your practice for periodic checkups, so should your practice conduct its own wellness examinations about service. I recommend that, annually at first and then perhaps biannually, the practice retrace its steps through the process described in this book. An appropriate agenda for annual retreats, this kind of checkup should be linear from Step 1 through Step 16.

Check-ups are not all that you should do, however. *Check-ins* are also important. Rather than moving through the steps in a linear fashion, check *in* once in a while at whatever step in the process you choose to revisit. Periodic individual, departmental, and practicewide "How are we doing?" assessments, conducted by you and others, are helpful. Reminders of the lessons and rationale for service are worth exploring again. Looking inside and asking the hard questions will help you stay on track.

Whether engaging in a checkup or a check-in, considering each of the major divisions of this book will give you points of focus. Within each section are the important steps that need to be revisited if your practice is to maintain its course.

Part I: Preparing for the Journey: Reviewing the definitions of the key concepts will keep your journey on target. Reminding yourself of the rationale for starting this trip in the first place can renew your commitment to it. Revisiting the lessons about service learned by others can prevent a sense of isolation. These three steps started you on the journey, and they can bring you back to the underpinnings of its meaning and purposes when you might need them.

Part II: Focus on the Customer: Redefining your primary and secondary customer populations on an ongoing basis can maintain your awareness of who they are, an essential part of being able to provide service. This process will also help identify any customer populations that might enter the picture or shift in importance. Revisiting the factors about customer feedback can help pave the way for the ongoing process of seeking input. From the informal point-of-contact interactions to the structured and formal shaping of your customer report cards, the process of inquiry must be maintained. You can never stop wanting to know what is important to your customers and whether you are meeting those needs.

Part III: Focus on the People: Daily attention needs to be paid to the communication skills that are essential to task performance and relationship building in the practice. The service responsibilities for each segment of the practice personnel should be revisited: Physicians need to keep examining how well they maintain the service-driven heart of the practice, office managers need continuous reflection on how skillfully they are leading the Total Service parade, and staff members should constantly be aware of how capably they are handling their service responsibilities. All need to revisit the commitment this practice made to work together as a team and reinforce those behaviors that demonstrate that commitment.

Part IV: The Systems, the Cycles, and the Processes: Systems, cycles, and processes must be constantly revisited and challenged. Since change is a given in the healthcare environment and it is part and parcel of who customers are, then the way things are done in the practice must reflect awareness of these changes. Key moments of truth must be reexamined on an ongoing basis. The doctor/patient interviews and the practicewide difficult moments of truth that can make or break customer relationships need continuous monitoring and appraisal.

Part V: Continuation: Service promises and personal service statements must be revisited, reinforced, and occasionally revised. All practice personnel must be rewarded on an ongoing basis, and daily acknowledgement for service performance is not too frequent! If people are to repeat service behaviors, then they need to know that these behaviors are valued and appreciated.

The most important part of continuing the process is to keep it alive in your heart, in your work, and in your consciousness.

Be Ever Observant of What Other Service Champions Are Doing

In the second in his series of books on service, *At America's Service*, Karl Albrecht cited 10 characteristics of organizations he would describe as Service Champions.[1] Let me share those with you.

1. They have the basics down pat. Just as with a Total Service Medical Practice, these organizations have been through a process of becoming customer-focused, even customer-driven. The steps in the process have become a part of who they are. They have reached that point of instinctive-service responses.

2. They believe that quality service drives profit. In Chapter 2, I talked about the rationale for becoming a Total Service Medical Practice. All of the practice development reasons that are offered, impact the bottom line: Quality service in your practice will attract new patients and retain existing ones. It will also attract and retain a loyal staff, eliminating the expenses of hiring and retraining new ones. Quality service also reduces the likelihood of malpractice suits, and additionally, it makes the practice more attractive to important sources of income, such as groups and networks. Finally, quality service reduces the stress for all concerned, thus also reducing costly stress-related absence and illness in the staff. When a commitment to quality service comes first, the profits will follow.

3. They know their customers. These organizations have undertaken the process of inquiry similar to that described in Chapter 6. They know who their customers are, what they want and need, and have an ongoing awareness of the organization's ability to meet those needs.

4. They have a Moment of Truth focus in their operations. Not referring to surgery here, Albrecht is talking about the attention each person in the organization gives to his or her contribution to the total service experience. When each person manages each moment of truth effectively, quality service results.

5. They have a "whatever it takes" attitude. These organizations are focused on what they *can* do, not on what they *can't*. They are willing to go that extra distance that may seem risky or even foolish to the casual observer. An example I will offer later in this chapter describes a program at Chicago's Lake Forest Hospital which took such risks, and the results have been overwhelmingly positive.

6. They recover skillfully from the inevitable blunder. As I have said, since service is provided *by* human beings *to* human beings, things will not always be perfect. The key to a Service Champion organization is that they have mastered the art, if you will, of handling those difficult moments of truth discussed in

Chapter 14. They know mistakes will happen, and they are poised to correct them when they do.

7. Service happens inside the organization as well as outside. Remember, in Chapter 4, I identified the key customer populations of your practice: Internal customers headed the list. There is a direct link between internal and external service. If, in your practice, you are treating each other as valued customers then you are going to be able to provide quality service to those outside. Office Manager Deborah Goodyear described such an environment in her practice: "We don't live in different stratospheres around here. Doctors can't see the patient without the staff, and the staff can't have a job without the doctor. So we all need each other. We meet together. We laugh together. We stay together. I've never been in a practice like this one." Perhaps Ms. Goodyear's practice is already a Service Champion.

8. They see management as a helper and a supporter. The role of management in a Service Champion organization is to remove obstacles and make decisions that will allow staff to provide quality service. They are also there to back them up when they need it. As we know from Chapter 8, the medical practice is somewhat different in structure. Everyone who works there is on the frontline, dealing with the customers directly. Thus, the distinction between management and the frontline staff can sometimes become blurred. However, rather than relieving management in a medical practice (physicians, managers, and supervisors) from the responsibilities of decision making and support, their frontline contact is an additional duty. They still must function in the management role when it comes to making decisions and supporting their staff. Tina Butler, the manager of the department of pediatrics at Harvard Pilgrim Health Care in Providence, Rhode Island, beautifully demonstrated the spirit of this characteristic. During a workshop I was conducting with her unit, one of the participants said, "What do I do when I am alone at the front desk, everyone else has gone to lunch, the phone is ringing off the hook, and I have a patient who needs my undivided attention?" Without hesitation, Tina spoke up: "That's what my beeper is for. I wear it all the time. You hit a situation like that, you let me know. That's why I'm here." I believe that Ms. Butler is an excellent example of a Service Champion.

9. They care about their employees as well as their customers. Earlier in this book, I cited Hal Rosenbluth, the author of the book *The Customer Comes Second* and CEO of Rosenbluth Travel. The premise of his book is the same as this ninth of Albrecht's Service Champion characteristics: In order to provide good service to those outside the organization, the people inside must feel valued and appreciated too. Mr. Rosenbluth talked about management's responsibility to the employees.[2]

While Mr. Rosenbluth's philosophy is an essential one and sets the tone for what I have said before and will say again, I want to take it even a step farther. I believe that *each* person needs to feel valued and appreciated. That means doctors, managers, and supervisors as well as all members of the staff need to go out of their way to convey to each other how much their efforts are appreciated. A Service Champion organization will let the praise and thank-you's flow. And so should yours: horizontally, vertically, and at all levels throughout your practice.

10. They are perpetually unsatisfied with their performance. What Albrecht is talking about here is the ongoing nature of service that I have been discussing in this chapter. The Service Champion organizations he is describing are not satisfied to sit on their laurels, saying, "We have arrived! We are there!" They will keep the process alive!

Sometimes being a Service Champion means making the ordinary seem extraordinary. As I mentioned previously, during the period of time I was writing this book, I fell, sustaining a major injury to my elbow. Not only did this accident interrupt the writing process, but it also gave me the opportunity to see healthcare, up close and personal, and I got to see the Service Champions in my PCP's office in action. The day after surgery I accidentally overmedicated myself on Percocet, and the receptionist responded to a telephone request to see my doctor by scheduling an appointment immediately. Even though his book was full, my physician saw me. When I complained of nausea, a staff member appeared with a cup of Gatorade. While I lay on the examination table, trying to clear my head from the impact of the powerful medication, another staff member assured me that I was not to move until I felt ready. "It's lunchtime anyway," she said, patting my good arm comfortingly. "You stay right where you are." The most memorable moment for me, however, was when Dr. Sullivan himself, taking part of his precious midday break, pushed my wheelchair through the office and out to the parking lot. He waited with me until my friends brought the car around to pick me up, and then he helped me into the backseat. "You call me if you need me, now, OK?" he said as he shut the door and hurried back into his busy life and full schedule.

Did I call him back to thank him for the sincerity of his concern, or did I send a letter to the staff praising them for making me feel so cared for during a time of vulnerability? No. I wish I had, but I didn't. Did they treat me the way they did because I am a uniquely special human being? Again the answer is no. Did they go right on extending to others the same kind of genuine caring and concern that I received? I'm absolutely certain that they did. I am grateful to have the opportunity to thank them publicly here in these pages. I am also grateful that they were there for me when I needed them. These people understand service.

Other times being a Service Champion means taking a risk and being creative, which is what Lake Forest Hospital did.[3] I believe, based on the criteria he articulated, even Karl Albrecht would agree that this is the story of a Service Champion.

Beginning in the mid-80s, Lake Forest Hospital implemented a most unusual program, especially for a healthcare institution. Called simply the Guaranteed Service Program, it was applied to the nonclinical aspects of patients' visits, such as waiting time. The hospital offered, on the spot, whatever solutions to problems that customers wanted. The staff was allowed to design the program and soon developed a great deal of ownership of it.

Once the service guarantee went into effect at the hospital's outpatient surgery department, employees were told that when delays occurred they were to go immediately to the patient or family member, acknowledge what was happening, and apologize. They were trained to listen to the customer to determine if he or she was upset, and to ask what they could do to make it right. If at all possible, that request was to be filled immediately by the employees. Sometimes patients were sent home with a check for dinner or to make up for the pay lost during the visit. However, most requests cost little to nothing. One staff member sang a gospel hymn on request from a patient who knew of her beautiful singing voice. Another went to the coffee shop to buy a patient's disgruntled spouse a hot fudge sundae. Under the guarantee, if something goes wrong the number one priority is to fix it or to get an acceptable substitute.

There are three keys to the success of this program, and it has been successful. First is that problems are solved on the spot if at all possible. William Ries, president of Lake Forest Hospital, said, "You can't fix a matter . . . five or six days later with a call from a supervisor, or worse still, when the bill arrives at the patients' door. And even if you do address a patient's concern at that time, it doesn't have the same effect as when a person can walk out the door with the situation resolved." Second, this program empowers employees to resolve problems without fear of reversal. Employees were given the power to fulfill requests. First the patient was challenged with the question: "Are you sure that's fair?" But if the answer was *yes*, then the employee had the power to do it immediately, including demands for refunds. Ries explained to me in a telephone interview, "Now employees have the tools with which to handle difficult situations. We've told them, 'Whatever you decide—we'll back you up.'" Third, because of their empowerment, employees feel more in charge; they do not wait for patients to complain. In most cases, they can see a problem as it is brewing. Gail Okon, RN, manager of the post-anesthesia care unit of the day surgery department, said, "This makes employees happier in their jobs. Because they have more control over addressing problems, they encounter less aggravation." Nipping problems in the bud also makes customers' requests much more reasonable. A minor irritation will result, in most instances, in a request for a song or a hot fudge sundae.

How much has this program cost the hospital? Since implementing it, the hospital has been giving away between $2,000 and $4,000 per month to patients who were dissatisfied with some aspect of service, usually unexpected delay. There's no question it's a lot of money, but keep in mind that Lake Forest's total operating budget is around $90 million dollars. Ries commented, "We believe that patient satisfaction is worth it." He also pointed out that large sums are spent each year on promotional campaigns that *may* pull patients in. The money-back guarantee satisfies and keeps customers they already have. This is exactly the thinking behind Nordstrom's legendary customer service guarantee, and there can be no disputing the success of that philosophy for that organization. At Lake Forest, the long-term goal of the program is to reduce the amount that must be given back: It helps them pinpoint problem areas. They want their service guarantee to put the money-back guarantee out of business.

What impact has this program had on patient satisfaction? It has increased it, pushing a hospital that was already receiving high ratings on the Press Ganey Patient Satisfaction research instrument into the 99th percentile! That is about as close to perfect service as any organization can come.

Get That Old Time Service Religion!

In no way do I intend to be sacrilegious with this statement. I make it only because many people who talk about service seem to find the best parallels in some important religious teachings. For example, consider the following:

The 10 Commandments of Service Excellence.[4]

Commandment 1: Don't act as though the customer is causing you an inconvenience.

Commandment 2: Don't treat customers as if problems are their fault.

Commandment 3: Don't ignore your customer.

Commandment 4: Work with your customer to come up with a mutual solution.

Commandment 5: Follow up by asking whether your customers are satisfied.

Commandment 6: Know your business, services, and products.

Commandment 7: If you make a mistake, settle the situation as soon as possible. Apologize and offer to make amends.

Commandment 8: Understand what your customers want, need, and expect.

Commandment 9: Create a service strategy.

Commandment 10: Treat your customers the way you'd wish to be treated.

Also, consider one of the best rules for dealing with people ever written: *Do unto others as you would have them do unto you.* In Chapter 14, I mentioned the nurse who said she handled difficult situations by just thinking, "Pretend it's me. How would I want to be treated?" Dr. John Egerton, M.D., broke that concept down into the golden rules of patient interactions.[5] Although specific suggestions for a specific population, they are worth including here.

Rule 1: Always greet the patients promptly and treat them courteously and discreetly.

Rule 2: Don't blame someone else for mistakes.

Rule 3: Never criticize another doctor (or any other practice employee) in front of patients.

Rule 4: Never do anything you're not qualified to handle.

Rule 5: Dress appropriately.

Rule 6: Protect patients' privacy.

Rule 7: Keep personal phone calls brief and quiet.

Rule 8: Don't eat or drink in public areas.

Rule 9: Treat each patient as a person, not as a diagnosis.

Rule 10: Treat each patient as if he were you or your family.

Ah yes! There but by the grace of God, go you!

Dr. Bernard Strauss, a urologist in West Orange, New Jersey, summed it up this way: "After a quarter of a century in practice, I've found that 'do unto others' is a catch phrase for success. If you combine your pleasant demeanor and genuine concern for people with strong clinical and communication skills, a topflight medical practice is virtually guaranteed."[6]

Actually there is another rule, specifically designed for service, that stems from this familiar and valuable one. Called the Platinum Rule, it brings our focus back to the customers: Do unto others as they would have themselves done unto. How can you know what others want done? You have to ask. And you have to keep asking. And you have to always, always listen and respond.

In the preface to this book, I referred to the story told by famed trial attorney Gerry Spence about the dude who road into town astride an elegant leather saddle placed on the back of a ten-dollar horse.[7] The meaning of the story makes the last point that I want you to remember: the spirit of service has to be in you. In your heart and in your soul. If it isn't, then your service efforts will be just like that dude and his ten-dollar nag. Remember, all of the methods, the techniques, and the steps that I have to offer will lead nowhere without that commitment, dedication, and belief in the intrinsic value of service.

Also at the beginning of this book, I told you the story of Amy, the workshop participant whose deeply felt reaction to what I said provided the impetus for writing this book. It was my purpose to do as she had asked of me: to find a way to share these thoughts with others who might need them. I have done that. I have completed my task. The rest is up to you.

As you implement these steps and keep the process going, making service a way of life for your practice, please remember that you aren't alone. My good wishes are there with you, and I'm as close as the telephone, fax, or E-mail. If you get discouraged or even overwhelmed, try to hear my voice in the background saying, "You can do it!" How do I know this is true? Because if you've had the dedication and motivation to reach this, the last line in this book, then I know that you are the thoroughbred needed to carry the Total Service saddle across the finish line . . . and far, far beyond.

END NOTES

1. Karl Albrecht, *At America's Service* (Homewood, Illinois: Dow Jones–Irwin, 1988), pp. 38–42.

2. Hal Rosenbluth, *The Customer Comes Second* (New York: William Morris, 1992).

3. "Patients Aren't Happy with SDS? Offer Money-Back Guarantee," *Same Day Surgery* 18, no. 4 (April 1994), pp. 47–50.

4. "Ten Commandments of Service Excellence," *Nonprofit Management Strategies* 11, no. 3 (November 1991), p. 18.

5. John Egerton, M.D., "Ten Rules We Don't Let Our Assistants Break," *Medical Economics* 71, no. 12 (June 27, 1994), pp. 66–68.

6. Bernard Strauss, "Tips From My 25 Years of Successful Practice," *Medical Economics* 70, no. 3 (February 8, 1993), p. 72.

7. Gerry Spence, *How to Argue and Win Every Time* (New York: St. Martin Press, 1995) pp. 5–7.

A P P E N D I X

FORM 1:

SAMPLE FOCUS GROUP/DEPTH INTERVIEWS QUESTIONS

Focus Group Questions: Patients

1. When you think of the nonclinical aspects of your experience with your physician's office, what is important to you?
2. What is the best example of service you have experienced in a medical practice?
3. What is the worst example of service you have experienced in a medical practice?
4. What do you like best about your doctor?
5. What do you like best about the staff in your doctor's office?
6. If you could change one thing about your doctor, what would it be?
7. If you could change one thing about the staff in your doctor's office, what would it be?
8. Thinking of all the people who work in your doctor's practice, what one last thing would you want to say to them?

Depth Interview Questions: Referring Physicians/Office Managers

1. What is important to you about the specialist's practice to whom you refer your patients?
2. How would you rank these items in importance to you?
3. From your perspective, what characteristics would the ideal specialist's practice have?
4. What is the most common problem you encounter when dealing with specialists' practices?
5. What criteria do you use for deciding where to refer patients?
6. If there were representatives from specialists practices here in this room, what would you say to them?

FORM 2:

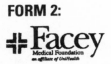

PATIENT SATISFACTION SURVEY

Dear Patient:

As part of our commitment to providing high-quality healthcare, we'd like to get some feedback about your experiences with Facey Medical Group and more specifically, your experiences with one of the doctors that has recently treated you. **"Your doctor" in the questions below refers to the doctor listed above in the right-hand corner of this survey.** Please check the responses that best indicate your opinion about the service you received. If a question does not apply to your situation, check "Does not Apply."

Once completed, please return the questionnaire in the postage-paid business reply envelope. Thank You!

Overall Care:

In terms of your satisfaction, how would you rate each of the following?

	Excellent	Very Good	Good	Fair	Poor	Does Not Apply
	5	4	3	2	1	0
1. Overall quality of care you received	☐	☐	☐	☐	☐	☐ (12)
2. Respect, courtesy, and sensitivity show by **your doctor**	☐	☐	☐	☐	☐	☐ (13)
3. Respect, courtesy, and sensitivity shown by the nurse	☐	☐	☐	☐	☐	☐ (14)
4. Respect, courtesy, and sensitivity shown by the receptionist	☐	☐	☐	☐	☐	☐ (15)
5. Amount of time **your doctor** spent with you	☐	☐	☐	☐	☐	☐ (16)
6. Explanation by **your doctor** of what was done for you	☐	☐	☐	☐	☐	☐ (17)
7. Time spent waiting in the office to see **your doctor**	☐	☐	☐	☐	☐	☐ (18)
8. Ability to speak with **your doctor or nurse** on the phone	☐	☐	☐	☐	☐	☐ (19)
9. Time between making an appointment and the day of your visit	☐	☐	☐	☐	☐	☐ (20)
10. Convenience of office hours	☐	☐	☐	☐	☐	☐ (21)
11. Ability of **your doctor** to coordinate your care if you had more than one visit or consult	☐	☐	☐	☐	☐	☐ (22)
12. How well the nurse was able to answer your questions	☐	☐	☐	☐	☐	☐ (23)
13. The cleanliness of the treatment area	☐	☐	☐	☐	☐	☐ (24)
14. Likelihood of recommending **your doctor** to others	☐	☐	☐	☐	☐	☐ (25)

Please Tell Us:

1. Do you have confidence in your **doctor?** ☐ Yes ☐ No *Please explain* _____

_____

_____

2. What most impressed you about your **doctor?** _____

_____

_____

3. How could Facey Medical Group improve its service? _____

_____

_____

THANK YOU FOR HELPING US SERVE YOU BETTER!

FORM 3:

SAMPLE SERVICE-QUALITY QUESTIONNAIRE

You have been a patient in our practice for over a year now and have had occasion to visit us several times. We value your overall opinion of the service aspects of our practice. Please respond to the following questions, trying not to focus on any single visit to our office, but relying on your collective impressions. Feel free to make comments or explanations in the appropriate blanks.

1. How would you rate the overall attitude of the clinical providers (physicians, nurse practitioners, physicians' assistants, nurses) with whom you have dealt?

   Excellent   Very Good   Good   Fair   Poor
   Comment: _____
   _____

2. How would you rate the overall attitude of the nonclinical staff members (receptionists, scheduling clerk, billing clerk, and so on) with whom you have dealt?

   Excellent   Very Good   Good   Fair   Poor
   Comment: _____
   _____

3. How would you rate the handling of any waiting times that may have occurred during your visits?

   Excellent   Very Good   Good   Fair   Poor
   Comment: _____
   _____

4. How would you rate the ease with which you have been able to make appointments?

   Excellent   Very Good   Good   Fair   Poor
   Comment: _____
   _____

5. How would you rate our overall ability to accommodate your desired appointment times?

   Excellent   Very Good   Good   Fair   Poor
   Comment: _____
   _____

6. How would you rate the telephone communication of our office?

   Excellent   Very Good   Good   Fair   Poor
   Comment: _____
   _____

7. How would you rate the overall facilities of our practice

   Excellent   Very Good   Good   Fair   Poor
   Comment: _____
   _____

8. How would you rate the billing/collections procedures of our practice?

   Excellent   Very Good   Good   Fair   Poor
   Comment: _____
   _____

9. How would you rate the insurance coordination provided by our office?

   Excellent   Very Good   Good   Fair   Poor
   Comment: _____
   _____

10. What other item would you like to bring to our attention, and how would rate it?

    Item:_____

    Excellent   Very Good   Good   Fair   Poor
    Comment: _____
    _____

Thank you very much for your assistance! It's through your feedback that we can honor our commitment to put service first.

FORM 4:
ORIENTATION OF NEW EMPLOYEES

Preorientation Packet
Before the new employee arrives, he or she should be given an orientation packet containing the following: a letter of welcome from the doctors or medical director and the office manager, the directions to the office (even though the new employee has been there before), an indication of exactly where to arrive on the first day and at what time, and a schedule for the day-by-day orientation period.

Day One
The office manager, the medical director, and when appropriate, the immediate supervisor, should greet the new employee and make him or her feel welcome. Discussion for the day should be conducted by the office manager or the supervisor, and should include the key items in the Practice Handbook, the job description and exactly what the new employee will be doing, specific instructions on how to work with the doctors in the practice, and clarification of expectations and the values of the practice.

At the end of the first day, the medical director, office manager, and, when appropriate, the immediate supervisor should spend time talking with the employee to inquire as to how the first day went and if the employee has any questions. A similar conversation should be held at the end of the first week. The new employee should be told directly how important his or her role is to the operation of the office and how glad the practice is to have him or her on board.

Days Two through Five
The new employee should be introduced to his or her first "buddy" or "mentor" (designated individuals in each part of the practice who will explain their respective areas to the new employee). Anywhere from a half day to a day in each area should be allowed. The purpose of this detailed tour is to expose the new employee to the total operation of the practice and begin cross-training. The designated buddy or mentor in each area of the office will introduce the new employee to coworkers, explain what happens in his or her area, and allow the new employee to observe for a specified period of time. (The productivity of the buddy will probably be reduced during this period, but it is well worth the temporary lag.)

Days Six through Ten
Training on the job: After the "buddy visits," the new employee should return to the area where he or she will be working. Now specific training will begin. A checklist of what the new employee should learn during this period should be shared. The trainee should be encouraged to assume some ownership of this learning process by checking off the items as they have been covered and understood. The appropriate supervisory personnel should meet with the new employee at the end of the first day and again at the end of the week of on-the-job training.

FORM 5:

STEPS IN THE AFFINITY PROCESS

Step 1   Spend 15 to 20 minutes in silent, individual brainstorming. Group members may be given specific categories in which to respond, or they may merely be asked to address one central question, allowing their thoughts to come forth in a totally unstructured manner. Each team member is given a packet of Post-it® notes and is asked to write one idea on each note.

Step 2   Again in silence, the individuals post their notes on the wall. Sometimes these notes will be placed under the categories indicated in Step 1. Other times the notes will just be placed on the wall in no particular order. Allow only about five minutes for this step. No one should be reading notes at this point.

Step 3   Again in silence, the team members rearrange the notes, linking together any that seem to be expressing a common theme. Participants may move any note or linking string of notes. Allow approximately 15 to 20 minutes for this process.

Step 4   In this step, group members may talk to each other. By now most if not all notes will be linked with at least one other. If there are single ones left, put them in the "bone yard" to be examined later. Using partners or groups of three to four people, label each of the linked combinations. At the top of each linked combination, post a new note with the label written clearly. Examine single notes that may exist in the bone yard to see if they might fit with any of the combinations, and, if so, move them to the appropriate spot. If the single notes do not seem to belong with any of the combinations but merit attention, hold them for later discussion.

Step 5   Have someone from each pair or group read the combination of notes. Do not worry about duplications at this point. Discuss the implications of the list and identify any that seem critical.

Step 6   If these lists raise problem issues, make a commitment to discuss solutions. The Affinity Process can also be used for brainstorming solutions to these problems, or a less structured process can be used.

Step 7   Have a team member commit to taking notes from the wall, typing them, and distributing them by a specified date.

FORM 6:
STEPS OF CREATIVE PROBLEM SOLVING

Step 1   Define the problem.

What is the issue being discussed?
Whom does it affect?
How long has it existed?

Step 2   Discuss the extent of the problem.

How serious is the problem?
How many people are affected?
How much money does it cost?
What are the harms?
What are the causes?

Step 3   Determine the critieria for a successful solution.

What would have to happen for any solution to work?
What would a successful solution look like?

Step 4   Brainstorm possible solutions.

List any and all solutions to the problem. (Do not evaluate any of them at this point.)

Step 5   Evaluate the solutions created in Step 4 by the criteria determined in Step 3.

Step 6   Plan the solution that best meets the criteria.

Identify what needs to be done.
Decide on the first step to be taken.
Lay out the remaining steps: Who? When? What? Celebration?
Specify how to celebrate the successful completion of the first step.

FORM 7:
STEPS FOR CREATING YOUR DREAM TEAM

Step 1   Have every member of the practice, or in a large clinic have representatives of each department, complete the following sentence: "Six months from now, we will be . . ." This sentence should be completed with words and phrases that describe how the team members would like to be working together.

Step 2   Go around the table, having each person share his or her list and have one person recording the items from each list on a flip chart. When an item is mentioned on more than one individual's list, place a slash mark beside it so the frequency can be counted.

Step 3   As the members hear words or phrased they like, these can be added to their own lists and read when it is their turn.

Step 4   From that combined list, construct a Team Commitment statement. "We, the members of the _____ Practice Team commit to work together in the following ways:" List the items, combine and reword items, but ultimately come up with a list of ways the team will work together.

Step 5   Begin each meeting, for a while, by reading the Team Commitment. This will help reinforce the promises made and will keep the team focused on the kind of behaviors it agreed were desirable. After a period of time, read the agreement once in a while, and always upon request by any member of the team.

Step 6   Give every team member a copy of the agreement. Some practices do this by reproducing the agreement on wallet-sized laminated cards, others place them on a larger piece of paper to be posted next to desks and in staff areas. Some practices have each member of the team sign a copy of the agreement that is then posted in a high-traffic staff area.

This strategy was created by gifted management consultant Stanley R. Wachs, founder of Wachs Associates in Los Angeles, California. Dr. Wachs specializes in dealing with conflict situations and is the author of *Confronting Difficult Issues*. His e-mail address is: stanley@wachs.com.

FORM 8:
STEPS FOR PRODUCTIVE CONFLICT MANAGEMENT

Step 1   Label the problem as yours and express your need to talk about it: "I have a problem that I need to talk about."

Step 2   Set a time and a date for the conversation.

Step 3   Describe your problem and unmet needs.
   a. Label the situation: "I have a problem."
   b. Describe the behavior of the other that is troubling you.
   c. Describe the effect the behavior is having on you.
   d. Describe your thoughts.
   e. Describe your feelings.
   f. Suggest a solution.

Step 4   Be sure that you have been clear by asking your partner to paraphrase what you just said.

Step 5   Solicit your partner's feedback.

Step 6   Express your understanding of your partner's needs.

Step 7   Negotiate a solution.
   a. Generate a number of solutions.
   b. Evaluate the solutions.
   c. Decide on the best solution.
   d. Follow up to see how the solution is working.

FORM 9:

COLLECTION & BILLING TIMETABLE
GUIDELINES

Time	Example	Do This	And This	Tips:
Month service is rendered	July	Send statement	Nothing	Is it itemized clearly? Have you enclosed a self-addressed colored envelope? Hospital consultations — enclose patient booklet. Have you indicated that the account can be paid by credit card?
Month	August	Send statement	First Reminder	Handwritten reminders on the statement are very effective. Computer messages should be reader friendly.
Before mailing of September bill	Middle of September	Phone call	Review age-analysis report and patient chart with registration form	Objective: To find out why payment has not been made and to secure commitment of payment. LISTEN! TAKE NOTES!
Third month after service	September	Send statement	Second reminder	Send in plain envelope. Only indicate your return address on envelope — not the name of office.
Before mailing October bill	Middle of October	Phone call	Review collection messages on the account.	Be specific. Why wasn't payment received? When can payment be expected? Offer solution. KEEP NOTES!
Fourth month after service	October	Send statement	Third and Last Notice	Check with Dr./Office Manager before sending. Send in plain envelope, like second reminder.
Fifth month after service	November	Turn account over	Wait until November 15	Send to collection agency, attorney, small-claims court or write off. Note action taken on account.

Note: These guidelines should be modified to accommodate your practice's special needs.

TIPS:
- Continue to send monthly statements, even though waiting for insurance payment.
- Best times to mail statements, either the 10th or 25th of the month.
- Cycle bill if high volume or for better cash flow.
- You are paid for results not effort.
- Copayments—how cost effective is it to bill for accounts less than $10?

palmer ASSOCIATES, INC

(For Insurance Patients—put on practice's letterhead.)

CUSTOMIZED FINANCIAL AGREEMENT

Patient: _____

Person responsible: _____

Address: _____ City: _____

State: _____ Zip: _____ Phone: _____

Description of services to be rendered:

_____

1. Estimate of Fee for Services $_____
2. Estimate of Insurance Benefits $_____
3. Estimate of Patient Portion $_____

_____ **I prefer paying 100% of the patient portion of what the insurance does not cover on the first (   ) appointment.**

_____ **I prefer paying 50% of the patient portion on the first (   ) appointment. The remainder to be paid within 15 days after the insurance has paid its portion.**

Please apply to my:
___ **Visa**   **Card #** _____
___ **MasterCard**   **Card Expires:** _____
___ **American Express**   **Amount: $** _____
Signed: _____   **Telephone:** _____
Print cardholder's name: _____
Address _____ **City & State** _____ **Zip Code** _____

In the event the account should become delinquent for a period of thirty (30) days, I hereby acknowledge that I will be responsible for all the balance, interest, court costs and/or attorney fees.

_____

I hereby certify that I have read and received a copy of the foregoing disclosure statement this _____ day of _____, 19____.

Signature _____
              Responsible Party

palmer ASSOCIATES, INC

FORM 11:

(For Non-Insurance Patients—put on practice's letterhead or when Insurance has paid their portion.)

CUSTOMIZED FINANCIAL AGREEMENT

Patient: _____

Person responsible: _____

Address: _____ City: _____

State: _____ Zip: _____ Phone: _____

Description of services to be rendered:

_____

1. Fee for Services $_____

2. Down Payment/Previous Payments $_____

3. Remaining balance owed $_____

_____ I prefer paying the full amount on ( ) and receiving a 5% bookkeeping allowance.

_____ I prefer to pay 50% on the first ( ) appointment and the balance in two equal consecutive monthly payments.

_____ I prefer to pay 1/3 on the first ( ) appointment and the balance in two equal consecutive monthly payments.

Please apply to my:
___ Visa   Card # _____
___ MasterCard   Card Expires: _____
___ American Express   Amount: $_____
Signed: _____   Telephone: _____
Print cardholder's name: _____
Address _____City & State_____ Zip Code _____

In the event the account should become delinquent for a period of thirty (30) days, I hereby acknowledge that I will be responsible for all the balance, interest, court costs and/or attorney fees.

_____

I hereby certify that I have read and received a copy of the foregoing disclosure statement this _____ day of _____, 19___.

Signature _____
            Responsible Party

palmer ASSOCIATES, INC

FORM 12:
STEPS FOR WRITING A SERVICE PROMISE (OR STATEMENTS OF GOVERNING PRINCIPLES)

Step 1   Identify the customer population for which this promise is designed.

Step 2   Each individual in the group should write a sample service promise.

Step 3   Each person should read his or her promise aloud to the group twice. While the readings are going on, the other members of the group should close their eyes, allowing them to concentrate on the words and how they sound.

Step 4   At the end of the second reading of each promise, the group members should note in writing the key words or phrases that they liked in the promise just read.

Step 5   A group list should be made, usually on a flip chart, based on the sharing of the above favorite words and phrases of each individual.

Step 6   This group list should then be analyzed for recurring words and phrases and for those that are especially compelling to the group, even though they may have been mentioned only once.

Step 7   A discussion of the meaning of these words and phrases should be conducted, including how they would be demonstrated structurally and/or behaviorally.

Step 8   Each group member should now write a service promise using the words and phrases that the group just found appealing.

Step 9   Repeat Step 3.

Step 10   The group should then reach agreement on the promise statement that comes the closest to what they would like to, and be willing to, implement.

Step 11   Refine that promise until all are happy with it.

Step 12   Test the promise by making certain that all know what is meant by each key word or phrase, and that any problems with the implementation are listed and discussed.

FORM 13:
STEPS FOR WRITING PERSONAL SERVICE STATEMENTS

The following steps will result in effective personal service statements:

Step 1   Identify a cycle of service or internal process in which you play a part.

Step 2   Identify the customer who is the immediate participant or recipient in the cycle or process.

Step 3   Identify the moment of truth or the step in the process that you are responsible for.

Step 4   List the important service factors that can and do impact this moment of truth or step in the process.

Step 5   List corresponding behaviors that you need to demonstrate to create a positive service experience for the customer.

Step 6   Write your own personal service statement, based on all of the above.

INDEX

DATE DUE

MAY 0 5 1998			

Demco, Inc. 38-293